The work of Alfred Tomatis, the French physician, psychologist, and educator, has had a revolutionary impact on our understanding of the ear, opening the way to a transformation of human listening and a breakthrough in the improvement of learning, communication, language, music, creativity, and self-esteem.

This is the first English translation of his famous autobiography, which has sold over 50,000 copies in Europe. An intimate account of the life and work of an indisputable genius and a veritable Renaissance man, it brings us up close to both the personal and the scientific process of conscious change — and the inevitable resistance to that change. The Tomatis Method, together with his patented invention called the "Electronic Ear," has achieved considerable recognition in Europe where his theories and method have generated both controversy and acclaim. Dr. Tomatis brings to bear the discoveries of many domains: education, psychology, audiology, speech/language, medicine, intrauterine life, music (including music therapy), and engineering. He addresses some of the most difficult therapeutic/educational problems now facing us, such as stuttering, autism, dyslexia, motivation, balance, and motor-control integration, and shows how they are affected and controlled by the ear.

The Tomatis Method is used in over 180 facilities in 15 different countries. Children, adolescents, and adults experiencing language, learning and communication difficulties from very mild to severe have benefited from this method.

The
Conscious Ear

The Conscious Ear

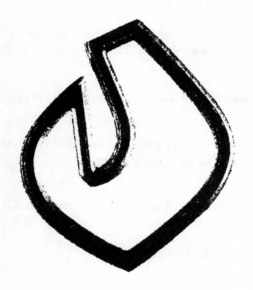

My Life of Transformation Through Listening

Alfred A. Tomatis

Station Hill Press

Originally published in French as *L'Oreille et la Vie*, copyright 1977, 1990, Editions Robert Laffont, S.A.

Editing and final translation draft by Billie M. Thompson. First draft translation in English by Stephen Lushington.

Published by Station Hill Press, Inc., Barrytown, New York 12507, and Sound Listening and Learning Center, Inc., 2701 E. Camelback Road, Suite 205, Phoenix, AZ 85016.

Distributed to the trade by The Talman Company, 150 Fifth Avenue, New York 10011.

American Cataloguing in Publication Data

Tomatis, Alfred.
    [Oreille et la vie. English]
    The conscious ear: my life of transformation through listening /
Alfred A. Tomatis ; translated by Stephen Lushington ; editing in collaboration with Billie M. Thompson.
    p. cm.
    Translation of: L'oreille et la vie.
    Includes index.
    ISBN 0-88268-108-7

    1. Tomatis, Alfred. 2. Otolaryngologists--France--Biography.
3. Audiology--Research. 4. Language disorders. I. Thompson, Billie, 1943-
. II. Title.
RF38.T65A313   1991
617.8'092--dc20   91-21610
[B]   CIP

To my parents
I am indebted —
to one I owe my existence,
to the other I owe my life.

For you I will achieve the
mission entrusted to me.

Acts of Apostle, XX, 24

Other Books by Alfred A. Tomatis

Contents

Foreword

I first heard of Alfred Tomatis through Sandra Seagal, an American psychologist with an unusually sensitive ear. Tomatis, she said, is a dynamic researcher and inventor living in France. "And he's a lovely man," she added, not a compliment given lightly.

The Conscious Ear is the story of a life and a pageant of discovery. In the tradition of Buckminster Fuller, Emanuel Swedenborg and Nicola Tesla, Tomatis is an irrepressible pioneer. He has dedicated himself to exploring the workings and purposes of that mysterious labyrinth, the ear.

This search led him to the eerie conclusion that the primary importance of the ear is to *charge* the nervous system. From this discovery he has fashioned tools for healing and enhancement that someday may help millions.

"There is no such thing as a genius," Bucky Fuller once remarked. "Some of us are just less damaged than others." If this is so, Tomatis is one of the less damaged. The happy and unhappy factors in his life have been the warp and woof of his achievement. Or, as he put it in describing his family members, "Such were the characters who threw upon my childhood their heavy shadow and their dazzling light."

Those intrigued by the role of early influences will enjoy Tomatis' descriptions of his colorful childhood. His family lived in an apartment adjacent to both sets of grandparents. He tells us about his mother's lack of interest in him, her language difficulties and his father's gift of listening intently.

During a hard-to-diagnose childhood illness he was influenced by "a certain Dr. Carcopino....a man who belonged to that tiny and select group of people who truly know how to listen." Unlike previous doctors who had examined him, Carcopino said, "I don't know what's the matter with him. I must search for the answer." *I must search for the answer* became the motif for Tomatis' life. And he decided to become a physician.

He had his father's support. Because Umberto Tomatis was often on the road singing and acting, he decided to stabilize Alfred's education. At age eleven Tomatis was living in his own apartment in Paris. His efforts in school, his experiences in World War II, and his ill-considered first marriage -- shed further light on his work and motives.

Umberto's singing career indirectly led to Alfred's unique specialty. In 1947 he was asked to treat opera singers who were losing their voices. He guessed, and confirmed, that their own loud voices had damaged their ears. They could not sing because they could no longer hear in their singing range. "A person can only reproduce vocally what he is capable of hearing."

Eventually he found that he could restore singers' voices by means of an "electronic ear," which filtered for certain frequencies. His account of "Caruso's fortunate deafness" reads like a detective story.

He also discovered that people differ in their range of hearing according to the language(s) they learned in childhood. For example, French people (1,000 to 2,000 Hertz) have considerable difficulty in learning English from the British (2,000 to 12,000 Hertz) but not from Americans (750 to 3,000 Hertz).

The Electronic Ear breaks through this barrier. By enhancing certain frequencies it enables the user to learn new languages with the fresh ear of a child.

Tomatis describes the events leading to his unique therapy for the autistic. "Sonic birth" replicates the universal passage from *in-utero* hearing (amniotic fluid) to the experience of airborne sound. He also describes his theory of the approach to stuttering.

A prophet is not without honor save in his own profession. Tomatis tired of responding to charges of unprofessionalism from fellow doctors and eventually gave up his medical practice to devote himself wholly to research, development and writing. *The Conscious Ear* is in many ways the story of persistence and transcendence. To many he may have seemed a fool, but has lived in the tradition of "holy fools," of natural spontaneity.

Tomatis concludes with the passion that moved him. Tomatis makes the point more than once that he has been profoundly supported by Léna, his second wife and inspiring collaborator. His movement toward the spiritual, his ever more frequent references to God, could be attributed to the aging process and anxiety about death. That would be a mistake. Tomatis had already experienced death —— or near-death.

His turning toward the spiritual is the natural unfolding of a life devoted to listening. "Finally," he says, "everyone knows that the soul sings and that, in this world, everything is done to prevent it. As age advances, the soul sings naturally." This book is an adventure and an invitation to sing.

Marilyn Ferguson

Marilyn Ferguson is the author of *The Aquarian Conspiracy* and the editor of *The New Sense Bulletin.*

Preface

"Do you mean the ear grows the brain?" That was my first direct question to Alfred Tomatis in Paris in 1985. For years I had been visiting centers in Canada and Europe observing the most unique and specific process of sound application for mental, linguistic, and musical improvement.

Nowhere in my life as a professional musician, teacher, and researcher had one person, one theory, or one technique set my ear on edge as his had. I had already completed two books, *Master Teacher: Nadia Boulanger* and *Introduction to the Musical Brain*, when I met Dr. Tomatis. Ironically, they had prepared me to meet him.

Tomatis came from a musical family. His father was a major performer at the Paris Opera. I was thirteen in 1960 when I entered the *Boulangerie,* a group of students studying with the most important woman in the history of Western music and composition, Nadia Boulanger. It was within a mile of the present Tomatis center, across from beautiful Parc Monceau, that I studied with her and another of the world's most renowned musicians, Robert Casadesus.

During the late seventies and early eighties, I had researched the use of multi-sensory integration in music education. I realized little attention had been given to the ear or the role of sonic stimulation by music teachers or music therapists. Performing artists had little more than a teenager's knowledge about the ear, the nervous system, or vestibular function.

When I first read his autobiography, published in French as *L'Oreille et la Vie (The Ear and the Life),* I was stunned by all the associations and connections it made with music, learning, and language development. My experience of "ah-ha" was so frequent as I read the contents that it took years to assimilate.

In the last 40 years, Dr. Tomatis' first basic theory has been tested with over a million clients worldwide: **The voice contains only what the ear hears.** In other words, the larynx emits only the harmonics that the ear can hear. To the musician and music teacher this ignites a genuine curiosity about the very laborious "ear training" methods being used in music classrooms and studios. To speech therapists, reading specialists, and psychologists, this basic theory has dozens of other important implications.

From simple techniques like the observation of ear dominance to the most complex applications for stroke and comatose patients, Dr. Tomatis insists that we listen with acute attention to the new dimensions now being discovered and tested in neurology, audiology, and holistic health. Through his very specific Method of using filtered and unfiltered sounds of Mozart, Gregorian Chant, and the mother's voice to learning how to sing "through the bones," Dr. Tomatis challenges every ear to listen with greater facility.

The Conscious Ear is the unfoldment of a unique life. It is an insightful autobiography describing the transformation of life even as Dr. Tomatis comes to terms with his own ability to listen—personally, professionally, and artistically. I am sure this book will serve to father and mother our modern ears!

And yes! Now I understand how the ear grows the brain.

Don Campbell

Don Campbell is the Director of the Institute for Music, Health and Education in Boulder, Colorado, and the author of *Music Physician for Times to Come* and *Rhythms of Learning*.

Introduction

What is this symbol?

Dr. Alfred Tomatis, noted French physician, psychologist, and educator, says it represents the fetal ear. The ear, he says, is much more than an appendage on the side of the head. What you see externally is only the tip of an amazing organ from which language, verticality, and laterality are born, all of which distinguish us as being human.

This symbol also represents Tomatis' lifelong search to know, to be, and to connect with self, others, and the cosmos. It is the logo for his life's work, the development of a method to improve the focusing ability of the ear so that one can listen, speak, and learn well. This book tells his story. It is an update from the Éditions Robert Laffont 1977 and 1986 publications, *L'Oreille et la Vie*, and an edited and extended version of Stephen Lushington's original English translation completed but not published in 1986.

"I must search" are words that have guided Dr. Tomatis since age nine. His search takes him through a lifetime of discoveries about the roles and functions of the human ear and its relationship with the rest of the body, beginning in the fetus.

Professor Tomatis, or Tom, as friends call him, is seventy-one years old. His eyes are kind and wise. His voice is pure and vibrant, filling a room with energy for himself and those who listen. He speaks French, Niçois, English, and Spanish. He is a Greek at heart, an Italian by descent, and a lay member of a Gregorian sect by invitation. His partner in everything for the past thirty-five years is Léna, his wife.

Like a Sherlock of the ear, Tomatis unwraps layer by layer the mysteries of one of the most amazing organs of the human body. To read this autobiography is to know his pains and gains and "ah-ha's." It is to connect his observations to his insights, his questions to answers, and our own ability to listen to the ability to learn. He acknowledges the influence of his family, education, external events, and personal search for love and meaning.

The Conscious Ear is an intriguing story for those who work with people and who, like Tomatis, are searching for ways to assist others to discover more of their potential. If you like a good mystery, this book will take you on a tour of the ear, our natural labyrinth, to discover its functions and its impact on what it means to be human. It introduces listening as the foundation for language, social communication, and learning. We listen, speak, read, write, and sing with our ears. It describes the Tomatis Method, used in many centers, schools, and organizations throughout the world by professionals from such diverse backgrounds as education, psychology, speech/language pathology, medicine, audiology, performing arts, occupational therapy, and foreign language instruction.

The curious will find in Tomatis' story fresh insights to old continuing problems not yet solved. That is how I came to be involved in this work, by looking for effective programs to offer others who want to improve or accelerate their learning. My "listening" for these programs led me to the Tomatis Method. Now I routinely hear adults describe the changes made by their children or themselves following participation in the Tomatis Method. I am continually amazed, as they are, at the transformations, each so individual, so liberating and supportive of the person to learn and expand. The parents of Chris, 14, and Cindy (pseudonym), 8, share their experience as follows:

> Two weeks after completing the program, Chris aced his science final. (He had been failing science.) The following semester he did his homework on a daily basis without fail. He stopped skipping classes. He actually read two books for pleasure! Chris has raised his grades from .8 to 3.5. We are so proud. More importantly, he is proud of himself....Our only wish is that every parent who has a child with a learning or behavioral problem could know that there is a non-intrusive way of helping their child find help and happiness."

(Parents of Chris)

> "I'm amazed at all she can do now —— reading so well, directions, puzzles, everything. She just *does* it. She has not had to learn anything. It was all there —— this large vocabulary, sense of humor, reasoning —— she hasn't had to *learn* it. It all was covered up and just had to be uncovered. How this must feel to her must be incredible and a little scary. That's how we felt about it —— it's a little unsettling to have a new person in your home, and that's what she is. It's so wonderful. This is what I've been dreaming could happen to her. I knew there was more in there, but so many people have told me not to worry, she's fine, and she does well in school. But at such a cost —— so much effort and how she feels about herself because she knew there was so much more, too."

(Mother of Cindy)

These stories are common for those who complete the Method and continue to use the techniques of good listening. The success I see with this work keeps me active in helping it develop in the English-speaking world.

I believe this autobiography will assist others in discovering how much the ear has to do with problems of language, learning, motivation, and life in general. Some will delight in the new insights while others might feel challenged by the departure from what they have previously been taught. Whatever the response, I invite all readers to wonder what could happen if people were able to listen and speak in the comprehensive way Tomatis shows us.

Billie Thompson, Ph.D.

Billie Thompson is the Director of the Tomatis Center in Phoenix, Arizona, and the co-editor of *About the Tomatis Method*.

THE CONSCIOUS EAR

1

Life Begins —— Just!

"It is useless to bother with him. He's dead."

These were the first words my ears heard when I left my mother's womb, though I certainly did not understand them. I was a premature baby of six and a half months, weighing just under three pounds. I was such a wretched specimen that the midwife seized me by my right ear, leaving a mark I still bear, and discarded me in a basket. She could do nothing more for me, and I would undoubtedly be dead if my father's mother had not been present.

My grandmother, a quite remarkable woman, was greatly experienced with pregnancies, having given birth to 24 children herself. While everyone else cared for my anguished mother, my grandmother approached the basket where I lay helpless. All alone on the sideline of the main event, she revived me. I owe her my life. In other ways, too, this woman was destined to profoundly influence my childhood.

I am convinced that the conditions of my difficult birth greatly determined the direction of my work investigating prenatal life. It was not mere chance that guided my research over many years to reconstruct the remarkable developmental stages of the fetus. My vocation of "searcher" began as a premature baby seeking a nirvana from which I was shut out much too soon. Could I by understanding prenatal existence reconstruct something that was removed by chance from my actual experience? What would I have discovered if I had not been deprived of those last two and a half months in the womb? These questions and others arising from them gave real meaning to all my efforts to study what happens in the primordial period of the life of the fetus.

My arrival in the world does not seem to have been expected, much less hoped for, by my 16-year-old mother. I have never known if my mother's marriage to my father was welcomed. The birth seemed to pose a problem for everyone in the family, and no doubt they were eager to get rid of this unexpected baby quickly and with little fuss. Remarkable compression efforts were used to prevent this pregnancy from being noticed; the corsets of that past age, so strongly supported by unbending whalebones, readily helped. My mother's body responded to her psychological distress and, of its own accord, brought about contractions which no doubt induced my premature birth. The compression also apparently influenced my need during the first 40 years of life to live tightly swathed in clothes, with a body belt that cut me in two, and restricted also by narrow and confining shoes. At night, I did not sleep unless at least eight blankets were piled upon me. Though I was not cold, I needed to experience this pressure of the world around me to reproduce the vital conditions I had known in my mother's womb. Throughout those 40 years, I also felt compressed on the inside of my body. I had the constitution of a thin man, but I was padded with a dense fat and weighed 264 pounds. The meaning of all this became clear one morning as I flew to Canada to discuss my research on this very subject, life before birth and filtered sounds. As we flew along the coast of Labrador at dawn, the light, sounds, and special atmosphere in the plane submerged me into the long-ago conditions of my mother's womb. I immediately felt once more the oppression of some enormous weight, pressing closely upon me, cramping me. From that moment I understood the origin of my need for compression, and I never needed to experience it again.

I have an unshakable intuition that my work and speculations are deeply bound up with the conditions and events, feelings and sensations, conscious and subconscious thoughts, basic needs, and secret desires which surrounded my entry into the world and then put an indelible mark on my infancy. I only discovered ultimately who I am through a consideration of everything I have experienced in my long and complicated journey. My desire to share my experiences led me to write this autobiography, not a desire for exhibitionism nor the pleasure of looking once more at the events of my life. It is a journey all of us make in search of our humanity while being guided by the underlying controlling thread of the Being who beckons.

Here then are the facts: I was born in Nice on the 29th, 30th, or perhaps the 31st of December, 1919, half an hour before midnight. I am sure of the time, but the exact birth day is in question. The civil service official was told that it was possibly the first of January, 1920. My family decided to tell this little white lie for reasons connected with a census return.

We lived in the old quarter of Nice at 6 Rue St. Joseph on the first floor of a building that no longer exists. My father was born two doors away at No. 10. I eventually saw this house of ours pulled down, cracked and tottering, but still so beautiful. It was an Italian style dwelling which once sheltered a court justice and was often the scene for meetings of famous people. Our kitchen was set up in the old council chamber. I always remember a wall cupboard at the back of which I discovered some secret doors. This was a fabulous house for a child; it was not merely a place to live, but rather a place of mystery and dreams! It was replaced by a building with no character and no soul, one among many. Unfortunately, Old Nice carried within itself the seeds of its own destruction. The decay of the buildings and the lack of interest taken in them by the city's restoration services gradually caused the old quarter to lose its unique identity. In a few decades, not only the buildings, but also the spoken dialect of Old Nice, which had remained absolutely intact since the fifteenth century, virtually ceased.

When I was a child, my family and neighbors all spoke the Niçois dialect. The few rare old Niçois who also spoke French had to learn it like a foreign language. That is what my father did, and what I myself did later with the very greatest difficulty. Speaking the Niçois dialect quite clearly emphasized our particular character to a far greater extent than most people imagine; it was not merely a question of "any" dialect from southern France. Communication with those people who expressed themselves in Provençal was very laborious. It was much easier to communicate with the Italians of the Lombardy Riviera since the two dialects belonged to the same speech group, that of the Ligurian languages. No doubt this explains the relatively large number of marriages between members of the two linguistic communities. Such was the case with my parents.

My mother was Italian, born unexpectedly on a trip to Monaco in the house of an uncle who was Vice-Consul in the city. Her family lived for a long time in Forli in the province of Romagna.

My mother's father, Alfredo Raggi, attended high school with a forceful and unruly fellow who created an influential and famous newspaper that soon spread beyond the walls of the school. All Forli was shaken up by the increasingly widespread movement led by this man. His name? Benito Mussolini! It was because of him that my grandfather found himself in prison for a day. The future Duce was experimenting then with that well known technique of creating a vacuum around himself in order to be the leading figure in his circle. My grandfather had the good fortune to escape Mussolini's influence and immediately chose the path of exile. If he had not, my mother would never have met my father.

My father, Umberto, was 20 when I was born. His father, a man of Herculean stature from the Piedmont and a true Gaul from this side of the Alps, had wanted to name him "Dante." The town hall clerk was officially opposed to it, so Dante became his middle name. Umberto Dante Tomatis was very young when he left childhood behind and threw himself into the real world. He often helped his mother, who worked with Dr. Pilate, a member of one of the city's great Protestant families. Eventually he became a printer for the newspaper *L'Eclaireur de Nice*. His health was weak because of lung trouble, which was the disease of the age in the South of France. Several of his brothers and sisters died of it. Umberto was well-built, slim, and possessed a lordly air. His face, solidly constructed, was dominated by eyes of steel blue and topped by a head of thick, wavy, almost blond hair. He displayed considerable energy, often working day and night. I once saw him single-handedly work three consecutive day and night shifts. When he was not engaged in manual work, my father immersed himself in the French culture. Without help from anyone, he learned to speak, read, and write French. He mastered the language so well that his epistolary style became a model of its kind.

This man rarely rested. To watch him always at work convinced me that a

normal adult life was nothing more than a breathless and relentless succession
of tasks and endeavors. This strange idea was destined to shape my entire
existence. Today I still live the life of a relentless worker, not out of duty but
because this sort of frenzy has become my natural rhythm. Without work I feel
lost.

When the war of 1914 broke out, the Niçois organized a banquet to celebrate
the occasion. Like many French people, they were sure Berlin would fall in
three weeks. Plus, the front seemed so far from the shores of the Mediterranean
that they felt they could devote themselves without a second thought to patriotic
exultation. During the dessert course, everyone had to sing a song. My father,
then 14 years old, had never sung in his life. Afraid of making a fool of himself,
he reluctantly got up and plunged into the Marseillaise. He did this in such a
thunderous voice that everyone was impressed. When he finished, Garibaldi, the
managing director of the newspaper, took my father aside and told him that he
would personally pay for music and singing lessons for him. Umberto accepted.

The realization of his gifts did not go to his head. As usual, he worked with
great persistence. It was only when he turned 21 that he began to make stage
appearances, and even then he remained at the newspaper where he had become
an editor. But this long apprenticeship bore fruit. A success from the start, he
soon began to sing in other towns and quickly established an international
reputation as a "Basse Noble."

I always considered my father an exceptional being with whom I communi-
cated well and shared a close understanding. I can never overestimate what I
owe him. He had a rather difficult childhood and was nicknamed "Tol" (the
Sulker). He worked hard so that I might escape the anger and sorrow he
experienced as a child. He was born into an enormous family as the seventeenth
child and grew up believing himself to be unloved. Real or imaginary, this lack
of love left scars on him. He wanted better for me. Throughout my childhood,
my father was a precious ally in the family quarrels which occurred almost
daily. And even more than that, he was an "ear," a listener who was always
ready to hear me with true attention.

Communication with my mother, on the other hand, was never easy. All my
attempts at intimacy were repulsed. Besides our deep incompatibility, any
communication with my mother was riddled with technical difficulties. Like her
own mother, mine never really assimilated either the French or Niçois languages.
In addition, like so many expatriate Italians, she gradually lost the mastery of
her native tongue. Her struggle with language produced a genuine blockage. She
was essentially walled in by her state of ignorance.

My mother's parents, it is true, did not bother to provide her with the
slightest cultural background. Their only ambition was for her to be a good
housewife and, especially, a marvelous cook. Toward this end, they sent her to
board with an aunt in Bologna. The Bolognese are like the Lyonnais of Italy ——

they hold proudly to their culinary traditions and their love of good food. The Bolognese cuisine is rightly praised throughout Italy. In her cooking classes, my mother showed remarkable talent; in my aunt's home, she spent most of her time in the kitchen simmering delicious and special family dishes. Polenta was a favorite of my grandfather who consumed enormous amounts without ever tiring of it.

My mother's cooking earned her a double advantage in life. First, it provided her with a remarkable means of attaching my father to herself and ensuring his return home. Women were very attracted to him, and his career kept him on the road. So my mother had the anxiety of constantly having to bring him back to her. Fortunately, he fervently admired his wife's cooking. In fact, it was difficult for him to keep himself going when she could not prepare his meals, short of preparing his own particularly choice dishes.

Second, my mother's culinary skill was obviously what psychologists today would call her "compensation." With her incontestable superiority, she could invest her psychic energy in cooking without fear of ever being reprimanded. In short, it was among the casseroles that her life regained its meaning. She had no other opportunity to be proud of herself. She was always suffering and I, her only son, gave her nothing but disappointment. No doubt my rebellious attitude towards my mother caused me to never express any interest in what she cooked for me. We had an almost permanent state of antagonism and constantly squabbled.

Our relationship might best be described as a "rivalry." In the eyes of my mother, my mere presence prevented her from joining my father in his travels. She blamed me for loosening the emotional ties between them and for causing my father to lead this shallow and hurtful "artist's life." I clearly sensed this deep resentment and settled down, without fully understanding it, into a fixed position of rivalry. I resisted her. I stubbornly opposed her. I refused to yield. I never shed a tear in her presence, and it was this that moved her most. To her, my stoicism underlined my fundamental ill-nature. Since she was reluctant to look after me, my father had to make sure I was cared for. In fact, from infancy on, he was the one who really looked after me.

My contacts with my mother were extremely tense. Moreover, my Grandfather Raggi, her father, took a malicious pleasure in pouring fuel on the flames. Pleasure? Actually, I do not really know what his attitude was about me. He was thoroughly ambivalent. On one hand, he overwhelmed me with presents. On the other, he hastened to tell my mother all the lies I had told, or that he thought I had told, so that I was regularly punished. This duality, or rather this duplicity, in the character of one and the same person presented me at the time with enormous problems. In the long run, it made me wiser. Trying to understand my grandfather helped me to understand human nature.

All the same, this Alfredo Raggi was an odd fellow! Lachrymose, crafty, and with a strain of naive mysticism which bordered on superstition. He always prayed because he was frightened of what awaited him after death. And he always strayed from the path mapped out by his religion because he was incapable of resisting the smallest temptation. Grandfather Raggi let himself be tossed about by life, at the mercy of a grumbling fatalism. When he reacted violently, it was nearly always against me. In particular, he could not bear it if I were not silent as soon as he opened his mouth. This claim for the privilege of speaking, exercised at my expense, struck me as a monstrous injustice especially since I was automatically in the wrong just because I was a child.

Why shouldn't I be able to say what I wanted to say, just like everyone else? One day, during a meal, I rose to speak my mind and, in return, received a memorable thrashing. Only my father knew how to listen to me and understand my point of view.

What did my Grandfather Raggi do? Nothing. He let my grandmother manage things. Like her daughter, she was walled in by language difficulties. She rarely opened her mouth, still less her ears, so it was nearly impossible to communicate with her. In addition, her sight had deteriorated to near blindness. To get rid of her (and allow himself some flirtations), Grandfather Raggi frequently sent her off for walks in the mountains, far from home.

Sometimes I followed my grandmother on her walks. We did not speak, but we were together. Today those mountains seem thoroughly commonplace, but then they seemed like paradise. On our walks, I met little Italian children, and all day we ran about barefoot and happy. Our playground was a vast one, the surroundings of Baus-Roux in the region of St. Martin-du-Var. When we were thirsty, we seized a goat and drank straight from the udder.

Alfredo Raggi wept a great deal when his wife died, but what exactly was he weeping for? For the love that he had not known how to give her? Or, more prosaically and egotistically, his own loss of comfort? Her death reinforced his loneliness still further. His deceitfulness continued and was resented by everyone around him. He gradually created an emptiness around himself. It was the irony of fate that at the end of his life, I was the only person he could still turn to. I was the only one capable of bringing him a shadow of emotional and physical comfort.

I christened my two grandmothers with special names. The one who strode about the countryside became "Nena della Montagna" or "Mountain Granny." The other was "Nena du paillon," or "Paillon Granny," because she washed her linen in the Paillon River which flows through Nice into the Mediterranean.

Paillon Granny was a little scrap of a woman, full of vitality. I was convinced that she was immortal. Her mother had lived to the ripe old age of 103 and her two aunts to 105 and 108. In fact, Granny Paillon lived to almost 90. She was carried off finally by a bronchial infection following a severe bout of influenza. My emotional ties with her were always very deep; I owed her my life, and I was, to some extent, her child.

I loved my paternal grandfather very much, too, and he loved me. When we lived in Nice, we were hardly ever out of each other's company. The three couples I have talked about all lived together in our house, sharing the first floor; my parents lived on the right side, my mother's parents in the middle, and my father's parents on the left. This arrangement aptly reproduced in the space available the structure of a southern French family. It also led to a dense accumulation of psychological problems of all kinds, especially since Grandfather Raggi liked to tell tall tales.

Grandfather Tomatis was my playmate. When I was three or four years old, we would get together for Tarot parties. The cards were huge, and I had the greatest difficulty holding them. But that was not the chief problem; what was really troublesome was that neither he nor I knew the value of the cards, much less the rules of the game. To top it off, we were equally set on winning — I because I was only a child and he because it was an idiosyncrasy of his character. I brought him to the verge of despair when I claimed to win a game. He would almost cry over it and then throw down his cards, while complaining to my grandmother, "But all the same I won. I won and that's all there is to it!"

He was one of the most gentle persons I have ever known. Yet he was a mountain of a man, a colossus, a force of nature! In the Piedmont, where a man's strength was gauged by the number of opponents he could tackle by himself, it was judged that he could only fight honorably when he had six or seven opponents on his back. He would accomplish prodigious feats, too, when he split wood. What is more, like several of his sons, he was a voracious eater. It would be more accurate to say that he was a man whose appetite could never be satisfied!

When a stranger commented on his appetite, he would smilingly indicate a finger's length and say modestly, "I only eat this much bread." While it was true that he ate bread in very reasonable quantities, pounds of polenta did not daunt him!

I cherish memories of my grandfather's unlimited generosity. He possessed a warmth that very few people have. I recall, too, his inborn talent for song, as compared to my father who never sang before being obliged to do so at the age of 14. Grandfather, by contrast, expressed everything in song: his joys, his woes, his cares, his dreams. He possessed what people called "a fine instrument." Above all, the volume of his voice was exceptional. When he began to sing, we were obliged to protect our ears. He could be heard four streets away! Many years later, after my father had heard on the theater circuit the greatest voices in the world, he told me that no voice was equal to my grandfather's. Though my father himself was famous for his vocal power, he could not hold a candle to my grandfather whose voice was a true river of sound. It possessed such a range and flexibility that he could sing in nearly every register. When he found

someone to sing with him, he could always take the complementary part —
tenor, bass or baritone — and sing it to perfection!

Such were the characters who threw upon my childhood their heavy shadow
and their dazzling light. To complete the picture, I must sketch in two more.
They were a little less close, but the presence of my Uncle Victor and Uncle
Clement had a real presence in my childhood.

Although deaf, Uncle Victor was in no way cut off from the world and other
people. This bundle of love was nicknamed "Bellessa," or Beautiful One, not so
much because of his physical appearance but for what one might call his inner
landscape. He was the image of my grandfather, and when grandfather died,
Uncle Victor quite naturally took his place in my heart. What a marvelous,
gentle man! Though I was only a child, he treated me as an equal.

Besides his great generosity, what struck me most about Uncle Victor was
his gluttony. He was particularly fond of sweets. When he arrived home from
work, my grandmother's only task was to open one of those metal candy boxes.
He crunched away as he read his newspaper, and every day, without exception,
consumed a whole two-pound box.

Uncle Clement was different from his older brother. Last born, he was the
spoiled child whose two great passions were motoring and sports. He often took
me with him while driving through the Alps or the Pyrenees in his Rosengart,
which at that time was considered quite a novelty. With him I experienced
exceptionally beautiful daybreak trips in the mountains.

So the days of my childhood flowed by at Rue St. Joseph, days of anger and
happiness, of deep tenderness and endless confrontations. The long thrilling,
crackling days of youth provided an unbroken chain of drama and excitement
where there was never a place for apathy. Echoing and mingling in my head
were the lofty songs of Grandfather Tomatis, the endless lamentations of Grandfather Raggi, my mother's scoldings, and my father's silences. Those silences
meant "I am here, I am listening to you" and were, in the end, often more eloquent than words of love. Already I was fighting to be heard, although I was
often defeated as children are who are so painfully victimized by the famous
duty to be seen and not heard. But I knew that at least one sympathetic ear
existed which was ready to understand and help me.

Other conflicts which did not concern me directly enlivened our household.
Alfredo Raggi's attitude was at the root of the latent antagonism between my
father's parents and my mother's. About one subject, however, they were in
complete agreement: the war. Neither couple understood it at all, particularly the
Tomatis's who saw most of their sons leave for the front in France and never
return. The system capable of giving rise to such tragedies appeared to them an
abominable and cruel absurdity. They professed a savage antimilitarism which
my grandfather himself espoused as a reaction against Mussolini. My father, too,
shared these pacifist ideas.

Beginning in 1923 or 1924, my father was offered very interesting singing engagements which forced him to leave Nice for a six month "season." I sometimes accompanied him on his travels, particularly to Belgium where two things astonished me: the care with which they polished every thing, including the pavement, and the enormous size of the slices of bread and jam!

Every passing year strengthened my father's reputation in the world of singers. The quality of his voice was such that in France he had no rival during his 41 year career, and he was one of the best paid artists in his profession. There were, however, difficult moments because my father was exceptionally generous and would sometimes give away all the money he earned during the season. That would sometimes create a crisis at home, so he had to regularly build up his savings again in order to meet family expenses.

I was often reminded that I was a particularly difficult child to bring up. The problem began very early, even when I was only an infant at the breast. It seems I was one of those children who would bawl, crying all day and weeping all night. Finally my father, exasperated by all this racket and tired of having his evening studies disturbed, had the bright idea of hanging me up outside in exactly the same way as the household linen was hung out to dry! I wonder sometimes if the symptoms of vertigo from which I suffered later did not originate from this unique method of keeping me quiet.

I was ill for a large part of my childhood, in fact, from the time of my birth. No doubt having a mother who paid too little attention to her baby's problems and a father who was often away from home played their part in making my incorporation into the surrounding world a difficult one. Between my birth and my eleventh year, I suffered from every illness a child could catch. In particular, I suffered from a great variety of digestive disorders, which I now think were certainly psychosomatic and brought on by the lack of communication between my mother and me. In retrospect, I think that for a doctor with a passion for psychology, like myself, to have lived through such an experience was a blessing in disguise. I must even say, without the slightest cynicism intended, that my misunderstandings with my mother greatly helped me to penetrate the secrets of the psychology of personal relationships.

I was almost constantly in poor health, with the result that doctor after doctor came to my bedside. I have a very clear memory of one of these doctors. After vaguely examining me, he declared, "It's nothing at all. He's playing games with you. He's pretending to be ill just to annoy you." Unfortunately, this time my illness had nothing psychological about it, and it was only when they decided to take my temperature that they realized just how sick I was.

We had no thermometer in our house at that time. Instead, we used a special family technique — a primitive custom where a piece of silver was placed on the subject's forehead. If the coin fell off, the person was not ill; if it stuck, there really was a fever.

My coin stuck.

At that point the household broke into a panic, all the more so because I had fallen into a semi-coma. A number of doctors trooped in and then trooped out again, lost. It turned out that I simultaneously had typhoid, Maltese fever, and Typhus Murin. Incredible? Not really, considering the conditions of my life at the time. The typhoid was the result of the very hit-and-miss food hygiene which was often found in the homes of old Niçois families. The Maltese fever I caught quenching my thirst at the often unclean udders of mountain goats. As for the Typhus Murin (a disease transmitted by rats' fleas), that was a memento of my secret expeditions in the cellars. In brief, I was riddled with animal diseases, and I can appreciate that the diagnosis was difficult to establish considering the complexity of the symptoms and the added confusion resulting from the natural course of each separate disease!

The doctors who examined me were at a loss, and they disguised their ignorance by saying whatever came into their heads. Then my parents appealed to a certain Dr. Carcopino. This doctor spoke Niçois, which made communication much easier. Also, his personality was such that people instinctively trusted his judgement and his ability. Even I, in my condition, sensed this. Here was a man who belonged to that tiny and select group of people who truly know how to listen.

Just like the doctors before him, Dr. Carcopino leaned over and examined me thoroughly and patiently. Then he straightened and spoke these simple words: "I don't know what's the matter with him. **I must search** for the answer."

Dr. Carcopino did search, and two or three days later he found the answer. He made his diagnosis and began to treat me. But more importantly, his words struck me in the deepest part of my being, penetrating the mists of my torpor and bursting in my head like a thunderclap: "I must search."

This phrase was to decide my destiny —— to become a doctor and "search" for what I did not know, like Dr. Carcopino. This ambition remained deeply anchored within me until I actually undertook my medical studies. Only for a few months during my last year of secondary school did I consider, and then not seriously, studying applied science and technology instead.

When I disclosed my intentions to my family, they were not particularly enthusiastic. At the age of nine they certainly did not take me seriously. In fact, they found my idea utterly ridiculous. Me, a doctor, when I had hardly even attended school because of all my illnesses? Me, looking after others when I was always ill myself? How absurd! They all shrugged their shoulders.

Except my father.

He understood that this was not just a child's fancy, a passing whim. For whatever reason, my father respected my decision and worked to help me attain my goal. Although I was almost incessantly ill for the next two years, as soon as I was back on my feet again, my father devoted all his efforts to arranging for me to pursue medical studies.

It was not easy. Far from it. I not only did not possess a basic education, but I had not yet properly learned the French language. To help me overcome these obstacles, my father took me to Marseille with him and placed me in a school. Despite my willingness to please him, however, I did not exactly shine in my studies. Indeed, I proved exceptionally incompetent, capable of driving the most blasé teachers to despair. I was overwhelmed by what was happening, but I did not lose heart. I reasoned that by working hard I should certainly one day at least understand the questions, even if I could not find the answers.

Unfortunately, time was against me. Like many actors' children who followed their parents from town to town without ever putting down any roots, I had to relearn everything at each new school I attended. Not only were the students and teachers different, but the textbooks and the syllabus changed, too. Each time we moved, it was as if I had been parachuted into an unknown country, a hostile one at that.

My father, whose solicitude never wavered in spite of these repeated setbacks, finally understood that I would never get anywhere like that. Something else would have to be tried. My mother suggested that he send me to a boarding school, but he made quite a different decision, in fact the only decision that no one could have predicted. It must have taken him no more than a split second.

2

Alone in Paris

"I have thought this over carefully," my father said to me. "My boy, if you really want to become a doctor — and a good doctor — you must go to Paris. We don't know anyone there, so you'll have to manage all by yourself, but you'll learn what life is all about, and that will certainly be of some use to you."

And so it was that at the age of 11, I was left in Paris to live by myself, not as a boarder in a school, but as a day-student, entirely responsible for myself. No parents, no friends, no contacts. There was no one to keep an eye on me or to help me if I needed it. Today, such an adventure would hardly be possible, but at that time, it was not quite so difficult. The risks to a child then were certainly more limited than in today's society. For one, the pace was a great deal less frantic and people were less self-centered. Besides, at that time a child had better defenses than nowadays, especially when he faced up to adult responsibilities so early. In any case, after taking everything into consideration, my family decided that this plan was less crazy than my desire to become a doctor.

My father set me up in an apartment in Neuilly at 9 rue Théophile Gautier. Neuilly, at this time, was still reminiscent of a village. My route from apartment to school skirted more gardens than business premises. Some of the teachers had also spent their childhoods in the area and told us that the Market Square was still covered with potato fields in their time and you could run into herds of cows.

My apartment included a sitting/dining room, bedroom, kitchen, and bathroom which I made into my study. The most difficult adjustment I had to make was in regards to the perpetually grey skies. I found the climate depressing. There are reasons why one is called "a child of the sun." I needed light. My later attraction to southern Spain must have been tied to my strong desire for light during my studies in Paris.

What astonished and saddened me most, in my new home, was to find that the Paris basin soil was not red. I was used to the fields of Midi; not to find red soil near my new home troubled me. I got over the discomfort, but even today I remain deeply attached to countries with red soil. This, too, was one of the reasons I travelled so often to Andalusia, a little village near Almeria.

So here I was at the age of 11, alone in a country not my own, or so it seemed to me. I was glad to avoid the daily confrontations with my mother, but I had to face many tasks that were quite new to me, such as washing, mending, cooking meals, and cleaning the apartment. My first weeks were very difficult because I had to invent solutions to all my problems with the means at hand, and without help. I hardly attracted any sympathy from my school friends — we shall see why presently. Later, after I forged ties of friendship with a few rare fellow students, things got much better. One of them, Jean Coti, remained a very dear friend and introduced me to his parents who often invited me to dinner. I also was lucky to find on my street the vice-principal of the Lycée Pasteur, my school. His name was Bonnet, and he was a fervent admirer of my father's voice. He regularly came to visit me at rue Théophile Gautier, giving me all sorts of advice and acting as my spiritual director. As he got to know and thoroughly understand my problems, he did everything he could to further my studies and my relationships with the powers that be. He granted me, I must admit, some unfair privileges without which I might have been sent home. For the first two years, I was far from being a satisfactory student. For example, if I were unable to meet deadlines, Bonnet authorized me to hand in my compositions late.

Why couldn't I meet my deadlines? Was I ill again? No. Although I was not bursting with health, I did not suffer any further illness severe enough to keep me in bed. Rather, I was working all day and for a large part of the night addressing envelopes by the thousands.

I got the idea that to thank my father for taking my vocation seriously I must not cost him a centime. At the beginning of each school term he handed me six thousand francs, which was a considerable sum at the time. I paid him back his money whenever he came to see me (he spent two months every year at rue Théophile Gautier taking advantage of his engagements at the Opera and of any free time between contracts).

Later, when I became a father myself, I understood what a mistake I had made in thinking this would give him pleasure. When he finally had to retire from singing and I tried to give him a comfortable life, it was an enduring sadness for him not to be able to repay me as I had once repaid him. Then how I regretted my youthful zeal! But at the beginning of the 1930s, there was nothing to stop me from earning this money and paying my father back as proof of my affectionate gratitude.

In any case, since I was now solely in charge of my life, I considered myself a young adult, and, as I mentioned before, I believed that adult life consisted of working with no respite and no rest. So nothing seemed more natural to me than to force myself to be continually busy. Where did I find the necessary strength to do so at the ages of 11, 12, and 13?

The question still puzzles me. But I am sure that the psychic energy which upheld me came from my profound love for my father and his love for me. Perhaps that was enough to give me the strength I needed. From my first day alone at Neuilly until I was 25, my father and I remained in daily correspondence (except, of course, during the times we lived together). I tried hard to bring my mother into this relationship. I began to write to her, but was repulsed once more; she made no attempt to answer me apart from a few clumsy words.

In fact, I worked those long hours not only to give thanks *to* my father, but with thanks *for* him. I dedicated all my efforts to him, and I imagined that he expected this of me. I actually thought that by working like that, I would put myself in tune with him. I only realized much later that my father, though by no means idle, was no longer such a glutton for work as he had been in my early childhood. I was a grown man when he confessed to me what torture it was to live at my pace whenever he came to stay with me at Neuilly! Believing that I was following his example, I acquired the habit not only of going to bed late but of getting up early, about four o'clock in the morning. When he was visiting and I lit the lamp, invariably the light which filtered under his door woke him up. "Wretched child!" he would say to himself. "Already up, when I am just settling down to sleep." However, he never waited long to join me. By about five o'clock he was at my side. What I did not know was that when he was not "on holiday" with me, he seldom rose before seven.

Of course I longed for more sleep. Like all children, I needed rest. I used several tricks to keep myself awake. For one, I learned my lessons by reading aloud. Even today, I prescribe this technique to everyone who comes to consult me. Reading aloud offers a great number of advantages, and, in particular, it improves one's retention considerably. It worked especially well for me; memorization had always been my weakest point. At this stage my memory was almost an infirmity! However, after some time, the benefits of reading aloud became apparent. I was able to begin assimilating certain facts which enabled me to remember others as well, and so on. I began to move forward in class in a spectacular way. In the seventh class I was perfectly useless; in the sixth I wasn't worth much; but by the fourth, I was already tops in all scientific subjects and well placed on the arts side. In the third class,[1] I won nearly all the first prizes. It was only in gymnastics that I did poorly. Since my fellow students laughed at me because of this, I decided to go all out —— in my own way —— for the gymnastics prize. I fiercely and systematically focused all my energy on this goal. I had a bar fixed in the corridor outside my apartment and worked out on it for two hours each day, doing all the exercises that would develop my muscles. There, too, persistence paid off. I actually won the gymnastics prize! A few years later, I even became university gymnastics champion. Once more I was merely following in my father's footsteps. Despite lung troubles, he was a real athlete. At one time, along with his singing and other activities, he was also a gymnastics instructor.

---

[1] The North American equivalents are: seventh class is grade five, sixth class is grade six, fifth class is grade seven, fourth class is grade eight, third class is first year high school.

My early successes taught me that man is never limited by what he appears to be. There exists within him all sorts of possibilities which allow him to surpass himself again and again. That is a very obvious discovery —— but what luck to make it when one is still a child! Nietzsche's famous command "to become who we are" really is an exciting proposition. Still, we certainly need a driving force in order to achieve this. The more I think about it, the more I am inclined to believe that the circumstances surrounding my birth provided my driving force. As a premature baby, I had to make extraordinary efforts just in order to survive; from the start I had to vehemently and repeatedly register my desire to live. Since then simple existence has, for me, been indissolubly linked to a generous and almost permanent investment of energy.

So no one will be surprised that I left behind me, at the Lycée Pasteur, the reputation of a fierce and tireless contender. I was almost the only one not to realize that my hard work and desperate eagerness amazed, exasperated, and discouraged my fellow students all at the same time, and it certainly did not help to make me popular. At the beginning, since I spoke French so badly, I had enough trouble just being accepted. Later, I made two or three firm friendships (firm enough to withstand the test of time), but all the same I remained isolated, on the edge of things, not within the bosom of the class.

Add to this the type of life I led. It forced upon me an outlook much different from that of my fellow students. I looked at the world and conceived of life in a different way than they did. For example, play hardly attracted me at all —— more precisely, I felt no pleasure in taking an active part in it. I was content to be a spectator. Such was the case with cards. I always preferred to observe a game of cards rather than to be one of the players. When I was 11, I was outstanding at pinochle. The day I became aware of my own mastery of it, the game lost all interest for me. From this point of view I have not changed: as soon as I know the rules of a game well, it immediately ceases to hold my attention. I realize that it does not lead to anything else but itself, and I find it difficult to understand that it can still create interest in anyone. To go round and round within some self-evident situation, which seems threadbare as it is, seems to me not only frivolous but also desperately boring.

In any case, like most emotional people, I am a born observer. I am most happy when watching and analyzing what is going on around me. This outlook has been of enormous help to me both in research and in the clinic. It fits in with my temperament, but it is also the result of the fact that I have been more often in the company of adults than of boys my own age. As a child, I got along much better with adults. Since they found my shyness entirely natural, the generation gap being what it was, I could observe them and listen to them at my leisure. When I was with my contemporaries, my reserve was inevitably taken as scorn. It often happens that way with timid children; others interpret reserve as conceit or aggressiveness when it is really a symptom of modesty or feelings of inferiority. I was not just a little timid. My timidity was outrageous, colossal, monstrous. My relationships with others were troubled by this, deeply and durably.

Now that I was rejected by my fellow students, I tried to compensate by working harder, which only served to widen the gap between us. In several subjects, the pace of my studies became too slow for me. I went ahead and tackled upcoming chapters that had not yet been assigned. My reading aloud was doing wonders and I was storing away a considerable amount of knowledge. At the same time, I grew intellectually stronger. In the first class [Grade 12], I was able to give an immediate translation when Tacitus was read aloud to me in Latin. The teacher was so delighted by this that he ended up designing his course solely for me. He read Latin to me by the hour and did not concern himself with whether the rest of the class was following or not!

In mathematics, I worked all the harder because I did not have the innate talent that some students have. If I had not worked hard, I would have been a thoroughly mediocre mathematician. Then I concentrated all my energy on bending my mind to mathematical thinking. It seemed to work. One fine day my father received a letter from the Lycée. The headmaster asked him to be kind enough to come and see him the next time he was in Paris. I was absolutely terrified although nothing in my grades or behavior justified such a reaction. I imagined that I must have committed a serious offense. Some time later, my father arrived. The headmaster met him, accompanied by my mathematics teacher who almost fell on his knees before him.

"Mr. Tomatis, Mr. Tomatis, you can't believe this. I said one day to the students in your son's class that if any of them wanted to do one or two extra exercises I would be pleased to correct them. This is a proposal I make every year to all my classes and which, up to now, has met with scarcely any response. But your son, Mr. Tomatis, your son listened to me, and since then I must spend all my breaks and part of my free time correcting these wretched optional exercises! He overwhelms me with them. Please do something! At least ask him to use a little moderation, for pity's sake!"

That is where timidity and the way one compensates for it leads: I had pushed this fine fellow, whom I remember as an exceptional teacher, to despair. All the same, I never became outstanding in mathematics (a fact which turned me away from technical schools and finally crystallized my desire to become a doctor), but I became skillful enough to prepare for the baccalaureate in elementary math together with philosophy.

I had not yet finished with my inhibitions. I passed the second baccalaureate at the age of 19. During this period, my shyness prevented me not only from having female relationships, even platonic ones, but even from being in the company of females. There were no girls at my school and I had few opportunities to meet any as I spent my life in classrooms or at my apartment. Also, I had no sister. Finally, the violent lifelong conflict between my mother and myself certainly did not help to normalize my relationship with girls.

In these circumstances, my rare conversations with girls were limited to formal and perfectly conventional exchanges. My father was disappointed that he could take no pride in seeing me make conquests. He always wanted to set up dates for me, no doubt in the hopes of making me "normal."

My father was distinctly more successful in getting me to meet, or at least hear, the great singers of that period. During the holidays we went together to the Garrier Palace or to Vichy. I can still see and hear them, their voices echo in my head — Chaliapine, Lorentz, Melchior, and that immense, enormous Wagnerian, the Flagstad.

When my father came to Paris I was bathed in music, saturated but happy. While I went about my business, he sat down at the piano and worked. In this way, little by little, I was able to absorb his entire repertoire. Ever since then, I have worked to the sound of music. When I write my books, when I fling my theories onto paper, or meditate pen in hand, I always fill my study with Mozart or some Gregorian chant. I need this acoustic recharge. Moreover, my studies have enabled me to understand music's workings and appreciate its effects in the most objective way. To some, it may seem to be a whim, but I recommend surrounding oneself with music. It energizes you, just as reading aloud does.

My father passed on to me not only his repertoire but, alas, his wardrobe and shoes. From the age of 14 to 23 I wore clothes which were neither my size nor suitable to my age and, above all, not to my taste. Like many artists, my father dressed in a rather eccentric manner. For me, "King of Cowards," it was torture to walk about clothed in these disguises which inevitably drew attention to my appearance and sometimes jeers. But my father seemed terribly put out when I suggested that the prospect of wearing these garish hand-me-downs did not make me faint at my good fortune. So I was ordered to wear out all the suits, coats, and shoes of which he was tired. The trouble was that as they came from good tailors and shoemakers, they were absolutely "unwearoutable," and impossible to finish off.

I particularly remember two pairs of shoes, one buckskin and the other of yellow straw-colored leather, the sight of which at the foot of my trousers filled me with horror. I did everything possible to get them rated by my family as "no longer serviceable." I played football in them and, at rugby, I craftily let them slip under the soles of players with great metal studs. You have never seen anyone so keen on the idea of wearing out shoe leather. At last I took them back to Nice to make it clear how unusable they had become, but all my mother had to do was a little work with a brush and a cloth and they looked quite new again! I was appalled. Finally, I forced my father to accept that I could no longer wear these terrible yellow shoes. Do you think even then that he would get rid of them? Not at all. He used them as part of his costume in a play. For years I still had to endure the pain seeing of them.

I must have been a sight during that time. Impossible yellow shoes, expensive theatrical clothes whose sleeves either entirely covered my hands or else rode up above my wrists, and to complete the picture, waistcoats, shirts, and socks washed and mended in my own hit-and-miss way!

From time to time, when a theatrical season kept him at the other end of France and he missed me too much (or I missed him too much), my father made me come stay with him. Sometimes it was for a month or two, sometimes for a whole school term. So I often left the Lycée Pasteur for another secondary school in Nice, Marseille, Toulouse, or elsewhere. The teachers of Neuilly made the greatest impression on me. I was lucky to have them, and several who taught me were most remarkable: the historian Auguste Bailly, for instance; another historian, also a writer, whose name was Mr. Peliot, but who signed his books Daniel-Rops; A.M. Debey, my mathematics teacher for elementary math, the same man whom I had condemned to forced labor by making him correct extra exercises and to whom I am grateful for having taught me how to work and shape my thinking as nobody else did.

On the other hand, I had a teacher who, in spite of his fame and charisma, did not influence me at all. Of all that he told us, and God knows he spoke fluently and copiously, I understood nothing. It would be more accurate to say —— using terminology which the reader has already guessed is dear to me —— that I heard nothing. Some years later, after I finished my medical studies, I picked up my old notebooks and happened upon the one for his courses. On the first page, in the margin, I had written: "I have had Jean Paul Sartre as teacher of philosophy. I believe I've had the bad luck not to understand anything he has said to me."

An exceptionally brilliant man, Sartre was obsessed with the obligation he had imposed upon himself to become an existentialist, which he was far from being at the start of his philosophical career. He expounded on Heidegger throughout his course, however, without quoting his sources and without following Heidegger's thinking to its conclusion. Sartre ignored the German master's move towards essentialism, which, rather than existentialism, is the basis of Heidegger's philosophy. The liveliness and brilliance of his mind and the vigor of his improvisations made Sartre convincing even when he spoke without preparation. And he could do so on any subject whatsoever. He was so impressive that one part of the class, taking everything he said seriously and literally, sank into despair. Searching for a solution to their agony they turned to drugs or even, in certain extreme cases, suicide. The other part of the class, to which I belonged, did not "bite" as far as philosophic language and thought went. For us, all these refined theorizations, this new type of reasoning, represented the height of the absurd. I remember one day I had written on the blackboard, as a joke, three utterly bizarre subjects. I still remember their titles: "There is no curtain without a curtain rod"; "Love among the Negroes"; and "The thoughts of a raw cutlet." When Sartre entered the classroom, he glanced at the blackboard and told us to deal with the exact three subjects written there! Personally, I was even more put off by this style of teaching because, in my elementary math and philosophy classes, the very same questions were introduced by another professor, Bastide, who was vigor and logic incarnate.

Actually, I did happen to grasp a few things in Sartre's remarkably rich lectures. But these ideas turned out to be the very opposite of my own. Sartre's metaphysics — it was the era of his famous book "*Nausea*" — were too devoid of hope to be attractive to me in any way. All the same, professor Sartre was, by virtue of his vitality and insight, exceptional.

I was not able to be a follower of Sartre because I was then what I have always remained: a believer and an idealist. I often had mystical experiences although my upbringing was hardly likely to have predisposed me to religious feelings. First, the whole South of France was the freehold of what was then called "radicalism," and the followers of little Father Combes were very numerous there. Second, my father had embarked on his singing career at a time when it was almost compulsory to be a Freemason (an international secret fraternity). He joined not so much in order to find work, as to keep in close touch with others and to be allowed to join in the group rituals. This was necessary so as not to set oneself apart. In fact, membership was more like a corporate password than the expression of any real philosophic conviction.

It is also important not to disregard the unpleasant taste of Paganism which flourishes everywhere in the South even within the Christian faith. It is well known that the strongest believers of the region are more likely to invoke local saints, hallowed by folklore, than to call upon Jesus. The cult devoted to the Virgin of Gue, in particular, could well appear to be an amalgamation of Christian symbolism and a more ancient folklore, pagan in origin. This phenomenon is in no way confined to the region. One only has to travel round the world a bit — as I have, thanks to my profession — to observe that spiritual mixtures exist in many places. It is an almost uniform characteristic of the western civilizations within the Mediterranean Basin.

I grew up in an atmosphere of superstition where some of my close relations, without going so far as animism, were involved in all sorts of unorthodox beliefs. For example, some of them believed in witches or "Masca," as they are called.

My father was a Mason, but his mother was a sincere Christian who was, at the same time, particularly susceptible to local beliefs and superstitions. When I was quite small I accompanied her on the pilgrimage to the shrine of the Virgin of Gue, a journey which everyone was obliged to make at least once in his or her life. We had to walk about 20 kilometers (12.5 miles). It took hours and, for me, this pilgrimage took on the proportions of a prodigious crusade. As no one had taught me about it, the faith of those around me seemed very mysterious. The mystery itself, however, attracted me, and I felt deprived at not having received the same initiation as other boys my age.

Although I had been baptized — mainly to please my grandmother — I had not made my First Communion at the usual age. I regretted this deeply and was keenly frustrated. I wanted to go with my friends to the catechism class, mostly because I was fascinated by the priest, an old man with much vigor whom I would see walking down the streets of old Nice with his ample white beard like Moses or God the Father himself!

One day I could not contain myself any longer and hid behind a pillar at the far corner of the rear sacristy where he was giving the catechism lessons. I had not entered this part of the church since my Baptism. At the time, I was quite ignorant of liturgy and dogma. The priest began to explain at length the symbolism behind the sign of the cross. I lost track of what he was saying very quickly for want of the elementary knowledge which would have enabled me to understand him. I dozed off, noting vaguely that he was teaching others in a very detailed and sententious way to tell the difference between their right and left hands. That was not surprising as we were all more or less dyslateral. This was soon demonstrated. As I daydreamed, stunned with the ideas of "right" and "left," I suddenly saw coming at me a black cassock with a large white beard above it. A voice, warm yet serious and a bit angry, ordered me to lift my right arm so the other children could judge whether I had listened carefully to the lesson. Without hesitation, I raised my left arm (an ironic touch on the part of a future specialist in laterality whose work emphasizes the preeminence of the right hand). I was immediately chased out of the catechism room forevermore with a solid kick in the behind. After that I stayed outside when the others went in to listen to the preacher.

My Paillon grandmother took charge of my religious education. What she provided was more mystical than orthodox. When she took the wash to the Paillon river I accompanied her on her long walk, a walk which seemed shorter thanks to the endless stories she told me. She was an untiring storyteller. In the evenings, she would weave stories for hours until her voice sank and faded as she drifted off to sleep — so unaware was she that her hands continued to knit even as she dozed! A haunting picture! But was it less so than those which arose from her words? My grandmother knew strange and wonderful things about the preacher-magicians of the Hinterland, those simple-minded and saintly men of miraculous powers who prophesied, gave new life to the faith of their audience, and tracked down and cast out evil spirits. She knew of one man in particular who talked every night with the stars. She had been present many times when he addressed the heavens. He had the reputation of being a great prophet. Such supernatural powers were ascribed to this priest that some of his parishioners began to have doubts as to whether they could all be true. They decided to put his gifts to the test.

To question the stars, the priest settled himself on a rock, always the same one. One day, unknown to him, someone slid a sheet of newspaper under this stone. According to my grandmother, the people thought that, in this way, the soothsayer would be disconnected from the earth and his behavior would change if he were not playing tricks on them. That evening, the priest took up his place on his rock and declared to the dumbfounded assembly, "I don't know what is happening, but this evening I feel a great change. Either heaven has drawn nearer to me, or earth has drawn nearer to heaven."

My grandmother also told me, as if she had witnessed the event herself, the following story: One day a sinful soul of old Nice fell seriously ill. In despair, he implored one of these preacher-magicians to exorcise his illness. The preacher came to the man's bedside and dutifully said his office. When the man died, something indescribable was seen to leave the house, pass down the street, and dig a great hole nearby. I was impressed by this story, all the more so because the hole was still visible a few hundred meters from where we lived. Every time I passed near the hole in her company, my grandmother, unruffled, recounted her story.

Thanks to her I also was initiated into the realm of children's fairy tales, myths, and legends. In bringing up her many children my grandmother had gathered an enormous collection of books, as many in French as in Italian although the language was of no importance as she could not read. These books were illustrated with drawings in the style of the period —— Dantesque to say the least! She herself arranged a large number of these fantastic pictures in a sort of anthology, which I spent most of my evenings looking at, not even stopping to eat if we were alone, and all the while she would comment on the pictures with never-failing patience.

So it was that I learned a great many medieval legends and archetypal myths. As all children do, I made the acquaintance of Little Red Riding Hood, Tom Thumb, Puss-in-Boots, and others. However, I got to know them through illustrations often rough, fierce, and terrible. For a long time this was my only culture since I remained illiterate for many years.

I have spoken about supernatural feats, demonic manifestations, terrifying stories and pictures. The reader might infer from this that I was a traumatized child, prey to all sorts of nightmares by day as well as by night. But nothing could be farther from the truth. On the contrary, my failure to recognize or understand fear was one of the most outstanding features of my character, so much so that if I did suffer any psychological shock, it was not caused by the events and stories themselves, but by the strong reactions and emotional upsets they provoked among the grownups.

I have already mentioned the extent to which my mother's father, Alfredo Raggi, was burdened with talismans, riddled with superstitions, preoccupied and haunted by atrocious fears (of dying, of living, of the next world, of this world, of other people, of himself, and of fear itself). This terror, for which there was no remedy, led him to spiritualism, and this brought him back again to fear. I myself experienced a great deal of unease and bewilderment from witnessing his agony.

In general, the restlessness, anxiety, and panic of adults upset me deeply. Above all, I was confounded by the contrast between their verbal heroism — the boastful harangues common among the men of Southern France — and the speed with which they collapsed at the slightest fright. These same people who glorified their own deeds and made terrible threats against others lost all courage in the twinkling of an eye when they had to face danger! I found this all the more difficult to understand because I had never experienced either fear of the night or fear of being alone (or, especially, fear of being alone at night). Yet God knows that I had every opportunity to feel lonely in my little bed what with a traveling artist for a father and a mother who either followed him in his journeys or paid very little attention to me when at home. But I have no anguished memories of my nights alone. I only remember a warm and friendly atmosphere, ultimately a protective one. My bed was sometimes set up very near the stove, and I can look back on myself at age four or five daydreaming or sleeping peacefully there.

I maintained this peacefulness, this unshakable calm, throughout my childhood, adolescence, and adult life. There was never a moment, to my good fortune, when life seemed "difficult." Life is a complex business, of course, and demands constant and sometimes painful efforts, but it is not difficult and it certainly is not something to be dreaded.

Even when I lived alone at Neuilly I was never afraid. I realized later that, in this respect, I was very different from certain adults. I recall one anecdote about Alfredo Raggi, himself a coward beyond description, forever kissing and sucking holy medallions so as to ward off the anger of the powers above. A spiritualistic seance took place in our apartment. I was six years old at the time, and they started by sending me to bed. Then those taking part settled themselves round the table, ready to invoke the Spirits. My grandfather abruptly declared that he was tired and left to go to bed. In actuality, this slave of fear had decided to terrorize the assembled company. He located a loaded revolver and returned stealthily to a position just outside the seance room. When my father's sepulchral voice pronounced the ritual phrase, "Spirit, are you there? If you are there, tap once," my grandfather pulled the trigger.

The violent explosion shook the whole house. I jumped out of bed to see what was happening and found a beaming, laughing Alfredo Raggi standing in the doorway of the now empty room! Or rather it appeared to be empty because everyone had taken refuge under the table. They were paralyzed with terror, and some of them kept to their beds for several weeks!

So my education did not take place just within the four walls of the classroom, and I did not gain all my knowledge and experience of life at school. On the contrary, I learned most of the things which have really formed my character during my holidays from school. This knowledge enables me, today, to follow a profession largely based on psychology. I constantly have the chance to listen to what people say and to notice what they do not say.

My father's backstage life was rich in lessons of all kinds for me. I assimilated not only his repertoire, but also the psychology of all the singers of that period who achieved fame alongside Caruso and Gigli (Escalais, Journet, Schipa, Tita Ruffo, Pertile, Del Lafuente, Fleta, Granier, Charrat, Monavelli, Carpentier). I also learned the psychology of their public. Theater at the time was very important; radio and cinema were still at a very primitive stage, and sports were not as popular as they are today. Lovers of bel canto and of opera, particularly in southern France, came from all the economic, professional, and cultural groups so opera audiences represented a true sample of the whole population. Some of them were so passionately interested in the opera that they were formidable experts; they knew the score note by note and could repeat the libretto word for word. More than once I was present when an artist had a momentary lapse on the stage and the correct note was uttered by one or more persons in the audience. To have been close to all these people, so different yet united by the same enthusiasm, unquestionably has played its part in forming my character.

Starting at the age of 11, I spent a few weeks every year at Saint Barnabé (near Marseille) with a family who still lived in accordance with the old Provençal traditions. The neighbors might have been called Fernandel and Raimu.[2] Each day's pleasure was mingled for me — city-bred as I was — with the exciting illusion of sharing in the farm chores. I am deeply impressed by these happy times, not only emotionally, but intellectually. They gave me a more objective view of patriarchal families than the accepted clichés.

Much has been written about the family dominated by an all-powerful patriarch in which the women are controlled, subjugated, enslaved by the men. Here is what I saw, even though I was still only a child.

This whole family assembled at meal times, together with the farm-workers, and, as was commonly supposed, the women were treated as inferiors. They were dominated and exploited. The father of the family took his place at the head of the table. Then the sons took their seats — the eldest on his right, the second on his left and so on down to the youngest. The farm-workers came next in order of length of service, and I came after them because I was the youngest of the whole company. Then I could see in successive stages the whole of this

---

[2] Fernandel and Raimu were famous French film actors well-known for their rustic and bucolic roles in Pagnol's movies.

social organization, portrayed and developed even as I watched, like a living organism where all the elements are arranged and coordinated by appropriate relationships. Standing behind us, silent, watchful, efficient, the women brought the dishes and filled our plates under the orders of the mistress of the house who stood in the midst of them. Nothing escaped her. Helped by her daughters, she had prepared the meal at length and with the greatest care. The meals were abundant, copious, Pantagruel-like![3] I could hardly manage to taste every dish. Everyone chewed steadily with a savage, ritualistic intensity. The father alone opened his mouth from time to time to let fall some truth: words full of his experience, of his past life, of his idea of work, of morals, of authority. They were full, too, of that light which the Provençal sun had caused to spring up in his whole being, for he was "somebody" whose worth was as notable as his ruddy complexion. Around the table his fellow eaters maintained an attentive and respectful silence, always ready to reply if the master directed a question at them.

The patriarchal family at this level existed just as it has always been described. But, as I was soon to perceive, this was only one aspect of reality. Thanks to my dual role of child and stranger, I was allowed in the kitchen when the men got up, either to go to their siesta or to leave for work, so that I was present, too, at the women's meal. The mother took the place that her husband had occupied; the daughters sat down in their turn. They ate what the men had left.

By seeing and hearing them year after year I was able to create for myself a more precise and accurate idea of the system. Little by little I understood the essential function, the prime importance, the fundamental position that these women occupied, so devoted, so submissive, so respectful towards the men, so involved in their mission to nourish the males. Before my eyes there gradually emerged what constituted the hidden substructure of the patriarchy, its roots, its foundations, the soil which allowed it to grow. This was the matriarchy.

During the whole time the men set at the table, serious, proud, dignified, tyrant-like, the women let the men say and do everything. They had fed them as children are fed; they gave them drink as one suckles an infant at the breast. They let the men believe that they dominated the household by the fluency and force of their speech. Once the men left, these same women who had been so busy serving the men, so reserved, so silent, were now enjoying themselves —— laughing, happy to be alive, exchanging a thousand little stories, full of those ideas which the men thought they had originated. In fact, it was the women who had put the ideas into the men's heads! Behind a tradition of obedience, which was a mere façade, they fulfilled their fundamental vocation of "governing" (in

---

[3] A character in the work of sixteenth century French author Rabelais known for his voracious appetite.

the highest sense of the term) the men. Not only was it they who ran the household, but it was they, too, who controlled the development of the business; again, it was the women who dominated and were the central pillar of family activities and politics. In a certain way, they formed the house itself, its beating heart, its strongly defined boundaries. Basically, the attitude of the men, including what is today called their "sexuality," was only what the women wanted it to be. As for the men's conversation, they raised it and built it up from foundations laid by the women. In brief, what was called the patriarchal structure of the ancient Provençal family (then part of the Greco-Latin family) was *not* a structure, but mere superficial imagery, a pure illusion kept in place by the women themselves. The truth which came to light from this revelation showed that the husband is never anything but his wife's eldest child. The loud, triumphant, masculine utterance was, in fact, only the bombastic echo of the original, gentle, feminine speech. I shall never forget this precious lesson.

I devoted another part of the long holidays to excursions in the mountains. With Uncle Clement and some of his friends crammed into a very small car, we travelled through the Alps where traffic was then almost non-existent. We stopped, camped, and walked a lot. At the beginning of the thirties very few people went camping or mountain walking. In most of the places we visited, we were the only tourists and could enjoy the magnificence of nature without restraint. The places we stayed in, isolated farms, gave me a chance to experience for the first time a way of life very different from what I had known in Old Nice, in St. Barnabé, or backstage in theaters. Just seeing the mountain ranges and glaciers helped to form my character, providing also a lesson in the appreciation of beauty and in humility.

Nearly always we went to the Alps of the Midi. Only once did we set out for the Pyrenees, and this trip was, to some extent, a failure. We were unable to visit Lourdes as planned because our mountaineering clothes were not commonly worn at that time and were not considered acceptable dress. Another plan to take a little tour in Spain was equally unsuccessful. This journey started in the summer of 1936; the civil war broke out on July 17th when the uprising of Melilla took place. Our only choice was to turn back.

After my baccalaureate I enthusiastically registered for the PCB certificate in Physics, Chemistry, and Biology, required as a prerequisite for admission to medical studies. My fellow students and I were the first to attempt this certificate, which had been set up only a year or two earlier to replace the old PCN (Physics, Chemistry, and Natural Science). My thirst for knowledge, my impatience, and my confidence in my capacity for work over a range of subjects made me think I need not confine myself to one certificate. I put my name down at the same time for the SPCN (Certificate of Sciences: Physical, Chemical, and Natural) and the MPC (Mathematics, Physics, and Chemistry) both of which were being given at the Sorbonne. This was not a mere affectation on my part.

My plan was to have as many chances as possible of being accepted one day as a candidate for the Entrance Examination at the Institut Pasteur, and so realize my childhood dream of becoming a doctor engaged in research. This was as yet only a vague notion, but I knew already that I should have to assimilate at one and the same time both specialist medical knowledge and general scientific knowledge.

I was living in Rue Théophile Gautier then, away from home even more than before. Finding my way between the Medical Faculty and the Sorbonne, I got to know the streets in the Latin Quartier well. We had lunch in the dining halls of schools such as Louis Le Grand or St. Louis; in the afternoon and evening we would dine in the clubs near Rue St. Jacques and Rue de l'Abbé-de-l'Epée.

Inevitably, I met girls during these meals and other students, in the lecture halls, who were fired by the same ideals as me. In this way, I became part of like-minded groups where each individual benefitted from the experiences of the others. I formed a particular partnership with a friend from Alsace, Emile Boutserin, and we divided our areas of study and various assignments. Boutserin was the acknowledged master of the sciences, especially the natural sciences. I became the acknowledged expert on medicine, physics, and math. We arranged regular meetings several times a week to exchange new knowledge and course notes. In this way we benefitted simultaneously both from our own progress and our partner's.

This workplan was efficient, but left us very little free time. This did not bother me since leisure had never played a great part in my scheme of life. When I had a free moment, I took an extra course in math, physics, or chemistry.

3

The War

Absorbed by our studies, we were like strangers in the city. Though most world events made no impression on us, we could not help but notice the public's concern with the international tensions and conflicts that would eventually lead to World War II. In fact, in 1939 and 1940 the clash of arms and conflict of opposing ideologies weighed heavily on every aspect of university life. "We could not ignore it." The great question was this: "Should we be allowed to finish our studies?" For once I experienced the same distress as everyone else (a distress which, curiously enough, included a feeling of euphoria caused by our participation in great events). While we waited, Boutserin and I thought it best if we redoubled our efforts to learn as much as we could as quickly as possible.

The war took a very bad turn for France in the spring of 1940 and that put an end to our frantic behavior. Students due for mobilization took exams early. I took tests for both the PCB and the SPCN in the same week. I was somewhat apprehensive when I went for the exam, but my preparation had been so eager and meticulous that I could answer every question. With 97 marks out of 110, I obtained the best results in the PCB. And though 32 of us took the written examination for the SPCN, I was the only one at the oral. After I passed the practical tests in chemistry, my examiner came up to me and said, emotionally, "Young man, I must congratulate you, and above all thank you. By taking this oral, you have saved my life." I was flabbergasted. He explained that because he had conducted my oral exam, he was not in his laboratory at the Renault factory when it was destroyed by heavy shelling and all his fellow workers were killed.

I passed the SPCN with a score of 210 marks out of 230. The results arrived at the same time as my call-up papers. My orders were to join up at Yssingeaux immediately. I was very surprised, even disconcerted, for this sounded like a Belgian or Dutch town, and I could not understand why I should be sent to an area which was entirely in enemy hands, particularly since my military bearing and fitness for war were very poor. Furthermore, I doubted I would even reach Yssingeaux because someone told me it was situated right on the Massif Central.

Nonetheless, I started on my journey. However, I was stopped on the outskirts of Clermont-Ferrand and ordered to follow one of the many columns traveling on the French highways. At Chazelles-sur-Lyon I stayed for some time with a group in a hat factory that had been requisitioned for lodging. Like all new arrivals, I underwent the usual selection tests. Recruits were classified according to their school or university qualifications. First, we were asked to raise our hands if we had the primary certificate of studies. All who did not were grouped to one side as illiterate ignoramuses. Then they continued through the hierarchy of diplomas.

Since I did not have the primary certificate because it was never taken by students at high school, I could not put up my hand and was turned over to the illiterate group. No one allowed me to explain that I had passed my baccalaureate and even held two university degrees.

To distinguish between simple dunces and the unteachables, those in my group were given dictation and elementary computation exercises. The dictation could have saved me — but the computations succeeded in ruining me! I have always been unpardonably careless in this area. Like many people used to abstractions, I am too absent-minded, or perhaps too attentive to other things. I made so many mistakes in my calculations that the Army considered me to be, if not totally illiterate, at least a perfect idiot. However, I do not regret in any way living through what was to be an exceptional human experience, one that certainly would never have happened if they had classified my abilities as superior.

Since I did not ask to be posted to the Medical Corps, I was drafted without further ceremony into the infantry. There I found among the alleged derelicts of intelligence — really the rejects of the school system — all sorts of picturesque figures and engaging personalities. Most of my fellow soldiers were originally from the suburbs of Paris. In civilian life they worked at difficult and lowly factory jobs. By knowing them, I began to realize how sheltered my own adolescence had been. They came to grips with life long ago, and not just through books and household washing! They bore the marks of that difficult life and extracted from it a certain philosophy of life, a philosophy of which I took advantage since it opened my eyes to a quite new and extraordinary universe. Until then, the circumstances of my life prevented me from experiencing or even exchanging views with any who had led such a life. Now I caught up, renewing my old role of observer, watching and listening attentively. These young workers, unbeknownst to themselves, became my teachers of psychology. My time in the Army did not make me a valiant warrior, but my personal encounters allowed me to recognize the true nature of social and psychological relationships; I discovered a rich assortment of living elements, snatched from living examples. I doubt that, later, I would have understood these on a practical level without having had the good fortune to experience them firsthand.

As far as the rest goes, from the day of my joining up to the day of my demobilization, I remained a soldier without conviction. Perhaps I recalled only too well the pacifist harangues of my grandparents. I proved to be a wretched soldier, so it was quite puzzling as to why I was assigned to be a light infantryman in reconnaissance patrols. In that capacity, I was rigged out with a machine gun that was much too heavy and clumsy for my taste. I awkwardly dragged it along as I marked double time, crawled in the mud, and hurled myself into the undergrowth whenever an imaginary enemy was signalled. I went through all the motions with no enthusiasm and no pleasure. The adjutant, a man most appropriately named Peste, noticed me right away and made my life a little harder each day. Perhaps not unreasonably, he suspected that I was a civilian who was incorrigibly insubordinate to the glories of military discipline. Alas! I did not have a military bearing and wandered, moonstruck, through this life so unsuited to my ambitions. I could not take my duties seriously because during my patrols I never saw even a hint of a German — even when the Germans were busy winning the first phase of the war! To me, it was "the phoney war," and I am not the first to observe that tragedy smacks strongly of tragi-comedy.

Finally, we found ourselves once more on the move heading toward Le Puy. I can visualize myself carrying my pack and that of a comrade who was even more worn out than I. From time to time we were made to clamber into a truck. We got down again in villages where, to our total amazement, we were greeted as saviors. We looked wide-eyed at these rapturous civilians, then resumed our strategic withdrawal toward the south. Our retreat, however, was noticeably slower than the German advance.

One day the trucks stopped in open country so we could learn how grenades worked. After the brief stop, we set off again only to be halted in a few kilometers. We were hastily ordered to get down from the trucks and take up positions in the ditch. An enemy column was in sight! I, for one, was completely confused, unaware of what was happening and unable to see anything except a few nearby grenade bursts. Almost immediately the Cease Fire order came. As it turned out, we had almost attacked our own allies, a detachment of Polish soldiers marching south just as we were and wearing uniforms not immediately recognized by our officers. Soon after, a column of Germans and Italians took all of us prisoners, Poles and Frenchmen alike. When we finally arrived at our goal, le Puy barracks, we were enemy prisoners rather than friendly allies.

Every day the narrow entrance gate at Le Puy admitted fresh prisoners. Thousands of us were imprisoned under a virtually symbolic guard — a few Italian sentries at the gate and an occasional airplane overhead. For some unknown reason we had been allowed to keep our civilian clothes in our packs; it seemed absurd to me not to escape under such lax conditions. I was astonished and disappointed to learn that only a handful of my fellow prisoners shared this thought. Most of my comrades greeted my suggestion with sarcasm, scorn, or despondency.

"Don't get excited, Tomatis," they told me. "The war is finished. No one is bothering us, and it is peaceful here in prison. Don't go looking for trouble. Let things be, my friend. Don't show too much zeal."

Only a small group of the more highly educated men listened to my arguments. When we knew that the rest would not change their minds and come with us, we decided to make our escape. It was not difficult. We left the barracks as one might leave a factory. No questions were asked, either inside or out.

We stayed around le Puy for a few days observing the barracks from a distance. No one else attempted to escape, although there were enough of them to have easily charged the gate and quickly overcome the Italian soldiers. This passive attitude cost them dearly for one day they were loaded into trucks and taken in whole convoys to prison camps in Germany, where they experienced prolonged captivity and misery.

As for us, we were listed somewhat paradoxically as deserters! This dishonorable nametag hung around our necks for a long time, but eventually we found ourselves once again in what may be called "The Youth Work Camps." I was lucky enough to be sent to a nearby camp situated in a marvelous village overhanging a valley. I lodged with a group of students, many of whom were from Alsace and did not speak French. For some unknown reason, I was appointed head of the barrack-room, a responsibility I could gladly have done without.

For some time I continued my psychological and social education by observing my companions. We lived in a sector of the free zone, leading the vegetative life of barracks-bound infantrymen until something happened which was destined to completely change my life: the work camp directors ordered the recall of men with certain medical qualifications.

The medical service at this time was utterly disorganized and chaotic. While many doctors were prisoners in Germany, others had been demobilized and returned to civilian life. Only one doctor remained with us, a captain who was on his own because his assistants were posted to sectors lacking any medical service.

Two of us, a pharmacy student and me, reported to this doctor. He told us that he would be demobilized himself in a few months and that, before leaving, he would try to reorganize the service by using our various talents and speeding up our training.

So it was done.

This captain, Doctor Eyraud, came from the Lyons region and, from several different aspects, was a quite remarkable man. He identified the huge deficiencies in my knowledge, due to only one year of medical study, and made me work day and night for his last three or four months in the camp. I quickly learned what was essential for any army or country doctor to know about emergencies and infectious diseases. Without the help of a single book or paper, this man explained the most complex problems. He did so with a clarity and relevance that I have only experienced from the very best medical faculty professors. His teaching talent was as remarkable as his vast range of knowledge. He gave me an exceptional opportunity to observe someone who was a master of his subject.

In record time my colleague in pharmacy and I were so well grounded in medicine that we were able to be of some use. On the day our captain said good-bye, we assumed the duties of battalion medical officers! What a strange situation I was in: second class battalion medical officer and deserter to boot — because no one had ever reported my presence in this sector of the army. I did my best in my new job, an appointment which lasted until I was posted to a labor camp in the neighborhood of Cluny, in Saone-et-Loire. There, two or three of us worked together under the command of a man who was later to become General Vinot.

We brought to our new assignment a small treasure, a railway train equipped as a mobile surgical unit. I had chanced upon it, and my two comrades and I managed to get it going. With it, we took on new roles: fireman, engineer, and switchman. When we arrived at the labor camp, we organized a hospital service which had all the necessary supplies and equipment along with an element of the picturesque. I took on still another role. For all the semi-idle young men who had interrupted their studies, I provided some education courses in a school where I was the only teacher. I poured out all the knowledge I had assimilated during my years of formal and informal study. My methods could not have been too bad since some of my students sat for and ultimately passed their baccalaureate.

Demobilized from the labor camps, I at last returned to Paris, now occupied, where life was not easy. I forced myself to start university life again. Thanks to my captain, my daily practice in the medical corps, and my personal habits of intensive study (I spent nearly all night studying, although the only light I had was driven by a hand-operated generator), I was able to reach the third year of medical studies in just a few months. So the war had not caused me to lose a single year.

However, I never forgot that the war continued beyond our frontiers and, in a less obvious but no less stubborn way, even within our own country. I wholeheartedly approved of the Resistance movement so I decided not to limit myself to a purely intellectual sympathy and looked for a more practical way to support it. I was again in touch with my father, and through him and certain fellow-members of the General Association of Students, I contacted a network and assumed responsibility for reception and rediffusion of intelligence to the west coast and to England. I became one of the many "baggage carriers" in the army of shadows.

All this time I pursued my studies without any insurmountable difficulties. I established my headquarters at the Sorbonne rather than at the Medical Faculty, and every year I followed the courses which produced more than one

Certificate of Higher Studies: General Physics, General Chemistry, Botany, Mineralogy, and Biochemistry. I renewed my splendid old partnership with my friend Boutserin, who had never left Paris, and we backed up each other as we had in the past, always keeping one goal in view —— to become researchers.

Shortly after my return from the labor camps, I passed the hospital's external exam and began to rotate into its different surgical departments. I particularly remember M. Sorel who was in charge of the bone surgery department. However, the teacher who most deeply and lastingly impressed me there, as much by his personality as by his teaching and conception of a doctor's role, was André-Thomas, one of the greatest neurologists in the history of French medicine. Once more I had the opportunity to be close to an exceptionally distinguished man. Though I could say a lot about him, perhaps what struck me most was his way of conducting a clinical examination, particularly those of children and infants. His power of observation and his delicacy of analysis were astonishing. He brought to these tasks not only an immense experience (he was very old at this time and lived to be a hundred), but also a most original vision of problems. This vision led him to make remarkably fruitful discoveries and fundamental contributions in the field of the motor effects of mental processes. He was one of the most complete doctors I ever met, at one and the same time a neurologist, physiologist, and anatomist. Over and above all this, he was a man of extreme gentleness who introduced a psychological dimension into his consultations; the effects of this were very interesting for a beginner to observe. Finally, his humility and modesty were incomparable, his good humor was unfailing, and his availability to us was limitless. He gave out his valuable knowledge with good humor and generosity, and his easy manner of teaching could not be easily equalled. In every respect he possessed that simplicity of greatness which I have always considered to be one of the most admirable qualities for a great man.

During my adventures in the Army, Boutserin, a brilliant student, had made his own way. He enjoyed a certain notoriety at the Sorbonne, not only among his fellow students, but also among those who taught him. As he was not liable for military call-up in 1939-40, he had devoted himself body and soul to his studies. He had certainly not wasted his time while I was playing the fool in the brushwood of the Massif Central and on the roads during the army's collapse. Professor Plantefol[4] (surely a name planned by fate!) employed Boutserin in his famous botanical laboratory and seemed to value his work highly. Besides this, Professor Combes, a most exacting man and a great authority on zoology, arranged for him to enter his own laboratory. Boutserin married a student he had met in the lecture rooms of the Sorbonne, and though he set up house with her

[4] The name means literally Plant-madness.

at Gagny, this did not interrupt our fruitful collaboration. We advanced by leaps and bounds and thought we might soon be accepted for the examination which would lead us to careers in research.

Sadly, fate decided otherwise. Terrible bombardments destroyed the east of Paris, and one day I was urgently summoned to Gagny to identify the bodies of my friend and his wife. They had taken refuge in a basement where they were killed by the blast of an explosion. Their bodies were absolutely untouched. Only a little blood could be seen, with some difficulty, at the edge of the mouth — a sign of a burst lung. They were stripped of everything, including their clothes; the corpse-robbers had lost no time. These are the turns of fortune in time of war, and I chose not to dwell on this subject.

Boutserin had kept me in touch with the non-medical aspects of science. When I lost him, I not only lost my best friend, but I also had to say good-bye to some of my most cherished plans. This was not the only drama I lived through during the bombardment of Paris, for while studying under the direction of Professor Bousser at the Bichat hospital, I experienced yet another loss.

Professor Bousser, with whom I had a long and personally enriching relationship, was similar to André-Thomas. On the surface Bousser was less communicative, but his silence concealed an equally great heart and spirit. When anyone actually dared to ask him a question, he cordially plunged into a series of always brilliant insights. Working with him was indeed a privilege, and I felt another loss when our relationship ended abruptly.

When the Allies landed in Normandy, the bombardment of Paris intensified. We began to receive more and more wounded at Bichat. At this turning point in the war, a most disconcerting thing happened: many of our staff deserted just when we needed them most. It seemed overwhelming for a young idealist like me. As more and more patients flowed in, more and more services were shut down. Under the direction of those professors who remained, we worked without rest for 12 days and as many nights. The devotion I witnessed was outstanding. Even when my idealism was at its strongest, I would never have believed it possible that one could give so much of oneself to relieve the sufferings of others. I learned that human charity could bring about real miracles, and I summoned all my energy to set myself at concert pitch. At the end of 10 days and 10 nights, we were, of course, thoroughly exhausted. Some friends came and made me return to my own house at Neuilly to spend one whole night in a real bed. After a few hours of sleep, I remounted my bicycle and, using some trickery to avoid the German army vehicles which were patrolling the streets, I returned to the hospital.

When I finally got within sight of Bichat, the scene was terrible. The hospital's entire right wing had been destroyed by the bombing during the night. The patients and comrades whom I left the night before trying to get a little rest or selflessly attending to their jobs had been crushed in the disaster. Besides me, only one hospital attendant survived out of the entire hospital staff. We had no time even to shed a tear for our fellow workers; we had to busy ourselves right away with the sick who had escaped this atrocity.

Even before this happened I had decided to do all I could to hasten the end of the war, redoubling my activity in the Resistance. Within a few days of this tragedy I rejoined the forces. At my request, I was assigned directly to the Medical Corps and once more donned an Air Force cadet uniform. I was posted to the 117th battalion under the immediate command of Captain Raboutet, an efficient and understanding man who would finish his career as Inspector General of the Air Corps. Since the battalion was quartered in Paris, he authorized me to continue my studies at Medical School. I was attracted to a specialty which I had always planned to add to my education, that of Otolaryngology (Ear, Nose, and Throat or ENT). Very early I became aware of certain difficulties encountered by singers who were my father's friends, and though I wanted very much to solve their problems, the medicine of that era was slow to find a solution. This was no doubt ambitious on my part, but it provided a fine way of showing my affection for my father, who always supported and inspired me during my high school and university studies.

In his exceptional kindness, Captain Raboutet even went so far as to introduce me to one of his intimate friends, Captain Cuzin, who was the chief ENT doctor of the Air Corps. He had me and another cadet named Clement help him organize a clinic requisitioned at Neuilly (which was not far from the American hospital). This was to be the center of ENT services for the Air Corps and also responsible for services to disfigured ex-servicemen. Captain Cuzin had received very advanced training in reconstructive surgery, notably in England. His abilities in the ENT field were considerable since he had been one of the brilliant assistants of Professor Aubry, who was also, under the title of doctor-in-chief, a consultant at this clinic. Under the leadership of such a man I enthusiastically launched myself into this new adventure.

We faced a tough situation. In 1944 and 1945, there was no lack of disfigured servicemen. Overwork was our daily routine, and when I say "overwork," I do not use the word lightly. Our stamina in the face of exhaustion stupefies me when I think of it today. Reliable witnesses confirmed that we established endurance records three times. Once I remained on my feet for 11 days without sleep; another time, 13 days. We had no choice; we had to respond to what confronted us. I learned an enormous amount while assisting Dr. Cuzin, who was an extremely gifted surgeon. Once again, I gained an accelerated education under the guidance of a remarkable master.

I lived only a few steps from the clinic. But this time I did not live alone, for I had at last married. However, this marriage represented only an adventure for me, not a final goal. Conversations with my wife were scarcely more profound or enriching than those from several years earlier with the young ladies to whom my father introduced me. "Conversation" is not the right word since both experiences typified a lack of communication. For a dozen years my first wife and I remained side by side without ever really meeting. We were as far apart as if we lived in different universes. With my wife I reproduced the failure of my relationship with my mother. I was hardly surprised. In hindsight, even at the time of our engagement, we could find no mutual harmony, and I already had an inkling of future difficulties. And with my past, how could I even imagine that real communication with a woman was possible?

Why then did I get married? Due to my inexperience with women, I believed that marriage was inevitable from the moment I asked this young lady to go out with me. We met at the hospital at Neuilly where I was an intern replacement. For one of my duties, I gave a teach-in at a patient bedside to a group of students from the nursing school. One of them attracted my attention. I talked with her more than I had ever talked with any woman and eventually asked her for a date. In my heart I already felt engaged and saw our destiny outlined: marriage and a shared life. But even then, when our conversations left strictly professional subjects, communication floundered. I must admit that I was not very talkative, but the little I allowed myself to reveal of my deepest aspirations, ideas about life, and varied interests did not awaken the slightest response in her. To be honest, I felt compelled to continue with the fiasco because, by inviting her to go out with me, I thought I had pronounced a sacred oath. The only thing left was for me to "do my duty."

Against the unanimous advice of my whole family and all my friends, we became engaged. With the confidence of youth, I still hoped to make this a successful union. I was wrong. For nearly two years we continued to look at one another without seeing, to listen to each other without hearing, and to spend time together without getting to know each other. Then we married and continued this emptiness for years. I obstinately tried to prove a loyalty which nothing and no one really compelled me to prove. We even started a family, which was, for me, the ultimate purpose of marriage. I had very set ideas on the subject: I wanted six children. We eventually had four: Marc-André, Patrick, Christian, and Evelyne. The first was born exactly nine months after our marriage, and each of the other three at intervals of two years. Though the births could have brought us together, they did not. My wife's attitude toward the children did not match my idea of a mother's role. I became more and more acutely aware of the failure of our union and eventually sought refuge in my work, something which had never disappointed me. The temptation to let myself become absorbed in my job was all the stronger because of my passionate interest in it. As I pursued my work at the hospital, the rest of my time was gradually taken up by private patients. Much more than consolation awaited me. In my intensive professional practice, I found my real reason for existence.

4

Occupational Deafness

I left the army and Captain Cuzin and entered the service of the Bretonneau hospital as a non-resident. There my training in ENT took on a phoniatric aspect. My chief was Dr. Maurice Lallemant, a man to whom I am enormously indebted. He introduced me to current practical work in this specialty and, most important, gave me his confidence, thereby enabling me to become an assistant without going through the intermediate stage of intern. I wanted to prove that I was up to the job and worked extra shifts every two or three days and, eventually, almost every day. After the birth of my second child I began to practice in the city in order to make ends meet. I administered injections, replaced or assisted doctors, and even practiced a little surgery. And to top it all off, I threw myself into my first research project.

Since I was concerned with the problems of disabled ex-servicemen, I kept in close touch with foreign reports on this subject, particularly American reports. I read many studies of auditory difficulties among subjects exposed to violent noises (for example, explosions caused by gunfire or the roar of jet aircraft), and the various possibilities of curing them. Since I had been a consultant physician to the Air Corps arsenals since 1945, I had observed many people who had been subjected to noise. In fact, several thousand employees of the arsenals worked in almost permanent conditions of acoustic assault. I obtained from the officer in charge of this district, Colonel Bourdon, authorization to study these people. At considerable expense, out of my own pocket, I had an audiometer sent from the United States and immediately set to work — unpaid, of course. My laboratory was a coal cellar which we fixed up as well as we could with a table, a few chairs, and a temporary lighting system.

I naively thought the workers would flock to my office to be examined. After all, my analyses would fill a gap in the infant area of industrial medicine. I was in for a rude awakening! It took interminable discussions to get even a few of them to admit that it might be in their interest to undergo my tests. But the majority stubbornly refused, not because they doubted my abilities, but instead because they over-estimated them. Many of these workers actually feared that, with my mysterious American machine, I would be able to read their minds, to force my way into the most intimate strata of their personalities.

I also heard a rumor that the audiometric examination would be used to weed out workers; all those whose hearing was unsatisfactory would lose their jobs. Picture their agony! By insisting, however, I ended up, in spite of everything, amassing a number of observations and measurements. But the results were not valid. I only understood why several years later.

In 1946, my chief, whom I scrupulously kept apprised of my research, encouraged me to continue in this field.

"Go on collecting results," he said to me. "When you reach solid conclusions, I will help you publish them. Why don't we present a joint paper on occupational deafness at the International ENT Congress?"

This was all the encouragement I needed. I decided, more or less on the spot, to set up a personal laboratory at my own expense that I could use both for my consultations and my surgical operations. But first I had to find adequate space, and that was not easy. I visited several suitable places. Finally, I learned that an elderly colleague, Dr. H., was toying with the idea of selling his space. But since he had only recently declared his intention, I was advised to proceed with great tact.

I went to his house during office hours and mingled with the patients in the waiting room. I was already uneasy, for it appeared that the apartment needed complete redecoration. I vaguely remembered Dr. H. He had cared for me as a child and also had been involved with my father; after being an army gynecologist, he went to Paris to specialize in treating singers. When it was my turn, I went into his consulting room. The room was so filthy that I recoiled. I remember, in particular, a dark greasy mark on one wall behind an armchair.

"Well, doctor," I began in the tone of one making a confession. "A mutual friend told me in confidence that you are thinking of..."

"I beg your pardon?" he interrupted.

He had not recognized me and had no idea what I wanted, which increased my embarrassment, errant coward that I was. I gathered my courage and started to repeat my explanation.

"I was saying that we have a mutual friend from whom I learned that you..."

"What's that? What did you say?"

Finally realizing that he was rather deaf, I was obliged to raise my voice although I was terrified that everyone in the waiting room might overhear. But he still didn't hear me. I began again even louder, but with no better result. Finally, I shouted into his ear.

"A mutual friend told me that you are thinking of giving up this set of rooms."

He replied very calmly, "Yes. Yes. I see how it is. Sit down, my dear sir."

As I didn't want to annoy my colleague, I took my place on the seat.

"We will arrange all this for you," went on Dr. H. "This will be nothing at all. Put your head back and open your mouth."

I obeyed and, in less time than it takes to say "otolaryngology," he squirted oil on my larynx. This was a commonly used treatment at that time. It was thought, no doubt, that the organ needed greasing like an automobile engine. Dr.

H. was a fanatic on lubrication. He put some oil on every larynx that came within his reach. The unappealing mark on his wall had been caused by all the heads that had leaned against it while he administered his oil treatment. I swallowed my dose of oil, paid, and hurriedly made off to look for a set of rooms somewhere else.

After finally finding a place for my laboratory and then equipping it, I still needed to hire some fellow workers, again at my own expense. From the start it was difficult to keep this little research unit alive. Overcoming my repugnance, I actually went and rang doorbells, soliciting clients. Sometimes I was taken seriously. I incurred debts and more debts, laboriously repaid by the fees earned from the first clients. Fortunately, we enjoyed a measure of success. At the end of a few months, I was taking out a large quantity of tonsils! But the money was only just enough. Research is so expensive; it is like a barrel with a hole in the bottom. However, it was a marvelously exciting time, and our progress repaid me for the financial uncertainty. Financing our research preoccupied us all the time since we received no subsidy of any kind. In this way, at least, my situation has not changed one iota in all these years. I will share more about this laboratory later. For now, let us turn to how I discovered that my early measurements taken at the arsenals were totally false.

The medical press and major newspapers gave some publicity to the ENT Congress that year, particularly to the subject of occupational deafness. In collaboration with Dr. Maduro and Dr. Lallemant, I published a paper on this subject. Now, at last, those working in the arsenals changed their attitudes. They saw clearly that not one of them who had been examined had lost his job. Some of them were examined regularly, which enabled me to study their development. Their mistrust was gradually defused. They began to tell themselves that perhaps these examinations, far from harming them, actually offered the chance to discover and develop countermeasures against the sonic attacks they had to withstand at work. Some of them even went so far as to speculate that poor results in the audiometric tests would entitle them to a pension.

In a few weeks our coal-bunker was literally packed with visitors. A line formed at the door and we had to distribute numbered tags! Over the years, thirty people came before me three times a week. Those who have some idea of audiometry will appreciate the work this involved.

Almost immediately, I noted spectacular changes in the results of previously examined subjects. It was as if psychological changes (a release from anxiety and, in its place, the hope of some bonus) had transformed their hearing. For all intents and purposes, their performances were the opposite of the previous ones. Unlike their initial considerable efforts when they tried to hear well, now they were doing everything in their power to understand nothing. The two scores were so different that my first reaction was to wonder if they were deliberately trying to make a fool out of me. Since I thought they were trying to cheat, I decided to keep a close watch on them. But my vigilance was to no purpose. When I thought it over, I finally concluded that perhaps this was an unconscious response rather than an intentional falsification. Motivated by the prospect of a pension, the subjects "cheated in good faith." They obeyed psychological laws of which they were oblivious, and their subjective response was observed by measurements which were alleged to be objective. I was surprised to discover that a perfectly sincere individual, but one who secretly wanted to be diagnosed as deaf, was able to lower his auditory threshold by ten, twenty, and even thirty decibels.

I confirmed my hypothesis when I tested members of the flying staff. Those who intended to get jobs in civil companies (where flyers are incomparably better paid than ground staff) achieved, as if by chance, audiometric performances always equal, or superior to, the required standard. From one test to another, from one year to another, no significant modification occurred in their hearing tests, whatever experience they might have undergone. In brief, their desire for a good salary lent them wings as far as their ears were concerned.

In these conditions, audiometry's claims to objectivity appear extravagant. Putting too low a value on factors which could not be measured totally confused the charts. I was embarrassed especially because, in the course of my medical studies, I had not received even a bare bones outline of the study of psychology. After undertaking many surgical operations, I unconsciously absorbed the ideas of the surgeons of that era who firmly relegated spirit and its influence to the merely incidental. I certainly needed to change my way of thinking. In retrospect, the scorn of the Medical Faculty for the discipline of psychology seems to me dumbfounding, all the more so because a very great doctor several thousand years ago had let drop a phrase which should have put everyone on the right road. I am referring to Avicenna, that Arab genius, a teacher of medicine from the age of sixteen, a disciple of Aristotle whose writings were permeated with neo-Platonism. He stated in his famous "Canons of Medicine" that in the art of healing words come first, medicine, second, and the surgeon's knife, last. In other words, medicine's first weapon, even before drugs, is the word. I had a lofty premonition of the importance of psychotherapy in healing not only psychological problems but also physical ailments.

Today the influence of subjective limiting factors in audiometry is scarcely contested. American works, notably those of Ralph F. Naunton, have thrown light on them in an absolutely unchallengeable way. It is acknowledged that the character of the test administrator affects the result obtained in the audiogram. Naunton goes so far as to consider it useless for one specialist to pass on to another the audiometric graphs which he obtained. They only have meaning in the unique relationship which is established between the subject and the test administrator. One is even tempted to add "and the apparatus," for even in changing audiometers there is a strong risk of collecting different measurements.

Some time later I developed a Listening Test which measured psychological dimensions, somatic data, and the quality of interaction between the person and his or her sonic environment. Taking all of these phenomena into account, I applied most of my efforts to finding a way to make audiometry more objective. That proved to be a long-term and exacting research project, one which still occupies me today. Actually, I am encouraged by its duration because I believe nothing is more stultifying for a searcher than to find "the answer" too soon. **Discovery** often spoils the excitement of a **quest**, which might be more fruitful if pursued longer. This same belief led to the excellent saying of an irreverent seeker of knowledge quoted by Bachelard: "Great scientists are useful to science in the first part of their life and harmful in the second half."

This research opened the field of dynamic audiometry to me. I found out, for instance, that subjects submerged in noise do not hear in the same way as those who are in a silent environment, that their hearing changes when they begin to speak, and that their hearing deteriorates when they eat (because it is diminished by the sound of their own jaws, allowing us to take literally the well-known saying "A starving stomach has no ears"). I made all these observations either at the laboratory, in the munitions warehouse, or at my own laboratory, which somehow or other survived the pressure of creditors. Fortunately, I began to acquire a private clientele. This enabled me not only to pay my bills, but also to put my finger on certain phenomena which advanced my work a great deal.

My dream was to somehow aid singers who damaged or lost their voices. But knowing only too well their difficult character and their prima-donna-like temperament, I did nothing to encourage them to consult me.

That situation did not last long. My father told his friends who were singers what I had become. They in turn passed the news to others, and many of them, deceiving themselves about my qualifications and abilities, promised to call me as soon as they passed through Paris. They knew I was familiar with the repertoire and imagined that I also knew the innermost secrets of singing and could accomplish miracles. This was far from being the case.

I began merely by making inquiries, and started to grope about in the morass of specialized literature, which brought me more bewilderment than knowledge. In my experience, very few areas exist in which authors whose names carry great prestige have published such a mass of inaccurate information out of pure and simple ignorance! For a long time one of my great diversions was to open and read at random a page in a book dealing with the vocal arts. I was guaranteed a good laugh. It appeared that singers had no idea how to sing well and, when pressed, would say almost anything at random. Not one of these books helped me, and I was still perplexed when a colleague of my father knocked on my door.

He was a great and acclaimed singer, renowned internationally. Though he was a famous baritone with a remarkable technique, unfortunately he had continuous problems with his voice. What problems are we talking about? Every time his voice rose on the scale, he produced, upon leaving E or E flat, a kind of squeezing effect which caused him to sing more and more off key. Above a certain threshold he always produced the same note regardless of what note was actually written. With great pride, he brought me the diagnosis of one of the most eminent voice therapists in Europe, Froeschels, who practiced in Vienna before he went to the United States. I was such a beginner that I did not want to cast doubt on the opinion of the great expert who had pronounced "Laryngeal dystonia" (false tone caused by larynx). He quite logically thought that if a person could not sing higher up the scale, his larynx was "out of tune."

According to the prevailing theory, vocal quality was under the strict control of the larynx, which had to be regarded like a musical instrument. In this particular case, Froeschels compared the larynx to a violin whose strings became over-stretched. The only problem then was to reset them. How? The classic remedy was to prescribe strychnine products, and that was what my celebrated Viennese colleague had done. I imagined that if the treatment had not worked yet, it was because the dosage was not strong enough. So I gave stronger doses in conjunction with doses of male hormone, whose tonic effects I began to appreciate in my daily practice in the arsenals.

Immediately I recorded some improvement. This encouraged me, so I increased the doses of strychnine still further until finally my patient "choked" on the stage....but continued to sing false notes!

Meanwhile, another friend of my father's arrived in my consulting room. He, too, was a baritone and he, too, improbable as it seems, was troubled by problems of hitting the right note. I prescribed strychnine and obtained the same results. He returned the next day complaining bitterly of having "choked" during the course of the previous evening's performance.

Puzzled by these two successive setbacks, and having no idea to what saint to pray, I decided to make my two patients take the same audiometric tests I gave the workers at the arsenals. Should I thank the goddess of Fortune or flatter myself that I had an intuition? This test, which apparently had no connection with their troubles, was destined to point me in the right direction at last. I observed when I studied their auditory curves that both of them showed a hearing loss at the same frequency level. Then I recalled the audiometric pattern of those suffering from occupational deafness because, strangely enough, their curves were similar to those of the singers. I was profoundly intrigued. How could this phenomenon be explained?

I ended up asking myself whether these two baritones had damaged their ears by singing. None of the accepted theories enabled me to confirm this hypothesis, and I myself expressed great reservations about its validity. Was it not outlandish to try to establish such a link? All the same, I could not get rid of the idea. To check it out further I, who had reluctantly allowed singers to consult me, did everything in my power to examine the greatest possible number of singers' and musicians' ears.

It soon became apparent that I was on the right track. I recorded, for instance, a positive correlation between the number of years a professional singer had practiced and the damage caused to his hearing. Just as the munitions workers became increasingly deaf the longer they were exposed to jet aircraft noise, so, likewise, the hearing of singers grew worse the longer they practiced their profession. This verification convinced me that the singers were themselves damaging their ears because they were their own first and nearest listeners. This last idea seemed like a truism, yet stating it forced open many doors that had been slammed shut by the old assumptions of ENT and voice therapy.

These two sciences scarcely made any progress because their approach was based on erroneous, paralyzing ideas. For example, it was generally believed, without any proper verification, that singers' voices never exceeded 80 decibels and that this volume was too little to cause injury to a human ear. Furthermore, who would have imagined it was possible to damage one's ear while singing?

I did what all researchers do: I ignored all previous discoveries and started again from scratch. Fortunately, I had at my disposal in the arsenals a machine which measured the intensity of sound — a Sonometer. I settled all singers who consulted with me at one meter's distance from the machine and then carried out a whole series of measurements. I was surprised to discover that good professional singers were emitting 80 to 90 decibels when singing at half strength. At the full extent of their powers, they easily reached 110, 130, and even 140 decibels! At a meter's distance, 130 decibels represents 150 decibels inside one's skull. By comparison, a jet engine like the Atar (which drives the Caravelle) registers only 132 decibels on the ground. These figures are all the more impressive since the decibel is a logarithmic value. Though the energy of a singer is not comparable to that of a jet engine, the intensity of the sound is the same.

Consequently, I was no longer surprised that these singers ended up deaf, or at least partially so. However, I had yet to discover why they simultaneously began to sing off key. Had I continued to focus my efforts on the larynx and its possible over-stretching, my search might have been quite long. But my observations led me down another road. In a relatively short time, I examined many perfectly sound larynxes of non-singers (some of them exceptionally well-developed) and, at the same time, another group of staggeringly successful singers with damaged larynxes. Obviously, the problems were not connected with the larynx. But then, where were they?

I already knew the answer, but was unaware of it. I needed to become conscious of it, and the extremely simple idea that a singer was his or her own first listener helped me. "I can hear the wrong notes I sing!" my patients told me. I mulled the problem repeatedly. If they were singing poorly, it was because they were hearing poorly. Because of this they were no longer able to control themselves. To sing well, the subject must have a special perception of the sound being produced. The poor quality of this "self-listening" was responsible for everything. In other words, it was not the larynx that was to blame, but the ear — that same ear on which I had been working now for several years.

Such are the happy coincidences of scientific research. By putting myself at risk in one of those areas about which I knew least (urged on by the very exaggerated confidence that my father's friends gave me), I found that the subject I knew best was fundamental to the problem!

From then on I set about gathering proof, abandoning without a second thought the accepted theory that the larynx was the principal instrument of singing. My intuition was confirmed well beyond my hopes. As one example among many, the following appears to me characteristic of my findings.

The specialized literature established a definition of voices which corresponded to the shape and size of the larynx: a bass voice corresponded to the largest larynx; a baritone voice to a medium sized larynx; and a tenor voice to a slightly smaller larynx. It was clear, neat, and easy to remember and apparently "logical." The voice was quite simply likened to a pipe organ. This "law of nature" was so plausible (and so convenient) that no one seriously took the trouble to face the facts. I wanted to fill the gap and find out where the wrong road had been taken.

I examined enormous larynxes belonging to tenors, and quite small ones whose owners were black singers with the deepest of bass voices. However, the connection was not systematic, for I also met tenors with small larynxes and basses with large ones. No significant relationship existed between vocal pitch and the shape and size of the larynx. On the other hand, I did notice a connection between vocal pitch and certain auditory qualities. The most widely "open" ears belonged to basses; those "moderately open," to baritones; the most "closed," to tenors. By the terms "open" and "closed," I mean that they have more or less connection with low-pitched notes. Here is another proposition which in fact contradicts "common sense." This assures us, with characteristic naivety, that a bass singer sings "low," the tenor sings "high," and the baritone sings somewhere in between. This is simply not so; the three types of voice have the same raised overtones. What distinguishes them is this "openness" to low notes of which I have just spoken. Let us say, to be more precise, that a tenor sings in a band between 800 and 2,000 or 3,000 — even 4,000 to 6,000 Hertz for powerful tenors. But a baritone also sings within this band. The difference is that he adds lower notes. A bass does the same as the baritone, but goes down lower still. We are talking of the same voice more or less, cut off from the lowest frequencies. A bass without low notes is a baritone; a baritone without medium low notes is a tenor. What is significant, among other things, is that a bass is at the same time bass, baritone, and tenor. By this reckoning, this type of voice represents a sort of perfection. This accounts for its rarity.

Once more, the ear appeared to me to be the fundamental instrument of utterance. I could easily verify experimentally that the scotoma, indicated as a loss on the subject's listening test, always corresponded to a loss in the range of frequencies he could utter. I then formulated the proposition which was destined to be the starting point of all my observations and of all my subsequent discoveries: "A person can only reproduce vocally what he is capable of hearing." Since I have a taste for elegant formulations and paradoxes, I will express this newly discovered law in this simple phrase:

"One sings with one's ear."

This was in the year 1947.

5

The Fortunate Deafness Of Enrico Caruso

When I think about my life during the early 1950s, I realize that I must have appeared to others to be a somewhat strange fellow —— a glutton for work and a most irregular husband and father. I recall an assignment given by my Fifth Form (comparable to seventh grade) teacher, Auguste Bailly, asking us to identify ourselves with the judges of ancient times. My essay was read in class, not because it was better than the others, but because my point of view was so strict and inflexible. For the slightest wrongdoing, heads would roll! I was a harsh judge and could teach the most Spartan law-givers a thing or two. If others had applied my own law to me by using appearances as evidence, I would have been committed to the executioner's block repeatedly and frequently! However, only appearances could be held against me. As far as it is possible to know oneself and pass true judgement, I believe that I have always possessed two characteristics: a great fundamental honesty and an insuperable naiveté. These led me to innocently adopt attitudes which must have been harshly judged by outsiders, unless they also granted me the benefit of an incorrigible guilelessness.

My domestic relationships, in particular, ruined my reputation with many who witnessed them. What else could they see but a man who deceived his wife with his work and neglected his home to satisfy his personal ambitions?

And yet, I plead not guilty. I had too passionate a concern for my professional activities, it is true. On the other hand, my wife did not have enough concern and was, therefore, no help or support to me. As soon as I mentioned my research projects, which were so dear to me and yet caused me so much worry, she was bored to tears and showed it in the most explicit way. To her, I was an old graybeard with my gloomy stories about the larynx, the ear, and the audiometer. I found myself becoming a stranger in my own home, sometimes even an unwanted one. We might have talked about something else, but we found no common ground. There was no love because there was no communication; there was no communication because there was no love. It was a no-win situation. I know today that each party to a marriage discovers after the ceremony a partner that he or she was not expecting. The union can only succeed if the two individuals fulfill themselves and simultaneously become what the other wishes. In this way marriage is a contract, a sacred one. With my first wife, we remained two beings whose consciousness was totally impenetrable to the other even to the very end. We were light years apart, so it made no difference whether we were in the same room or not.

This first experience of family life was like travelling through a tunnel full of shadows. My wife did not experience any deep emotional relationships with our four children. It is tempting to think that, if she had, that would have brought them closer to me. But the psychological reality flatly refuted this very much over-simplified mechanistic explanation. All my efforts to make contact with my children were met with complete or partial repulses. I found it difficult to consider myself a real father; this was not the image of me they sent my way. Then, I understood nothing of what was going on in them and in me, and I lost more ground every day.

At one time my children admired me; at another, they rejected me. All this, you must understand, was because of what they heard spoken about me, or what they heard "thought" about me (for I remain convinced that children "hear" what adults think). When they told me they wanted to become doctors, I guessed that they identified with me. A little later, when they cast doubt on the value and usefulness of medicine, I understood that they were once more keeping their distance. But what was to be done?

One is not a father merely as a result of bringing children into the world. One *becomes* a father. And one can only become a father to the extent that one is assisted by the mother. Since this was far from my situation, I was a mere shadow of a father in spite of all my good will and fine principles.

Dissatisfaction at home drove me to my laboratory where I expanded the observations, measurements, experiences, and directions of my research. In particular, I sought an answer to the question "What differentiates a bad voice from a good one?"

I relied heavily on my "sonic analyzer" to tell me. I manufactured this machine myself, and it allowed me to take genuine photographs of the voice. The analyzer enables one to project on a cathode ray tube the distribution of frequencies of a voice. They are then spread out in the same way as a prism disperses the component parts of light in the spectrum of a rainbow. My analyzer was a hand-operated apparatus arranged in a series of filters. It enabled me to refute a fair number of accepted ideas. By this means I was able to give an account of how the speaking voice rises much higher than the singing voice. This was contrary to what was then believed. I expected that a singing voice would reach 15,000 Hertz. However, the finest singing voices in the world rarely exceed 7,000 Hertz. That of Caruso alone (studied by means of his records, despite the comparative inferior recording quality of his day) produced a burst of sound which ascended around 8,000 Hertz, a phenomenon which I have observed in no one else.

This machine did not help much in my search to find the distinction between a good and bad voice. The only significant differences that I recorded were those between trained and untrained voices, which was not quite the same thing. I realized I must attack the problem from another angle and discovered that a good voice is one which enables the body of the listener to experience pleasing vibrations. To listen to someone else singing is to enter into a partnership of vibration. Why? Simply because producing sound makes the outside air vibrate. The listener who is situated within this air space is going to find himself "sculpted" by the vibrations. To listen to someone playing, singing, or speaking is to let oneself be put in vibration with him. Inevitably we identify with the manner in which the person who addresses us uses his body. This explains why in the presence of a stutterer, sometimes we end up stuttering ourselves.

Mimicry can go even further than that. A few years ago in South Africa, I took part in a consultation which was very instructive. Seven or eight of us, including the interpreter, gathered around an extremely brilliant young stutterer who moved most curiously whenever he spoke. His body flung itself into a series of uncoordinated movements. After awhile, I noticed that all those present except my wife and I were, unknown to themselves, imitating every gesture he made. The most agitated among them was the interpreter, just as one might expect, since he was the most directly involved in the subject's words.

Two speakers face to face (or perhaps one speaker and one listener) are a little like two pianos set up in the same room: if one is being played and someone presses on the pedal of the second, it begins to vibrate. The founder of Taoism, Lao Tse, expressed this idea in the 6th Century B.C., using the example of two harps.

In any case, this theory throws light on many phenomena. If listening to a good singer gives us a feeling of well-being, it is because he communicates to us his own posture. Our countenance expands, and we begin to breathe deeply. In contrast, we easily become aggressive in the presence of a bad singer: we suffer with him, we tighten the larynx, and we strain, just as he himself is doing.

Nothing illustrates better the effects of this "placing in resonance" than the following anecdote. After I developed the Electronic Ear (which will be explained later) and was able to impose upon a subject the auditory curve that I wished, I did a simple but eloquent experiment with two monks. First, I gave them an identical listening pattern and suggested that they discuss together a particularly thorny theological problem. Next, I altered their listening curves so as to make them incompatible and made them talk about rain and fine weather. What happened? In the first case, they fell into agreement on every point in the discussion; in the second, they began to quarrel in less than a quarter of an hour! That opens a startling new perspective on the superficiality of some understandings and the shallow nature of some disagreements.

If a great singer is one who gives you pleasant vibrations, that suggests that he himself vibrated in them since the sound first "sculpted" the singer's own body before "sculpting" yours. In other words, the quality of the result depends largely on such parameters as the distribution, power, and flexibility of one's musculature and the thickness of one's bone structure. From this point of view, every person is like a musical instrument possessing its own qualities. Some of us are veritable Stradivarius's while others can only be compared to commonplace violins. People who knew Caruso well told me that when one tapped his skull, it returned a sound that was quite extraordinary. I believe it, for the celebrated singer had exceptional talents. But gifts are not everything. Anyone who seriously studies singing can establish, as the months go by, that his cranium itself begins to sing, to give out sounds far superior in quality to those it formerly produced. The thoracic cage also plays its part, by being a very large resonating box even before being a breathing box. Caruso —— always Caruso —— had no need to exercise his larynx much. In fact, this organ was probably in a state of total relaxation when he sang, at least during his great years before 1915. What sang was his whole body, and to the bones of his body he added his thorax, all of it. The latter was very much expanded, since Caruso measured 55 inches around his chest. Four liters of air passed through this great chest, although other singers of apparently less power took in up to ten liters of air.

I had no singing voice at all, but to more completely understand the problems of singers, I went on a pilgrimage to visit the singing teachers of Paris. Some of them who had seen me with my father knew me, but the majority were totally ignorant of who I was. I met the most incredible people, some of whom were absolute incompetents and impudent charlatans. Yet they had free rein. This profession is not organized in France as it is, for example, in Germany. Literally anyone can put on his door the notice "Singing Lessons." I met singing teachers who did not even know how to sing! I saw others who gave their students utterly crazy advice and who took advantage of their credulity and infantile fixation on their teacher. Though some of these teachers were men of good faith, that did not prevent them from telling enormous fibs about singing. Quite simply, they did not know what they were talking about. Generally they explained themselves by describing, as well as they could, the internal feelings that the student ought to experience in order to produce some note correctly. They tried to put into words their own feelings, forgetting that their complete subjectivity prevented reproduction of sounds from one individual to another, even if all else were equal.

Of all these men, the one I knew best was the one with the highest reputation. Let us call him "B." All the world came to see him in his apartment in the Pigalle area. He claimed to have practiced in all the top places of the vocal art, and, in particular, at La Scala in Milan. Such claims were all he needed to attract a crowd of debutantes and even experienced singers who wanted to improve their art. Photographs of celebrities he had helped in their path to glory covered his walls. A superb portrait of Campagnola was showcased in the middle of his apartment. This provided the unchallengeable stamp of his merits as a teacher, since Campagnola was considered the best singer ever, after Caruso himself. People murmured to each other in the wings of theaters that B.

had discovered the great secret of the art of singing.

I followed his lessons industriously, returning to the task two and three times a week, despite an obvious absence of natural aptitude. B. possessed genuine listening skills, some of which were indeed rare. I picked up from his teaching some interesting observations and even went on holidays with him to learn more. Things went wrong when I asked him to introduce me to Campagnola, his famous student.

"Impossible!" he cried immediately. "He is dead."

Clearly all I could do was to express my regrets, both for him and me. A short time later, I stopped seeing B., from whom I could learn no more to advance my investigations. I continued to lament the disappearance of Campagnola...until the day he walked into my office!

Somewhat bewildered, but not believing in ghosts like my Grandfather Raggi, I supposed B. must have been misinformed. To improve rapport with my client, I slipped into our conversation, "Do you know, M. Campagnola, that I know your master quite well?"

"My master!" he exclaimed with a sort of outraged stupefaction. "I took only two or three lessons with Nourrit. In fact, I learned to sing by myself with my guitar."

"But," I insisted, "I have seen your photograph in a prominent position in the house of...."

"Ah! I've got it! You mean that old bandit in Pigalle? I met him once or twice as a matter of fact, but that is absolutely all that passed between us. I've already been told that he uses that photograph as bait for customers."

After this misadventure, I did not spend much more time in the waiting rooms of singing teachers.

Meanwhile, I learned more about the self-controlling mechanism of singers. To say that "the voice only reproduces what the ear hears" in no way implies that a person is capable of giving out everything that he perceives. A good utterance, in fact, demands not only a good auditory receptivity but a good self-listening. To pass from one to the other is what distinguishes the good singer from others. The greater the singer, the more rigorous is the control which he exercises. Most of the time this control is automatic, but it is not unconscious. The structure of self-listening is only established gradually by means of the work that the voice does. As I have said, the instrument used is the ear. It was very easy for me to supply fresh proof of this, from the moment when, long before I got to know the work of Wiener and others on cybernetics, I discovered a set of cybernetic feedback loops.[5]

I showed that when blind spots (scotomas) are artificially introduced by a system of filters into a subject's hearing (it is easily done by installing deflectors

---

[5] Tomatis describes these in more detail in "L'Oreille et la Voix" (1987 p157-181).

which prevent a particular frequency from passing), then the vocal qualities of that subject are correspondingly modified. According to the position of the scotoma in the spectrum, one's voice may become more sonorous, more nasal, clearer, or warmer in tone. It was even possible to make someone temporarily lose his voice completely.

Pursuing my research in this direction, I soon perceived that, in matters of vocal control, the two ears are not used in the same way. Let us take, for example, the three successive stages of development of what is conventionally called "the musical ear":

(1) The ability to hear and appreciate music.
(2) The ability to reproduce it correctly.
(3) The ability to reproduce it, not only correctly, but with a degree of excellence.

At each stage, control is brought about by one ear alone —— the right ear. This is a vital point.

Philosophers have always asked why man was fitted with two ears. Zeno replied jokingly that he had two ears and only one tongue so that he could listen twice as often as he spoke. He was mistaken in this, at least insofar as we do not have one tongue alone, but rather two joined together by the median. We have also, for anyone who knows how to observe, two mouths, a "right" mouth and a "left" one. Adults speak nearly always with a preference for one or the other. In the same way, we have two eyes, two nostrils, two arms, two legs, two brains. But this very duality in humans involves, let us say, a functional lack of balance. We have two ears, but each fulfills a different function. The chief function of the right ear is to be a "director."

A functional distinction always depends upon an organic distinction. When one wants to produce a sound, the impulses which leave the brain can only reverberate at the level of the larynx. In man the larynx is a privileged instrument, but here again, we are in the presence of a duality: man possesses two larynxes. To be more precise, his larynx presents a lack of symmetry, and it is this lack of symmetry which reflects in some way the lack of symmetry of the ears. What exactly happens? The passage of the nerve impulses via the recurrent laryngeal nerves belonging to the tenth cranial pair (pneumogastric), from the cortex to the lining of the left larynx, is longer than that from the cortex to the right larynx. In the feedback loop of self-listening, which connects the hearing apparatus to the larynx, the right ear will be closer to the organs of speech than the left. I have deduced from this at the same time that the right circuit comprises five main stages (right ear, auditory center of the left brain, central laryngeal motor area of the left brain, speech muscles, and the passage from mouth to right ear), whereas the left circuit comprises six stages. In fact, from the left ear, sound goes to the auditory center of the right brain. To reach the central laryngeal motor area (which is situated in the left brain) a transfer of the left brain center is necessary; this transfer constitutes an element of delay, which can be measured. This delay varies, according to the individual, between 0 and 0.4 of a second. (Between 0.1 and 0.2 of a second, and especially around 0.15 of a second, the delay systematically provokes a stutter.)

The right ear takes charge of operations because it receives information more rapidly. This is an absolute: all great singers and musicians are "right-eared." In my whole career, I only met one exception to this rule — a baritone who was much admired for his technique, which he acquired first in Italy and then in France. This remarkable mastery enabled him to make a world tour, and yet his success was somewhat reduced everywhere he went. The majority of music-lovers found his voice colorless, not very lively, without warmth, and without an ability to soar. He seemed always to be slightly behind the beat. This was because he was "left-eared." The most curious thing was that in each hall where he performed, a small nucleus of unconditional admirers could be found. There was no doubt in my mind that they too possessed the characteristics of left ear dominance. No right-eared person could bear his voice for very long, for a feeling of weariness quickly supervened.

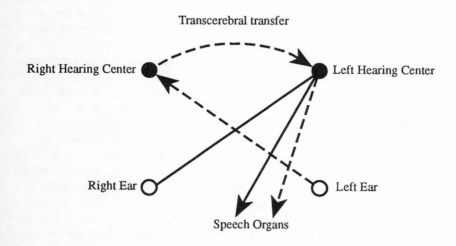

Figure 1. *Straight lines show normal trajectory of nervous impulse when the right ear is dominant: dotted lines show the trajectory with brain-transfer that a stutterer has (left ear dominant, with general lateralization to the right).*

Lack of balance between the two ears in self-listening is such that if you prevent a singer from hearing in his right ear by injecting noises or overloading sounds, his voice immediately becomes thick and loses color, fullness, and accuracy. Some individuals, when speaking, can be disturbed to the extent they begin to stutter. Musicians, when placed under the same experimental conditions, lose a large part of their potential, become unable to follow the beat, and cannot make their instrument give out its full sound. I had the opportunity to subject the great violinist, Zino Francescati, to this test; you would have said that his Stradivarius had been suddenly turned into a common piece of wood!

Without delay I needed to establish that what was true for music and singing was also true for language. When all these questions became more fashionable in scientific circles, some American colleagues declared that there was one ear for music and another for spoken words. I disputed the validity of this theory, especially since these researchers assigned musical perception to the left ear. This is quite impossible. The mistake arose, in my opinion, from a confusion between superficial amateur listening and the really accurate perception of sounds characteristic of music-lovers and musicians. The left ear is adequate for the first kind of listening, but only the right ear empowers the second.

In this respect, the auditory system coincides very accurately with the system of sight. When the eyes gaze into the distance, without focusing on anything in particular, without fixing on some point in the landscape, the dominant eye does not appear. But if one begins to read, it is the dominant eye which suddenly takes charge of the essential part of the work. The other eye only grasps the main shape of the book, the hands which are holding it, and the general setting. It is exactly the same with our ears: the dominant ear focuses on a precise sound, while the other is content to provide a general picture of the sonic background.

I was to rediscover this distinction between the two ears at different levels. Without getting too far ahead of myself, I can already say that the right ear "measures" the highest frequencies, while the left ear performs the job for the lower-pitched frequencies. This phenomenon is fraught with consequences. In fact, with the right ear, an individual may process wavelengths from 35 to 70 *centimeters*. But, with the left ear, the wavelengths may range from 35 to 140 *meters*! As a result, the left-eared person finds himself distanced by his ear. Not only is he a long way from the person to whom he is talking, but he is also a long way from his own body, since he cannot attune himself to the higher frequencies of his own voice. So, cut off from his own speech, his body becomes the prey of a "gaucherie" ("left-handers," "awkwardness"); he feels uneasy and somewhat clumsy.

Some of these considerations may seem to be abstract, but the reader who understands the point of my research must remember that, far from simply chasing pure ideas, I was busy finding the bases for an objective audiometry.

Besides, I was a doctor at heart. I have always considered myself a healer above all. What sustained me in my quest was the hope of perfecting a genuinely effective recuperative therapy for singers who had damaged or lost their voices. My eagerness to attain definite results made me think of constructing a training apparatus for audio-vocal education and re-education. But this is a long story which forces me to go back a little.

I became convinced that the voice can only produce what the ear hears. A listening curve allows us to make many predictions as to how an individual expresses himself vocally. Conversely, because of the existence of the self-listening mechanism, the voice translates and betrays the functioning of the ear. As a result, I had the chance, using recordings, to determine the listening characteristics of great singers whom I could not examine directly. If I could manage to impose these "perfect" ears on my patients, perhaps I could deliver them from their difficulties. This possibility was still very vague but, nevertheless, present. It was not to be ignored.

The greatest singer of all died in 1921, but he left behind a mass of recordings. Thus I began to take an interest in the case of Enrico Caruso. I began by amassing quite a collection of old records and even cylinders. I had plenty of help. Friends, and friends of friends, let me have recordings of the highest quality, even master recordings. The techniques of sound recording were very limited at that time, and it was vital for me to work on what had been the best —— that is to say, the least bad.

I took numerous extracts of Caruso's voice, following the chronological order of the recordings. My impression, derived from a review of the years 1896-1902, was that he certainly had a voice of great quality, but not one which seemed spectacularly beautiful. It lacked most of the characteristics which brought him glory. After 1902, however, the characteristics were all there, clearly apparent in the recordings. I noticed particularly that below 2,000 Hertz there was always a drop of at least 18 decibels per octave towards the low notes. It was as if Caruso had benefitted from a sort of filter which allowed him to hear, essentially, high frequency sounds rich in harmonics as opposed to low frequency fundamental sounds. In this respect, his ear presented intriguing similarities to certain hearing characteristics of people affected by a blockage of the Eustachian tubes. I asked myself if some sort of accident had befallen him.

Putting aside recordings for books, I immersed myself in his biography and finally discovered that at the end of 1901 or early 1902, he underwent a surgical operation in Spain on the right side of his face. The author said nothing more about it, but I imagined what might have happened. His Eustachian tube had been damaged, causing a partial deafness which resulted in his transformation from that a gifted singer to becoming the greatest vocalist in the world! It was only at this period that he began to achieve veritable triumphs. Following his operation, Caruso no longer heard the lower frequencies. My work confirmed for me that someone who has the good fortune to suffer from this failing, if I may call it so, possesses the means to sing better than another, all things being equal, because he no longer hears sounds of lesser quality and so cannot reproduce them. Caruso sang so remarkably well only because he could no longer hear except in the singing range!

Someone may ask if I had the right to found an entire theory on imperfect recordings and a biographical reference that could not be verified. Was I not playing a little too fine a game by aiming the spotlight at someone no longer alive who could not contradict me? I was the first to raise these objections, I assure you. To demolish the first was simple enough. Caruso was indeed dead, but another celebrity was thoroughly alive, Benjamino Gigli. I examined and assessed his listening test and was able to compare it with the one I obtained from Caruso's recordings some three years earlier. They coincided exactly.

As to the theory of Caruso's partial deafness, I received confirmation of this from the actual accounts of three singers who were my patients and also my father's friends. They performed on the same stage as the leading tenor of the Metropolitan Opera of New York (who had, as if by chance, obtained his post in 1903). Separately and of their own accord, all three told me that when they walked in the street with Caruso, he always asked them to walk on his left because he heard less well on the right, the side of his operation. His right ear was deaf as far as language was concerned, but it was more sensitive to song; more precisely, it was his "listening" that was sensitive to song. Instead of working through the defective external passage of the ear, the "self-listening" was carried out through bone conduction (cranium, thorax, etc.). I even claim that of all the great tenors, Caruso was the one who sang most "osseously," if I may put it so. He made his bone framework vibrate like nobody else. However, his act of listening through bone conduction is not an exception. All great listeners use this type of conduction, and we shall return to this later.

How do you make a skeleton sing? This is an intuitive technique that all great singers possess, particularly the Italians who adopt a position of utterance very different from that of the French. Italian and French voices, for reasons which will appear in the following chapter, present very different features. The French singer is condemned to force his larynx, to drive it powerfully, while the Italian singer, like Caruso, can sing with a perfectly relaxed larynx.

A French singer leans on his larynx like the mouthpiece of a trumpet. In this way, he obtains both quality and volume. The problem is that to accomplish this he sometimes has to use the flow of breath, with considerable force. Some French singers are always short of breath, even when they are drawing upon ten liters of moving air!

An Italian singer, by contrast, uses his larynx like a violin or a cello; the vocal chords draw near to each other and begin to vibrate. For that, a very small quantity of air is required. I knew a French singer who, as a result of an illness of the lungs, could only manage half a liter of moving air. She took up the Italian technique and became one of the most brilliant interpreters of Rossini.

It is not yet known how the vocal chords are stimulated. The question has often been raised of the natural resonators formed by certain bone cavities, for example, the sinus cavities among others. There again the idea seemed plausible, and I might have stuck to it if I had not, over many years, studied another most accomplished singer, the great international tenor André Burdino (who died in 1987 at age 97). He suffered from very pronounced sinusitis during the greater part of his career. So it was not sinuses that enabled him to sing well, since they were always blocked. What was it then? It was the conduction of sound through the bones. Burdino had no awareness of this himself, but in the technique called Italian, as well as in the German technique, the larynx supports itself on the spinal column. It plays the same role as the little piece of wood called the soul which in a violin enables first the base-plate to begin to vibrate and then the entire instrument. In the case of a singer, it is the body which becomes the instrument, like a violin. Besides, when a singer tries to explain his art, he often says that by preference he uses such and such a part of his body. Basses, for example, often claim to utter sound by means of their stomachs, quite simply because their vibrations essentially affect the area of the sacrum. The interplay of reactions, after the body has been set in motion by the voice, brings about the control of the voice by the body. In the art of singing, it is the entire being that is involved.

This simultaneous "listening" through the bone structure and partial lower frequency deafness resulted in Caruso becoming an exceptional performer. Realizing this, I decided to try to give, at least temporarily, a power of listening like Caruso's to subjects whose audio-vocal control was impaired. If my theory was correct, it was bound to produce some positive result. I put headphones over their ears and imposed this particular listening via a system of filters. The reaction was immediate. All, without exception, felt an increased sense of well-being. Even among those who were not singers, many confided in me that they felt like singing. I encouraged them in this, and established the fact that, provided they had the headphones in position and that I did not touch the setting of the machine, they sang incomparably better than at other times. But when I took away the headphones, everything once more became as difficult as ever.

So I was faced with a dilemma. My system of filters could develop into a machine to promote good singing, and hence into the apparatus for education and re-education of which I dreamed, but it simply was not possible to send people onto the theater stage wearing headphones. It was absolutely necessary to make this temporary improvement a permanent one. I examined in detail the words of Pavlov whose studies of conditioning had been definitive. I based great hopes on the repetition of experiments. Gradually, I thought, the subject would learn the self-control that a great professional singer has and would gain a similar listening capacity.

To a certain extent I was disappointed. The process of conditioning was laborious and the results weak. This was not the fault of the theory, but rather of the machine. The one I perfected at the beginning of the fifties was an invention made of bits and pieces. I thought of the design when I did a rather curious experiment with one of my patients, an accomplished French singer whom we will call T.

Fifteen years before he arrived in my consulting room, T. lost his voice and quit performing in public. His problems had even increased, for he could no longer speak. We achieved good results with the different kinds of therapy and he recovered his voice to a large extent. However, I heard him every day slaving away at a passage from "La Forza del Destino," where he came to grief regularly on "untrono." The first "o" of trono uttered on a "la" in B-flat seemed to be an insurmountable obstacle for him. He made a wild shot at it every time. I was all the more surprised because one of the most beautiful sounds ever produced on Caruso's records was precisely this one.

I plugged in my voice analyzer and photographed T.'s voice, then the Italian maestro's. In the first case, a signal on the cathode-ray tube was evident at the stage of this "la" in B-flat. But in the second, the picture showed nothing in an identical space of time. Put out, I repeated the test several times, always with the same result. I concluded from this that my machine was not working properly, or that it had been badly connected. I persisted in this for months, until the day when I abandoned the study of visual displays of the voice for the benefit of direct listening. Then I perceived that the utterance of the two singers was not at all the same! T. was forcing his larynx, and with the same thrust was blowing out the words "un trono" giving the impression that all the elements were continuous. Caruso, on the other hand, introduced a certain discontinuity by a "click," which I cannot define in the absence of any example from sound. One might have a clearer idea of this by learning that Italian singers call this process "the sob." When I asked Gigli what was the point of it, he replied simply, "That makes many things easier!"

I thought this was an interesting subject for study, so I applied myself to measuring the duration of this click, of this "gating" time which ensured better control and made better utterance easier. In terms of my previous discoveries, I thought that if a singer were producing the click, then it was a response to an auditory phenomenon which was therefore operating in the ear. From this came the idea of making singers who used the French technique hear it to overcome their difficulties.

My first machine was therefore built in such a way as to provide an effective "gating." I used manual circuit breakers, which had various disadvantages. At first, they made a lot of noise which in itself was an obstacle to data processing. Next, my assistants and I spent all of our time in manipulating these circuit breakers. I never succeeded in getting to the point where a single patient made the movement himself. I installed digital keys, and then I installed pedals without any better result. The rare singers who agreed to manipulate them did so at the wrong time (either too early or too late), which was dangerous insofar as they jeopardized not only the immediate, temporary condition, but also, in the long term, their chances of a final cure. In brief, it was not a question of playing thoughtlessly with the circuit breaker. I only solved this problem at the end of 1954, when I introduced into the system an electronic gating mechanism. I then christened the machine "The Electronic Ear."

Although it was far from perfect, the first machine caused much dismay in the slumbering little world of singing teachers and speech therapists. Alarmed, the leading practitioners rushed to my room and contemplated with the liveliest repulsion a machine which, they thought, was going to snatch the very bread from their mouths. As far as the second-rate were concerned, they pursed their lips, shrugged their shoulders, and made up their minds to laugh at it, which did not prevent them from building machines themselves which some years later bore a strange resemblance to mine! Most amusing was that they always continued to use their machines in their first form without acknowledging that the system of electronic gates revolutionized everything.

Contrary to what the public no doubt imagines, these petty pilferings are accepted as legal in the medical world. I had learned this the hard way, back when I was inspired by certain Russian works to carry out placenta sprays to improve the hearing of subjects affected by professional deafness. I designed the blueprints for a special syringe, which was a little like a grease-gun for cars, but reduced to quarter-size. I had some specially made for me and some colleagues in the arsenal workshops. A little while later, a traveling salesman came to see me.

"Are you in the ENT field?" he asked. "Have you heard about placenta therapy? I am going to show you something sensational!"

He opened his briefcase and triumphantly showed me a syringe that was an exact replica of mine. There was only one difference. This one bore the name of the inventor — only it wasn't my name. It was someone I knew very well, to whom I had offered my apparatus just a few months earlier.

But let us return to the Electronic Ear. Although it was not yet perfectly developed, its existence disturbed many people. I also disturbed them, quite innocently, for I was totally ignorant of certain laws of social behavior, so much so that I was thunderstruck when in 1952 Doctor Lallemant let me know that he was letting me go from his hospital service. What serious professional fault was I guilty of? None, but I had insolently contravened the most sacred practices of French officialdom. I had presented some of my own work under my own name; in particular, I had presented a paper to the society of speech therapists on the subject of this first machine. I had not, as the custom required, had it signed by my chief who had not collaborated in this for a single moment and, besides, was not even a specialist in speech therapy. I was the official specialist in this field! Maurice Lallemant had already taken offense because my name had appeared beside his on the cover of *Occupational Deafness* even though he had not written a single line. He had grudgingly allowed it to appear that way because Robert Maduro had insisted. But that a work should be published to my credit which did not even display his signature, that he could not allow.

After 1955, however, he reopened contact with me, and asked me to return to the hospital service. By then I had gained a certain measure of respect from colleagues abroad. Americans, in particular, began to take an interest in my work.

"You made your start in the hospitals, Tomatis," my old chief said to me. "We welcomed you and set your foot on the ladder. It is only right that your discoveries should spring from the French hospitals. Rejoin us. You will have nothing to complain about."

I declined his offer.

"Now that that is decided," I added, "I will gladly treat, for nothing, all the hospital patients that you care to send me."

In the years that followed, a certain number did come to consult me. However, my refusal to rejoin the hospital was the beginning of a series of misadventures with my colleagues. The majority of them could not accept that anyone else might display that spirit of independence which they themselves never had the courage to show. I say this without scorn and without hostility, but simply because the public ought to know why French medicine was in the process of dying and what were the roots of that sickness. All the pettiness, resulting from an outdated idea that is openly reactionary and anti-democratic on the part of the hierarchy, presented enough obstacles and delay to wear out even the best will in the world. Consequently, the momentum of medical research was largely blocked. The grotesque trickery that presides over the pursuit of a medical career, particularly at the university, diverts too much of the most brilliant students' energy. If we are seeing a veritable hemorrhage of researchers emigrating to foreign countries, it is not only because other governments offer better working conditions. It is also because the French bureaucracy is totally unbearable regarding human relations and insensitive and ossified regarding research.

Returning to the Electronic Ear, as its development continues to be refined to its final form, it represents one of the most important stages of my journey in the scientific field. It is solely as a result of this apparatus that I have made rapid progress in the matter of re-education and, as well, all sorts of discoveries to which I hardly paid any attention. As I said, the apparatus was both simple and complex — simple for anyone who has some idea of electronics, complex for anyone who is paralyzed by the mere word electronics. Figure 2 shows a simple diagram of its basic structure.

I will define its main principle before giving details of how it works. The problem was to auditorially condition and train the ear so it could take up a self-listening posture and create a quality utterance. This posture is brought about by a tension of the eardrum produced by means of regulating the muscles of the malleus and the stirrup (the two muscles of the middle ear). These muscles ensure the passage of sound into the inner ear along channels that are quite different from those commonly acknowledged. The inner ear is a most important turntable because this is where the analysis of sound information by the brain begins.

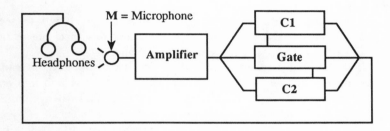

Figure 2. *Diagram of the Electronic Ear.*

The Electronic Ear comprises two channels (C1 and C2). An electronic gate joins them together and allows a subject to progress from a weakened power of listening to a better adjusted one. At the same time, another set of electronic gates or feedback mechanisms frees the right-sided auditory channel to act as the preferred one. The left channel is not eliminated, but unlike the right, it does not fulfill the function of focusing on sounds. Amplifiers operating on C1 and C2, a microphone, and earphones complete the system. The source of sound is provided by a magnetic tape fitted to a tape recorder. All these machines must be of very good quality.

Very well, the reader will ask, who will prove to me that this works? One cannot at the same time be a judge and a party to the case, so I suspect that my word alone carries very little weight. I shall appeal to the testimony of a third party whose honesty and integrity no one will doubt since we are speaking of André le Gall, Inspector-General of Public Education and at one time Director of Teaching in France. After an extended stay in my laboratory, André le Gall published his observations and conclusions in a memorandum entitled "The Correction of Certain Psychological and Psychopedagogical Deficiencies by the Electronic Ear Using the Tomatis Effect" (March, 1961). I quote these lines from the second chapter. The reader will grasp these better if he remembers that an emission "E" corresponds to an auditory signal "A" which brings about a vocal signal "G":

As a result of this, Dr. Tomatis shows that he has fixed the conditioning of the ear by obliging it to hear a sound in a particular way, as a result of the emission of this sound. In other words, the vocal signal which he will call G1, which results in an utterance of bad quality E1, corresponds, as we now realize, to a general hearing quality, A1. To change the indifferent utterance E1 and then the vocal signal G1, and substitute a vocal signal G2 and a true utterance E2, it is enough to compel the ear to make use of a method of adaptation...which determines the way of hearing A2.

It is enough then, in order to erase the signal G1 and to see appearing only the signal G2, to condition the auditory mechanisms to a new way of adaptation to the emission of sounds.

To deal with this conditioning, Alfred Tomatis has for several years made use of the following setup: a microphone, M, is wired into an amplifier, from which two different circuits lead; these two circuits operate two channels, which do not work at the same time.

For a given volume of sound, which may be modified at will, channel C1 alone remains open. This allows the subject being tested to hear himself as he usually does, so much so that for him nothing is changed. After the utterance of a sound on his part, as soon as he adds to the surrounding noise, which has always been there, a complementary volume of sound (which is merely what he is himself producing), channel C1 closes and only channel C2 is open. This second electronic channel will bring the ear under another method of control, which we have chosen, one which particularly corresponds to the utterance of a beautiful voice. In other words, the opening of channel C2 is brought about by a system of electronic gates, which automatically allows the transition from the A1 manner of hearing, which belongs to the vocal signal G1, to the A2 method of hearing which belongs to the refined vocal signal G2.

Once the vocal utterance is finished, the reduced volume rocks the system back again and C1 opens while C2 disappears. This cycle begins again every time the subject wants to speak, and the conditioning is very quickly apparent. From the first days of treatment, after a session of half an hour, a retention of about half-an-hour is established. At the end of some weeks, this retention remains permanent. Moreover, this play of gates can rapidly become a conscious phenomenon, and can determine at leisure the possibility of hearing whatever is desired.

The test proves that vocal conditioning (for example, speaking a foreign language) is not only something that follows auditory conditioning, but it is something that lasts....

However, this retention is not exclusive; the conditioning that sets it up may give way to other sorts of conditioning; a Frenchman may acquire —— either by long visits to England, or quickly by using the machine —— an excellent English accent; but when he returns to Paris, he will resume his French "listening" and way of speaking....

If the objection is raised that, under these conditions, the recovery obtained in these physio-psychological treatments is at risk of suffering a relapse and a return to the faulty method of hearing and speaking, our answer is that, in the therapeutic domain, the remedial conditioning is applied in a total way, not merely for the occasional use of a foreign language.... It is not juxtaposed; it is superimposed.

After the modification of phonation following the modification of audition, which is the principal discovery, the persistence of the recovery clearly constitutes a second and equally important fact. Because the conditioning is effective for both ends of the chain of listening and vocal emission, we might wonder whether this method could relieve the intermediate psychological phenomena from certain paralyzing or disturbing conditions and be reconditioned in the direction of freedom and effectiveness.

The reader will permit me to insist on this last point: The Tomatis apparatus in no way has the purpose of artificially conditioning the subject. It is not a machine for controlling the ears and the brain. On the contrary, it is an instrument capable of helping the individual, who is traumatized, frustrated, maladjusted, or blocked by some incident in his history, to rediscover by means of the full opening, that is to say, by the total liberation of his auditory perceptions, the positive freedom of his own nature, the freedom to act out his own destiny.

This therapy is indeed a conditioning, but it is a conditioning that liberates....

(André le Gall, 1961).

I do not know how to put it better and now return to some of the interesting learning experiences resulting from use of the Electronic Ear.

One day some young students whom I knew sent me an Italian of their age, a rather lazy adolescent who up till then was satisfied with daubing a few canvases without much conviction. He needed an operation for a cholesteatoma of the right ear. The problem was a benign tumor, which nonetheless had to be removed because in the long term it might cause a fatal abscess on the brain. If the auditory nerve is affected, or more precisely, if the inner ear is impaired, the next step is a total scooping out. On the other hand, if the inner ear is undamaged, a partial scooping out, which does not touch the osseous labyrinth, is considered sufficient. While I completed his listening test for the right ear to see if the nerve had been eaten away by the tumor, I was surprised to find that the pattern corresponded exactly to that of Caruso's ear!

If my hypotheses about self-listening and the reactions to it were valid, this boy should have the voice of Caruso. When I asked him, he told me that he had never sung in his life.

"What does that matter?" I said. "Everything has a beginning. I will start you off."

During the next week, I made him learn certain phrases from Caruso's repertoire and then recorded his voice. I kept the tapes. They take one's breath away! At moments, one could imagine that the master himself was singing.

I was overjoyed.

An hour later, T., who was making perceptible progress every day, came to my house. I was intent on making this great professional listen to the tape.

"Wait till you hear this," I said to him excitedly. "It's incredible! When you think that a few days ago this boy had never even sung!"

I switched on the tape-recorder and, beaming with joy, I awaited T.'s reaction, certain of his amazed surprise.

He listened for a few moments in silence, then looked at me suspiciously and spat out, "That's enough. He sings like an idiot, this fellow of yours!"

It was my turn to be surprised. I no longer felt that I understood what I was doing. When I recovered from the shock, I had another idea and said to T., "Wait, there is something here which I don't fully understand. Let me play you another recording. We will discuss all this afterwards."

"If you like," he answered.

I went to look for one of Caruso's records, one which showed his voice at its warmest as well as being one of the richest in frequencies — Verdi's "Louisa Miller." He had recorded it in 1914, at a period when he was no longer the very great Caruso of his maturity, but when his voice had a remarkable fullness. I put it on the turntable without identifying it for T.

"Who is it?" he asked me after a few moments.

"Caruso," I said.

"Just as I thought!" he exclaimed. "Really, I shall never understand how that fellow made the whole world talk about him. Listen, just listen! How awful! It's unbearable."

He was absolutely furious. It took me awhile to calm him down. I promised him that he would never again hear Caruso spoken of in my house.

When I was alone once more in my office, I brooded over this incident for a long time. My first reaction was to write this off as one of those examples of blind passionate hostility, such as too often sets two great artists against one another. But since I knew a little of T.'s psychology, I could not bring myself to accept this idea. I formed a different theory, which was obviously suggested to me by my current work: if he did not appreciate Caruso's voice as I did, perhaps it was because he did not hear it as I did.

I immediately constructed a filter to give me the same hearing as his; and, in fact, under these conditions, Caruso became equally "inaudible" to me. T.'s hearing and Caruso's were dramatically opposed, and such opposites occur more frequently than might be supposed. This happens often enough between a singing teacher and his student without either of them having any suspicion of it. And this produces real disasters. The master, by trying to force on his student a type of listening which contradicts the whole structure of the student's self-listening, may not only disturb this structure but, even beyond that, may upset his student's entire self. This was revealed to me when I asked T. as a favor to give some lessons to my young Italian. At the end of the third session, the damage was so considerable that the unfortunate beginner did not dare speak for three months.

The first thing to do before taking singing lessons, therefore, is to get to know one's own listening test pattern as well as that of the chosen teacher. Over a period of time, I amused myself by testing the ears (unknown to them) of all the singing teachers who visited my consulting room. I did this by playing a famous Louisa Miller recording (of which I knew all the frequencies) in the background and unobtrusively cutting out a frequency, then cutting out another one. By making a note of the exact moment when my visitor said to me "Wait a minute! That's changed!" I could easily determine at which level his own auditory "cut-off" was situated. More than once, I was bewildered, because I observed that I tumbled down five or six octaves without the "expert" in front of me having noticed anything at all.

From one person to another, the mode of listening changes, but not all modes are of equal use. Absolutely speaking, Caruso's listening was preferable to T.'s, particularly for good singing. And the proof is that, without telling him so, of course, I reconstructed T.'s voice according to Caruso's ear. His progress was so spectacular that when I sent a tape which T. had just recorded to Lehmann, who was then Director of the Opera, T. was summoned to his office and engaged on the spot. Unfortunately, he then thought that he could dispense with my services, and broke off the educational support from which he had benefitted. (A full recovery would have required lengthier training.) He subsequently had to abandon, only a few months later, a second career, which could have been as brilliant as his first. Later I treated a number of singers who, like him, did not continue right to the end, and they also lost all they had gained from the first sessions, even more quickly if their voice was full and of ample volume.

All this taught me many lessons from the psychological point of view. I already knew that the relationship between the patient and the therapist was at least as important as the effect produced by the action of the machine. This provided a new direction for research, one in which I was to be engulfed a few years later —— that of language and of the make up of one's very being.

Meanwhile, I found myself more and more committed to my idea that the utterance of sound —— the construction and effective realization of a suitable vocal signal —— was a question of the ear more than of the speech organs. And in this, too, I was fortunate enough to meet someone who helped me to prove it.

This time it was not a young Italian, but a young Spaniard. This man was perfectly conscious of his vocal talents. He even laid claim to some which he did not have, encouraged by an old lady for whom he was acting as a kind of general factotum and who had transferred her own desire to be a famous singer onto him. The trouble was that he experienced the greatest difficulty in uttering a sound because of a bilateral intracordal nodule from which he was suffering. This was a particularly serious type of laryngitis which transforms the vocal chords into wide spindles so they no longer can draw near to each other.

He made an appointment and described his case to me. This posed a particularly thorny problem. Usually nothing can be done in the presence of such an organic alteration, because to extract this nodule leads to the absurdity of removing the vocal chords themselves. It was clear that such a measure was to be avoided at all costs. He had to be told that he must give up the hope that he might one day recover his ability to sing. This crushed him and he complained bitterly of his fate.

"But how could I have caught that? Where does it come from?"

"From your ear," I answered, unguardedly. I should have led him little by little to this apparently bizarre idea after first explaining all that I had observed with other singers.

"From my ear!"

He looked at me with stupefaction, listened politely for a few more minutes, then thanked me and fled as quickly as possible to a colleague, furious at having wasted his time with a practical joker of my sort.

The colleague, who shall remain nameless, acted as chorus.

"Your ear! What idiocy! Why did you go to see that charlatan? Don't you know he's the only man in the world to uphold such absurd ideas? Come now, a little common sense. What do you suppose your ear has to do with your vocal chords? It's completely crazy."

He examined the young Spaniard and told him the source of all his trouble was his tonsils, which he took out without further delay, removing at the same time the entire soft palate for good measure. Alas! All this did was to transform a difficulty in vocalization into a virtual impossibility of uttering at all. In despair, the young man rushed to another colleague who suggested yet another diagnosis.

"Ah," said he. "It's a pity they've taken out your tonsils. A great pity, and quite useless, for the cause of all this lies in a deviation of the nasal passage. It's quite clear."

He seized his lancet, and attacked the source of the trouble. Undoubtedly he did so with too much ardor, and an awkward probe with the scalpel removed the mucous membrane. This did not improve the state of the patient at all.

The fourth surgeon to be consulted disassociated himself from the other three, declared that the osseous strips of the nose were to blame, and set about removing them with enthusiasm.

His nose was no longer a nose. It was a cathedral! Nevertheless, things went from bad to worse. Two years after his first visit, I found the young Spaniard in my waiting room once again. He told me in piteous tones of all his disappointments and declared that he now was ready to listen to me. I certainly could not put him into a worse condition than the one he was already in.

I explained to him what treatment under the Electronic Ear consisted of, and gave him an appointment. When he came for the first session, I was in the process of showing my laboratory to a group of colleagues who were from Marseille and led by Professor Appaix. As might be expected, they took an interest in this new patient. They asked for his case history and examined him closely.

Professor Appaix took me aside, saying, "Dear friend, you'll never succeed. What can you hope to do with a pharynx like that? It's like an entrance to the metro!"

"Sometimes I achieve results that astonish even myself," I said.

"I'm willing to believe it, but not under these conditions. Listen. You are going to speak at a conference at Marseille in three weeks. Tell us then what progress this man has made. I am convinced you won't have very much to tell us. Good luck all the same!"

Three weeks later, I got off the train at Marseille with my suitcase — and my patient. Not only had he become capable of normal speech, but he was even beginning to sing. This showed that a readaptation of the audio-phonatory structure may be effected, even when the speech organs have been profoundly damaged. When I use the term "readaptation," I am not referring to some approximate, superficial repair. The patient I am talking about fulfilled his dream (and the old lady's at the same time). He became a fine singer, whose job it was to understudy Luis Mariano for many years.

The unexpected success of this treatment encouraged me to dig yet deeper in this field. I abandoned certain parallel investigations for lack of time and, above all, lack of means. Earlier, I mentioned the therapeutic use of the placenta. This has given me great satisfaction professionally. By this method, in particular, the larynx regains part of its "tonus." In certain cases placenta therapy is sufficient for someone to recover their voice. Today, placenta has less therapeutic value because it is prepared in a laboratory. But at that time, used when it was fresh, it undoubtedly possessed regenerative powers, particularly on the ear. I imagine these powers are connected with the mixture of hormones which constitutes the placentary mass.

My earliest theories continued to be regularly attacked by my fellow doctors. The majority condemned them before they even had made an analysis of them. Others had the intelligence to behave a little more circumspectly; they were satisfied to ignore them. Only a few reserved judgement and waited for what I said to be confirmed or invalidated. There still existed in the medical profession in Paris a certain number of "free men." By "free," I mean above conflicts, class antagonisms, and personal muckraking.

Dr. Moulonguet was one of these independent men. I respected him a great deal. His particularly acute intellectual curiosity made him open-minded about numerous problems. Also, he was passionately interested in anything to do with voice disorders. One day he came to my laboratory and asked me to tell him all about my work. I did so with an eagerness which you can well imagine; he was the only consultant from the French hospitals who ever deigned to visit me in my lair! He was interested in an enormous number of things and, as usual, asked extremely pertinent questions. He was cordial when he finally left me.

For some time I heard nothing from him. Then one morning in 1957 while I was preparing to operate at the Alma clinic, Dr. Moulonguet, who was getting ready to operate in one of the neighboring theaters, met and talked with me in the antechamber.

"Tomatis, I think you will be happy about this. I have just presented to the National Academy of Medicine a method which bears your name!"

I learned then that in collaboration with Raoul Husson and the staff of the laboratory at the Sorbonne directed by Professor Monnier, he had undertaken the experimental proof of the laws which, in my view, regulated audio-phonatory self-listening. Scrupulously, he set up all the apparatus I indicated, and verified that the results, were indeed those I claimed to have achieved.

"The Tomatis Effect" was not only presented before the Academy of Medicine by Moulonguet and Husson, but also before the Academy of Sciences by Monnier and Husson. Moreover, it was formulated more clearly and more rigorously than before. My words, "One sings — or one speaks — with one's ear," caused much laughter and gossip. Those who were so generously responsible for the support and illustration of my thesis preferred phrases such as "The larynx only emits those harmonics which the ear can perceive." While this was perhaps less picturesque, it was certainly more diplomatic! And better received. At last people began to take me seriously.

6

An Acoustic Geography

My father continued to travel from place to place all over France. During the war he settled temporarily in the Southwest, not only because a singer could find more work in the Toulouse or Bordeaux areas, but also because he carried out most of his mission there serving the Resistance.

My mother rejoined him at Toulouse. When the war was over, she fell ill. The care she received was poor, and she worsened quickly. Neither the diagnosis nor the treatment was appropriate. I hurried by train to see for myself her deteriorating condition; the polio had ravaged her body.

I brought her back to Paris and immediately made arrangements to place her in an iron lung at the Bretonneau hospital. For four days I stayed constantly at her bedside. We had little hope of seeing any signs of recovery. I did not sleep at all those four days until finally, crushed by fatigue, I fell asleep, and she died.

Doubtless, my mother was bound to die, but I do not believe in coincidences. I am convinced that she did so at that precise moment because my own desire to see her live (reduced to a minimum by lack of sleep) was not strong enough to sustain her in her struggle. I believe in such transfers of energy. I believe that a deep enough emotional relationship possesses just such a power. To sit with someone seriously ill is not merely to watch over them; it is to connect them to forces which are the very forces of life itself. This connection eludes us insofar as it is not set to work consciously. Neither the sick person nor the person watching over the patient is aware of this transfer of energy. In my mother's case it was particularly clear-cut since she was in a deep coma. I have no other explanation for how she resisted death so long.

Some will say that I propose this hypothesis because I want to believe in the power of a son's love rising again, in this supreme test, after so many years of mutual misunderstanding. Though I freely admit this belief, much more objective evidence also exists. Right about the same time in the Bretonneau hospital was a baby whom everyone thought would surely die. Nothing could be done other than to watch him die. And yet, this little body was animated with an extraordinary will to survive. Day after day he resisted death. All the staff became part of his struggle. The hospital attendants petted and caressed him; the pediatricians kept trying new treatments, with no real hope for success.

I myself made the room where he lay my headquarters and passed the greatest part of my waking hours reading and working beside him. During the day I saw him whenever I had a moment. I did not know then how to pray, but

I gave him all my energy. I collected all my power to love in the hope that he might live. And he did live! As a result he was shown as the miracle-cure of the hospital service. But I am sure that the real miracle was an almost continuous presence and transfer of "will-to-live" energy. A miracle of love, if you like. Today I know, from my own long and difficult journey, that this relationship of love exists and surpasses our utmost hopes in its healing power.

My mother died in 1947. My father was so deeply affected by her death that he became completely disoriented. He lost his interest in singing and even in living. He went through a terribly difficult time and fell ill. His voice lost its vitality, and he refused contracts offered to him. His condition so disturbed me that I decided to take him into my own home.

It was then that I discovered his true personality — an anxious, uneasy, and very different one from what I had imagined as an adolescent. I realized that our relationship had existed essentially through our letters and that I had spent less time in my father's company than most sons. I loved him deeply, but I did not know him. It was almost as if I loved a different person.

I discovered — totally naive as I was — this basic truth: that living every day with someone is not at all the same as spending two or three weeks with that person once in a while. Before, I had idealized my father. Now I noticed certain weaknesses, certain less than admirable traits in his character. For example, I could not stop feeling rather annoyed to see him always behaving in real life as if he were part of a stage scene. This failing is common to artists, but I had not yet become conscious that it existed in him, too. A thousand little things irritated us both in our dealings with one another. This was especially true for me as his character soured after my mother's death and he virtually abandoned his career. Deprived of his work, he showed a certain tendency to play lord of the manor in my home. Things did not go smoothly.

He fell so ill that despite his lifelong love of food, he was unable to feed himself. His stomach rejected everything. My most difficult task was to make him take care of himself. He claimed that he had no confidence in medicine and let himself waste away. He soon became as thin as a skeleton. A collection of ulcerous symptoms brought him to the edge of serious illness. This illness was the very one which, according to psychosomatic experts, corresponds to the body's assumption of psychological troubles: an ulcer is the bodily symptom of "ulcerized" emotions. Finally, he agreed to be operated on by one of my friends, Dr. Champeau. His stomach revealed so many ulcers that it was necessary to remove the whole thing. Immediately after the operation, he recovered some of his normal drive.

For some reason, I had never told him about my efforts to re-educate singers. However, he soon learned of it. During his convalescence, the sounds of music from my study reached him daily. After a week or so, he said to me, "I know very well you have singers among your clientele, since I have sent some to you myself. But how do you make them sing? I have never heard of a doctor treating patients in this way."

When I explained, he listened, but made no comment. Despite his silence, he paid more and more attention to the sounds coming from my study. As he had no trouble in identifying voices, he soon got to know that certain patients, whose voices were very much impaired the first time he heard them, gradually recovered their accuracy, volume, and warmth. He considered the possibility that perhaps my unusual method did some good after all. Since he had recovered quite a bit of his natural appetite for life, he wanted to benefit from it himself. That is how I became my father's re-educator, a situation which posed some problems within the terms and conditions of the therapeutic relationship.

Despite difficult moments, both of us were amply repaid for our efforts. I kindled in him a voice that I have rarely succeeded in achieving with my other patients. My father was able to take up his career where he left off and even to enlarge the circle of his admirers.

He regained his old character and returned to set up house in Nice. This ended the sometimes tense situation created from the first moment we had to live together in the same goldfish bowl. The more I understand relationships which Freudian tradition calls "Oedipal," the more I am inclined to think that fathers and sons are animals that bear the same name, but who evolve as strangers even when they share the same house. Once life put us at a distance again, we rekindled the warm relationship of former times. We again took up our exchange of letters, which brought us just as much pleasure as in the past.

I always pressed my father to marry again, and he finally did. He married an exceptional woman with whom he found the happiness he had never found with my mother because neither of them understood the other. Neither was responsible for this failure. They were only wrong in not taking into account their insurmountable incompatibility. Although my father certainly suspected this, over the years it became apparent to me, perhaps because of my unique position. I was simultaneously outside their relationship and essential to it, essential in that my role was the one that was supposed to unite them —— certainly not a pleasant task for a child!

With his second wife, my father at last attained a level of communication and understanding which he never had reached with my mother. His life then became doubly reorganized, first on the material level, but also on the psychological level. This lead to mutual intimacy and openness.

I was now working with the Electronic Ear nearly every day. Although still doing surgical operations, I became busier and busier re-educating singers. The Ear was both a means of therapy and the privileged tool of my experiments. What I observed from this method launched me on numerous projects. Some of them led nowhere, but others proved extremely fruitful. I am thinking in particular of all that I discovered about the involvement of the body in vocal utterance.

I established that the physical behavior of my patients varied according to the frequency range they heard, that is, according to the type of listening which I imposed on them. Their attitudes and reactions to psychological stimuli of the same type and intensity were all modified when they passed from one mode of listening to another. I saw them collapse or puff out the torso, expand or retire within themselves, become enthusiastic or lose muscle tone. I decided to study these phenomena in more detail. From then on, I was no longer satisfied with drawing up audiograms and taking photographs of the voice. I carried out all sorts of investigations, many relating to the measurement of the human body.

My detailed studies were productive. I perceived, for example, that certain singers to whom I "gave the ear" of Mario del Monaco gained, in a year, four or five inches in measurement around the thorax. It was as if learning to hear and applying their audio-vocal control differently actually transformed their way of breathing. I was quite unable to explain how or why, but I made a careful note of all the facts. In the case of other singers on whom I imposed different types of listening, various different phenomena appeared. Some changed their posture, holding themselves more and more upright with their head slightly bent forward. Others manifested a quickening or a slowing of their heartbeat. Their entire neuro-vegetative life was thus revolutionized.

My observations of Zino Francescatti were interesting in this regard. When I cut out the high frequencies in his right ear, he always said to me, "That's strange, what you're doing. Not only does it disturb my ear, but I feel a strange discomfort when I shift my fingers on the strings."

When I filtered out frequencies a little lower in the spectrum, he said, "This time it hurts my arm!"

This was certainly proof that the ear affects a wide range of impressions on the body.

The study of the interrelationships implicating the body in the process of audio-vocal control took me years. Even twenty years later I was still not entirely finished with the problem. From the beginning, it promised to be particularly arduous since by attacking the *right* ear of the violinist I obtained a reaction in his *left* hand and arm. The whole complex question of laterality was posed, which we shall discuss later.

Other observations led me to formulate verifiable hypotheses more readily. This time, too, I was lucky. It happened that quite a few singers from around Venice came to consult me, all within a few months and all with the same problem: they could not pronounce the sound "r" with the tip of the tongue. This was particularly troublesome as Italian libretti are full of this phoneme. Instead of "r" they all said "l."

Having never studied phonetics or linguistics, I was puzzled and uncertain as to how to help them. Since my method succeeded in other circumstances, I told myself that I would be risking nothing if I put earphones on them and made them listen like Caruso. No sooner said than done. I set up the apparatus and turned to my first patient.

"You are going to repeat what I say."

He agreed.

I pronounced "r," and he repeated "r"! I achieved the same results with the other patients. So it became clear: if they had never uttered this phoneme, it was because they had never heard it. Their selective muteness was only a transmission of a selective deafness. A specific auditory handicap characterized the Venetians, but why them in particular? I could have searched for the answer to this question for a long time, but it occurred to me that perhaps each region of Italy had its own auditory curve, one which could not be reconciled with that of the others. The Venetians were deaf to our "r" sound made with the tip of the tongue, but perhaps the Milanese were deaf to a different element? And the Neapolitans? When this theory had been verified, I was proved right.

For each region there was not only a dialect (or way of speaking), but also "an ear" (a specific envelope curve which is highlighted by a preferred frequency band). Now a door opened to even bolder speculations. Why should there not be, at the next level up from this, a type of "ear" for each nationality: a French ear, a German ear, an English ear, and so on? This question drew my attention to the problems of learning foreign languages and became a new subject for research (already raised by André le Gall in the work I quoted earlier).

I want to mention one of the conclusions found in a student's thesis on "Language Laboratories," which was presented at the prestigious business school Ecole des Hautes Etudes Commerciales. The student discovered that, on average, learners in these language laboratories quit the course after the fourth lesson. One might theorize that such laboratories probably used teaching methods which were inefficient or boring. It might also be suggested (and this is, indeed, an accepted idea) that a Frenchman is less gifted for languages than, for instance, a Slav. The problem, however, is more complex than this.

Whatever the particular situation may be, the theory of teaching foreign languages is founded on a completely inaccurate assumption, namely that all people from all four corners of the earth hear in the same way. My experience with the Venetian singers suggested that the truth was just the opposite. I was able to prove that different types of hearing exist, connected with different geographical factors. In general, it truly can be said that a particular "ear" is associated with each and every language. Every ethnic ear can be defined by its spectrum of receptivity.

How may this be determined? Once more, I put my analyzer to work. I made Frenchmen, Italians, Englishmen, Germans, Spaniards, Americans, and others speak. The phonograms were collected according to the ethnic origins of the speakers. An envelope curve could be established for each group (Figures 3a through 3f), which is based on the average recorded values of all the frequency peaks found in the spoken language. I later called this curve an "ethnogram."

It was equally possible to establish the chosen area of the most used frequency combinations for any given language, and so for an ear. This is called the basic, or preferred, frequency band. The French ear, for example, hears essentially between 1,000 and 2,000 Hertz (Figure 3a). Meanwhile, the basic frequency band of the British English ear is between 2,000 and 12,000 Hertz (Figure 3b), and the North American English ear is between 750 and 3,000 Hertz (Figure 3c).

For the Germans the band which divides the low notes and spreads out to 3,000 Hertz is remarkably wide (Figure 3d); and that of Slavs is even more so, since it extends from very low frequencies to extremely high ones (Figure 3e). Spaniards are particularly sensitive in the low zone for frequencies between 100 and 500 Hertz, and higher up to frequencies between 1,500 and 2,500 Hertz (Figure 3f).

This does not mean that in each of these examples there is a deafness to frequencies outside the basic frequency band. But an undeniable sensitivity to certain frequencies exists which explains any under-use of other frequencies outside the preferred range (Figures 3a - f). Now it may be understood why it is so difficult for a French ear (1,000-2,000 Hertz) to hear a British English ear (2,000-12,000 Hertz). In contrast, North American English poses fewer problems because it presents a lower basic frequency band with a peak at 1,500 Hertz.

The very real ability of Slavs (Figure 3e) to master foreign languages is therefore the result of their wide-ranging auditory receptivity. The gift of languages is more an aptitude for hearing them than for speaking them. The ear which comes nearest to that of Slavs (Russians in particular) is the Portuguese. When a native Russian traveling abroad happens to hear Portuguese spoken (or vice versa), he pays attention, for he thinks he recognizes his own language. From this perspective, Portuguese sounds like Spanish that has been subjected to the audio-vocal control of a Slav ear.

When applying this outline of ear-voice relationships to the learning of foreign languages, success improves noticeably from the moment the student's way of hearing is modified so that his listening is adapted to the basic frequency band of the language being studied.

In Rouen, I undertook a series of experiments with a group of French schoolchildren of normal I.Q. who were obtaining satisfactory reports in all subjects except English. The results fulfilled my highest hopes: after re-education of the ear, these children caught up very quickly and reached the standard of the good students we had used as a control group.

As I was first and foremost a doctor, there was no question of my trans-

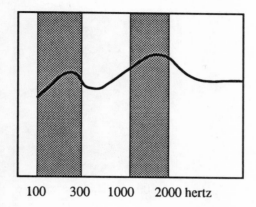

Figure 3a. *French language curve with range of selectivity from 1,000 to 2,000 Hertz.*

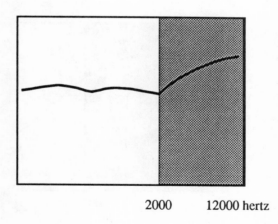

Figure 3b. *British English language curve with range of selectivity from 2,000 to 12,000 Hertz.*

Legend:

━━━━━━ *Envelope Curve* ░░░░░░░ *Basic Frequency Band*

Horizontal = Frequencies *Vertical = Intensities*

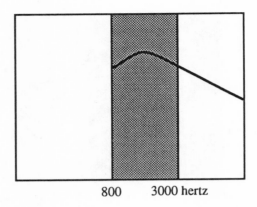

Figure 3c. *North American English language curve with range of selectivity from 800 to 3,000 Hertz.*

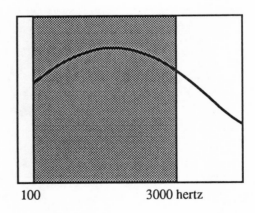

Figure 3d. *German language curve with range of selectivity from 100 to 3,000 Hertz.*

Legend:

████████ *Envelope Curve*   ▒▒▒▒▒▒▒ *Basic Frequency Band*

Horizontal = Frequencies   *Vertical = Intensities*

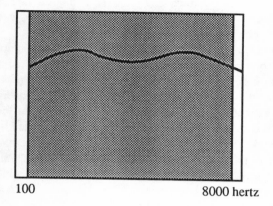

Figure 3e. *Slav language curve with range of selectivity extending from low sounds to very high sounds.*

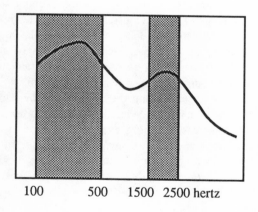

Figure 3f. *Spanish language curve with range of selectivity from 100 to 500 and 1,500 to 2,500 Hertz.*

Legend:

■■■■■■ *Envelope Curve*   ⣿⣿⣿⣿⣿ *Basic Frequency Band*

Horizontal = Frequencies   *Vertical = Intensities*

forming my consulting room into a language laboratory, regardless of these exciting discoveries. Nevertheless, I gathered numerous facts which supported my first observations, confirmed the correctness of my theory, and allowed it to become more refined and precise as the years passed.

For example, I had a German patient who came to Paris to perfect his French. He spoke his own language without difficulty and had absorbed English with a certain ease in the course of his schooling, but could not manage the French "s." If I was not mistaken, I had to repair a corresponding breakdown in his hearing brought about by an accident of some sort. In fact, this man had been a gunner in the war. The violent noises to which he had been exposed had finally impaired his hearing in the upper levels of the spectrum, particularly at that level where the control and integration of the French sibilants take place. A few treatments were enough to correct this difficulty. Learning French became much easier for him; the last barriers fell and he returned to Germany having attained his goal a lot sooner than expected.

This merely verified my original intuition. Other such encounters enabled me to advance and elaborate my ideas in more detail.

An experience with a professor at Sheffield University in England provided ample evidence of the compulsive effect of selective hearing. This man, whose French pronunciation and accent were very poor, wanted to record certain English texts to help some of his young trainee teachers learn to teach English better. When we finished recording, I suggested that he listen to the tape using the headphones of the Electronic Ear. I arranged the apparatus to impose a French ear so this teacher could hear his text just as his trainee teachers would. He put the headphones on and, to the amazement of us all, experienced enormous difficulties in understanding the phrases that he had pronounced so admirably just a few minutes earlier. When I asked him to repeat some of them, he was incapable of satisfactorily doing so.

I confirmed the interdependence of hearing and speech in the months that followed. One day I welcomed to my laboratory a score of modern language specialists on staff at the Hachette publishing house. They were escorted by the head of the department, a Russian by birth. He was a man distinguished by a great verbal fluency and aptitude for foreign languages, speaking four or five of them besides Russian and French.

At the end of our interview this gentleman agreed to sum up the results of our working session while wearing the Electronic Ear. Once the apparatus was fitted, he began a long speech. As he spoke, I discreetly modified the controls, imposing, one after another, different envelope curves with their basic frequency bands highlighted through the filtering system of the Electronic Ear. To the enormous bewilderment of his colleagues, we heard this man pass without warning from French to English, from English to German, from German to Russian, and so on. The best part was that he was unaware of it himself! He believed in all good faith that he spoke French throughout his summary.

I repeated this experiment shortly afterwards with Herr Lane, director of the foremost school for German interpreters. He, too, was an astonishing polyglot, and had a perfect knowledge of eight languages. During our various meetings, he moved naturally from one language to the other with equal fluency. To make things interesting, I asked him to read in succession several texts written in different languages which he knew while I modified the controls from time to time. As he did so, I heard him speak one language (that of the text) with the accent of a different language (that of the envelope curve imposed), such as German with a Spanish accent and Italian with an English accent. In brief, when dealing with a preconditioned person, it was possible to change the audio-vocal control at will by displacing, and so enlarging or restricting, the envelope curve and as a result, instantaneously modifying vocal utterance.

Mastery of a language becomes much easier by using the Electronic Ear to sensitize one to the prominent frequencies of the language to be learned. From one language to another the codes are certainly very different, but the brain and the nervous system present surprising possibilities of adaptation due to the relationship of the ear and voice (as verified by André le Gall).

I almost believe that absolutely everyone, except for those with congenital or pathological limitations, is in an equally good position to learn as many languages as desired. The only condition is knowing for each language the three basic parameters to which one's listening and speaking must adapt and conform to be successful. The three parameters which enable the character of a language to be precisely defined are as follows:

(1) The selective field, which is the opening of the auditory response so that it corresponds to the language's basic frequency band.

(2) The slope of this band, which is the curve which defines it (perhaps ascending, perhaps descending, perhaps presenting several peaks and valleys), such as those shown in diagrams on the preceding pages.

(3) Latency time, which is the time it takes for someone to listen to himself.

The concept of latency time requires some explanation and may be better understood if compared to that of visual adjustment. After gazing into the far distance, when we look back again to our index finger outstretched to the point of maximum convergence of the eyes, for a very short time we see not one, but two fingers. Latency time measures the interval necessary for visual adjustment. It is perfectly possible to speak also of "aural" adjustment. The ear, too, needs a certain time to pass from casual listening to an accurate appreciation of sounds. This latency time varies according to the language and corresponds to the average time it takes to utter each syllable. It governs the way that the speech organs (including the larynx) adapt and respond.

The Electronic Ear works in a similar fashion. It superimposes on a person's original listening pattern a way of hearing which compels it from that moment to focus on sounds according to one exact schema which is a function of (a) focusing hearing on the basic frequency band of the chosen language, (b) the slope of the envelope curve or ethnogram, and (c) the latency time inherent in the effort of adjustment. These three vary with each language.

This apparatus offers the chance of both grasping a message correctly and reconstructing it well, since utterance is strictly dependent upon the ear's perception. Every change marked at this auditory level will trigger a corresponding change in the parameters which define vocal emission such as tone, rhythm, and volume.

An adjustment takes place to create the conditions that prepare the ear to receive the stimulus of a particular frequency. The whole neuro-muscular circuit sets to work to make the body fit to listen, and then to speak in the desired manner. The retention effect does the rest; deliberate effort is gradually replaced by a genuinely automatic process. Permanent retention is gained at the end of a number of half hour sessions; the exact number varies between 50 and 100 according to the individual. From this point on, the subject is "condemned" to pronounce the elements of a foreign language well, whether he has models to imitate or he has to speak the foreign language with no other guide than his memory of what he has heard.

In this way, the opening of the ear to one *foreign* spectrum or another constitutes a sort of instant phonetic initiation —— an instantly perfect one. The student has no trouble acquiring it. Everything takes place as if the organs of hearing and speech and the related areas of the brain *ipso facto* adapt to the new idiom. What in the end is reestablished is the original auditory potential, the same innate conditions which enable us to learn our own mother tongue.

After studying several hundred different languages according to these three parameters, I concluded that all of them fall into one of twelve basic patterns of primary envelope curves. Of course, an analysis on a much wider scale (including still further languages), and a much more subtle one might well give a different result. The figures I put forward are only provisional, and I am sure that if a more complete collection of data were submitted to computerized analysis, we could refine the result if not correct it entirely. However, we cannot blind ourselves to the difficulties inherent in such a task. More than 4,000 languages exit in the world!

Before it became fashionable, but after the first pioneering works, I became interested in structural linguistics. I wanted to determine the characteristics which make a particular language an autonomous system. In the early 1950s, the Army asked me to examine a group of people who worked in counterespionage at Mount Valerian. They intercepted Morse Code messages sent by secret agents across radio waves. Nowadays, the interception of intelligence is done electronically, but then messages were picked up by men using headphones. Working conditions were all the more painful because a serious shortage of manpower compelled each operator to pick up two messages simultaneously, one from each ear, and have his two hands reproduce at the same time two different sequences of dots and dashes. I do not know how their brains succeeded in this disassociation, but I can bear witness that it happened. I was summoned because this incredible piece of cerebral gymnastics created problems, sometimes serious ones. As I observed these soldiers in action, I heard them comment on the messages as they came through, "Ah! a Japanese.... A German now.... Oh, here is a Russian...."

It was very impressive. Dash, dot, dash, dot, dot went the machine while the listener declared, "A Chinaman."

"You know Chinese?" I asked.

"Oh, no!" the man replied.

In fact, these operators scarcely spoke or understood any of the languages used by the different transmitters. Besides, they simply did not have time to decode the messages. They were able to identify their origins, however, by the rhythm of the dashes and dots. This was no virtuoso trick they were playing on me. Nor were they showing off. I verified their claims; they were accurate. These operators detected elements of rhythm which were linguistic pointers, the outlines of a structure that they *felt*, rather than theoretically defined. The essential scientific work remained to be done, but it was already possible, guided by the idea of rhythm and intonation, for me to compare the structure of a language to a sort of underlying music.

Whoever speaks of music speaks of an instrument. What then was the instrument which gave to each language its intonation, its timbre, its particular registers? To answer this question, I had to take into consideration the geographical distribution of the various ethnic ears. I did not have far to seek, for the solution was obvious. The reader who has been kind enough to follow me up to this point knows it already. The chief instrument for each individual is surely the air around him. Music (language) only changes because the instrument (the air) is changed. Far from being the same everywhere, the air around us varies in its function owing to a great number of factors, notably climatic ones. Let us call the whole of these factors together "the impedance of the area." This makes it easier, as anyone can verify, to speak English in England than in France, but easier in France than in Spain. In fact, it is this which determines the posture and adaptation of the ear. In humid surroundings (for example, on islands) the languages spoken are affected by the local impedance in the sense that a greater fluidity of speech occurs.

One must not be tricked by the apparent naiveté of this relationship between humidity and fluidity that seems to appeal to an archaic metaphysical interdependence. When I defended this theory, a professor at the Sorbonne made fun of it by saying, "According to Tomatis, it would be enough to go for a walk in the rain to learn to speak English!" His caricature was funny, but caricatures are not valid arguments. What this humorist took to be the whim of an isolated contemporary was, in reality, embedded in a tradition of thought already more than a century old.

More than 100 years ago, De Bekaer classified languages under such headings as "woodland" and "humid." One need not read his work to be convinced that this theory is well-founded. All one has to do is walk in summer in the D'Oc region from Toulouse to Marseille. If one listens carefully to the cicadas weaving a permanent background of sound, one will note that their song becomes more and more nasal the nearer one gets to Marseille. The cicadas, however, are the same everywhere; the way they utter sound is identical from one place to another. I will add, for good measure, that the phenomenon of nasalization is unknown to them. So it is not the message which has changed; rather it is our listening, and that can only have changed for one reason — we have passed from one type of atmosphere to another. The filter that controls our hearing is modified, and this brings about a change in the conditions of what we take in. I remember, too, that Zino Francescatti once told me that he always refused offers to play in Nice.

"Never will I go back," he confided to me. "I don't know what happens down there, but my violin refuses to play truly."

Are the acoustics at the Opera House at Nice deplorable? Not at all. It is a replica of La Scala at Milan. But the inlet of Angel Bay, the nearness of the sea, and other atmospheric elements bring about a local impedance unfavorable to music. This is so true that my mother tongue, Niçois, is one of the most discordant I know. In this country where Stradivarius refuses to play, words themselves truly cease to be melodious. Stradivariuses resonate just as badly in the middle of virgin forests; that certainly explains why violins were invented and built in Europe and not on the banks of the Amazon or in equatorial Africa.

Musical traditions are always in strict relationship with their environment. Races that practice polyphonic music live surrounded by forests full of confused murmurs and mingled noises while in desert regions like Chad the drum is the only instrument. Instruments, then, maintain a certain rapport with the impedance of the area. It is understood, of course, that these phenomena taken as a whole are much more complex as far as acoustics are concerned. Let us say that we are talking about *an atmospheric environment*, the action of which brings about a transformation. In connection with the particular psychology of the indigenous people, this atmosphere brings about a well-defined form of music. This form conditions how the whole human group listens and thereby influences all its other musical productions, with certain local variations. It is this process which explains why, for example, in France, Breton folksong and the boureé of the Auvergne are at the same time comparable (particularly in their rhythmic qualities) and quite distinct.

If the best way to learn a language is to go and stay in a foreign country, it is not only because we are immersed in a linguistic bath there, but also because we find ourselves immersed in a particular listening atmosphere which, by modifying the way we listen, helps us to adapt the way we speak.

From this point of view, the multiplicity of idioms and dialects within the same linguistic group may easily be conceived as a simple modulation of the original language according to the local impedance. This is why attempts to create a universal language like Esperanto always fail. To think that a single language may be widely circulated is an illusion, since its uniqueness is forcibly broken up when the impedance is changed. Take the case of English-speaking Americans of English origin. One of their characteristics is to nasalize when they speak, while British-English pronunciation repudiates all nasalization. The American Indians who were the original inhabitants nasalize enormously. If Neapolitans and Germans (to whom the phenomenon of nasalization is rather strange) are transplanted to the United States or Canada, after some time they too begin to nasalize.

Nevertheless, the majority of people who live abroad, even if they speak the language of their adoptive country to perfection, keep a slight trace of accent which enables a specialist to pinpoint their origin quite easily. In the same way, a Frenchman from the South or from Alsace who goes "up" to Paris and tries losing his accent always keeps a little of it, which shows despite his efforts at verbal disguise. This phenomenon is connected with the latency time which we defined earlier. This parameter provides a factor which individualizes groups and particular people within groups. Such a person speaks one language with the latency time of another.

This causes many important language modifications. Not only is tone affected, but also the organization of the speech apparatus, the use of the resonating cavities of the larynx which lie above and below, the contraction of the laryngeal muscles, breathing, and by repercussion, the act of mimicry. All are upheavals bound together by a reflex-firing process. Step by step they extend to an individual's whole morphological structure.

We transform the structure of our body when we speak, or essentially speak to it, since one's body is the first thing to be affected by the sound it utters. All the areas of the body are not equally affected. Little by little, speech sensitizes the sensory segments which detect the sound waves produced by the voice. The areas most receptive to this information obviously are located where the distribution of nerve fibers most sensitive to pressure is at its highest concentration. Moreover, each of us, according to what he is and what he has made of himself, centers his activity in one part of his body, and it is to this part that he speaks. That is his choice. That is why a champion cyclist makes his statements to the press in a hollow voice which is weak in sibilants —— he is talking to the center of his activity, almost the center of his life, which in this case is his legs. The use of voice centered in the low frequency range is necessarily bound up with the centering of interest in the lower part of the body.

The ideal would be for everyone to be able to touch, in a homogeneous way, the whole surface of the body. However, this is not impossible, as demonstrated by some Tibetan yogis who devote much of their time and psychic energy to this pursuit. After a certain amount of training, they succeed in speaking to their back as easily as to the palms of their hands. "True" sound does not come only from the lips, but from the whole body. Aristotle and Plato were right to declare that speaking or singing involves making the air which is outside and the air which is inside vibrate in harmony. But that signifies, too, that the full potentialities of language are not given to us right away: speech in its totality can only come as a reward for high aspirations and long training. We have much to learn from the wisdom of the ancients or, rather, to relearn. Through them we can rediscover all the old knowledge which we have lost.

To speak a particular language always means adopting a particular physical and psychological attitude. I experimentally verified this many times. By changing a person's aural reception, one leads him, though quite unaware of it, to change his posture. When I give a "German ear" to a Frenchman, for example, I see him raise his voice, force his words out through his throat, and stand up straight —— exactly what an actor would do when asked to play the part of an officer in the Wehrmacht.

To a certain extent, it also goes beyond language and influences one's mentality, way of reasoning and understanding, and fundamental ethnic attitudes to life. If you brutally deprive a person of his own way of listening, you will see him immediately entangled in difficulties, not only of expression but also of thought. He will lose his verbal fluency and mental flexibility. If he wished to continue speaking, his first reaction would be to snatch off the headphones that have been placed on him to carry out such an experiment. Once I played this dirty trick on some Chinese phoneticians. They became literally incapable of formulating a single thought or of articulating a single sound! Since their language was a tone language, they depended even more than others on their system of self-listening.

A chief advantage of using the Electronic Ear to learn a foreign language is to permit the student to assimilate corresponding mental attitudes at the same time as he is mastering the language. By this means, the spirit is acquired at the same time as the word. This is indispensable, since no one can claim to master a language till the moment when he thinks in it and exists in it. The Electronic Ear succeeds in helping learners to achieve a remarkably high standard, naturally and easily.

I have demonstrated to many people that it is not only an accent which impresses itself on the student's aural memory without any intellectual effort, but also phrase structure, grammar, and even to some extent, vocabulary. In a few sessions with the Electronic Ear, these elements become thoroughly learned, although it might take months or years under other circumstances.

With these new techniques, the whole structure of the language instills itself into the brain at one sweep, and with this a considerable part of one's national character. Behavior will be the first thing to be modified. If a Frenchman is subjected to a "French ear" and asked to draw a line, the line will be more or less horizontal. But if the same experiment is reproduced when he is listening with a "Spanish ear," suddenly he will draw the line in a descending curve! Each of the two lines corresponds to the frequency curve imposed upon the listener. This variation in behavior predisposes him to recognize (from the inside, as it were) the reactions of the people whose language he is studying. This enables him to understand them intimately and soon to be able to reproduce the same reactions. As soon as his brain is plugged in to "the foreign language channel," he will live these reactions spontaneously.

It must be emphasized that the Electronic Ear is never anything but a "tuning in" technique. It does not teach grammar, syntax, or vocabulary. It does make the acquisition of these things simpler and more lasting. But one can also count on — and this is the trump card — certain secondary effects, chief of which is the euphoria experienced by the learner. What is meant by this?

Motivation — the desire to learn, if you prefer — plays a basic part in learning and language. Very often the beneficial effects of this initial motivation are nullified after the first few weeks by the blockage of energy stemming from inhibitions. Fear of ridicule is the most common of these. The learner does not dare open his mouth because he is afraid he cannot reproduce perfectly the sounds offered as models. In other words, he feels his vocal self-control is faulty. Therefore, why should he wear himself out repeating sounds whose reproduction he can neither approximate nor control at will?

By immediately establishing effective vocal self-control or self-listening, the Electronic Ear lifts inhibitions and simultaneously makes the student more flexible and more confident, and then more enterprising. This produces marked progress which rekindles the desire to learn, and thus encourages further progress. This is what I mean by euphoria and its effect upon motivation. Moreover, this happens even more rapidly now that it is possible for us to play foreign language tapes in a manner which simulates intrauterine listening so that it brings out the language structure, and the structure alone.

At the Child Study Centre of the University of Ottawa, experiments carried out on a group of three-year-old children demonstrated the ease with which these children were able to learn French and English at the same time with the help of our method. The Electronic Ear enabled several foreign languages to be learned with the same facility — and very quickly. The whole secret is to separate the channels properly; if they overlap, failure lies ahead.

What do the terms "separation" and "overlap" of channels mean? Rather than provide a theoretical explanation, I will tell the following story. There was a time when young Spanish families settled in France in considerable numbers. The children enrolled in French schools where they seemed to do well. Then one day dyslexic problems appeared. This dyslexia affected not only their adoptive language, but also their mother tongue. The reason why soon became apparent.

To help their children, the parents had started to speak French at home. Their intentions were commendable. Unfortunately, their knowledge of our language was poor and they spoke it from within a frequency band that was not their own. For, unlike French teachers, they were using the Spanish ear to express themselves. In this particular case, the Spanish and French channels overlapped. It should be noted that in the families where the parents did not go to the trouble of speaking French, the children had no problems. For them, the separation of channels had been directly and quite unconsciously brought about in the children's brain mechanisms.

If the father were Spanish, the mother English, and the teacher French, the children could have learned all three languages at the same time without any problems — but strictly on condition that there was no confusion between the frequency ranges, that is to say, that each adult expressed himself in his own language. This is a condition I have always insisted upon with parents who have asked me to help their son or daughter learn a foreign language. When all these conditions are met, the results are remarkable.

I have known children ten-years-old who have mastered French, English, Spanish, and Arabic — not to perfection, but in a most satisfactory way. They were of normal intelligence. None of them was a child prodigy. The moral of the story is that, as far as language is concerned, no one who is himself in difficulty with language can help anyone else. Furthermore, all help coming from a person who is himself handicapped linguistically can only reinforce existing difficulties and might even raise additional ones!

One last point: the adaptation of auditory receptivity takes more or less time depending on the qualities of the patient's beginning audition. A damaged ear must first be treated. This will prolong the learning process by several weeks or months, according to the seriousness of the case. The personal factor must also be taken into account. The ethnic envelope curve is subdivided into regional curves, and these only represent the average of a whole collection of "strictly individual" curves. Each of us, in terms of personal history, character, and underlying personality, has a unique auditory curve. Our individual curve is not identical to any other. There are also illnesses and accidents. Many people, for example, are in a way *deaf* to frequencies above 2,000 Hertz. So how can they correctly reproduce British English sounds when they have only a foggy perception of them? Such troubles cause major difficulties to some business firms that want to make the staff of an entire department speak English, or another language, without first considering their listening. One or more of the group would probably have an imperfect ear and so be incapable of learning such lessons.

At the end of the fifties, these ideas had gained a certain notoriety. Many people attacked the theories based on their newness, being reluctant to make the intellectual effort to properly refute them. Some rejected them *en bloc*, before they even got to know them.

In 1960 at the Palais de l'UNESCO I addressed a conference on the subject of "The Role of Electronics in the Service of Foreign Languages," to which had been invited, in particular, the leading French interpreters. The head of the UNESCO interpreters, a man of irreproachable competence who possessed a great talent for verbal expression, did not want to hear anything about my theories. As I concluded my presentations, he came to the platform and, in front of the thousand or so present, made a virulent speech aimed at sweeping aside my arguments.

"Would you undertake an experiment?" I asked him.

"It is quite useless," he answered. "But, if you insist..."

"I am simply going to change your way of hearing," I said as I placed the headphones on him. "We shall see what happens."

The result was decisive. He began to splutter and stammer in front of everyone, and he did this in all eight languages of which he was a master. The audience was much amused. The most honest among them who were not previously convinced by my address decided that perhaps what I proposed deserved further examination. Several laboratories in France and abroad added the verification of these theories to their agenda. Some, of course, continued to ridicule me.

It is fair to say, however, that the evidence convinced the majority of specialists. I often met opposition and even open hostility, but in this area at least, people generally ended up giving me some credit. Gradually, authoritative circles acknowledged that the ear is indeed the vital instrument for learning foreign languages. Today this has become a recognized proposition, almost a truism. I cannot ask for anything more.

Back then only one language laboratory in Paris was equipped with Electronic Ears, although many more are now. Others have widely applied some of the principles I set forth. I do not ascribe any merit to myself. It is rather a sign of the times. Consider Marshall McLuhan's philosophy that in the West the civilization of the visual image is in the process of superseding the civilization of the written word. If a change is really taking place, isn't it rather an evolution towards the civilization of *sound*? To be able to ask such a question without leaving the realm of probability provides at least a partial answer. Even if we do not move towards the civilization of sound, we move towards one where sound holds an essential place.

Furthermore, if there is evolution or perhaps even revolution, it is more than the collective social realm which provides its origins, backdrop, and game plan. It is, above all, the person, he who is not at all isolated but rather caught in the complex network of psychological relationships. These relationships weave his uniqueness with the threads of his dependence and, in that radical otherness, make him a being who communicates. Let us leave things at that for the moment. I merely suggest that the new era we speak of can only come about if we rediscover the lost sense of ourselves. The giant steps brought about to build more sophisticated machines are nothing compared to the smallest flea's hop that our spirit (I would say "soul" if the word had not lost its resonance) accomplishes on this path, this journey of initiation.

Concerning language immersion, I established that the best results are obtained when audio-visual techniques and audio-vocal training are combined. The mistake made by too many, and which persists today, is an imbalance between audition and vision in favor of vision. We underlined this very point, my staff and I, in an article published through our center. It said, in part:

> Whereas on the visual plane the goal is achieved by permitting the student to verify by means of the image that represents the object being studied, on the auditory plane great uncertainty exists about how to integrate the oral message: one only has to verify the remarkable distortions in the mouth of the student who is doing a repeating exercise to calculate to what extent, by virtue of the laws that rule the relationship between what is heard and what is uttered, the message has not been properly understood.

At first these famous audio-visual methods seemed full of promise in comparison with techniques that were then in favor in French schools, the essence of which consisted of making students memorize rules of grammar and lists of vocabulary. But in reality, the dispute that they implied related more to form than to fundamentals. Too often these miracle recipes were only the pure and simple transposing of ancient crazes and old fashioned *a priori* teaching methods. Numerous systems lacked any scientific basis. In other words, they lacked what was essential.

A technique for language learning could be very valuable; nevertheless, it will remain unworkable *if the auditory apparatus has not been prepared beforehand.* In the same article, we reminded the reader that whatever ingenuity is provided to help the teacher serves no purpose if the entrance door of the ear remains closed to the linguistic message. It is necessary first to be sure that this door is completely open and that the ear is ready to receive the particular sounds of the language it has to learn.

The Electronic Ear takes charge of this preparation. It creates the environment for aural absorption indispensable for putting the audio-vocal control apparatus in place. By its relationship with the spoken word, it plays the part of the conductor of an orchestra. By adapting the student's listening to information contained in the language being studied, it regulates the volume of the voice, the tone, and the rhythm of the utterance. At the time of utterance, the ear, guided by the Electronic Ear until it is automatically regulated, controls volume, tone, intonation, and inflections. The act of teaching, which is not directly our domain, is complementary to this auditory training approach.

Certain fundamental rules must be followed to ensure success. It is preferable for the Electronic Ear to be used in a preparatory phase before the instruction proper. If one works with students who have already begun language study, it is best to start again from scratch — particularly if their pronunciation (and so their learning) is deficient. If, for some reason, it is undesirable to interrupt an already started course, half an hour a day should be devoted to conditioning exercises using the Electronic Ear.

One point needs emphasis. Many language laboratories lose customers after only a few months of training and yet, broadly speaking, their teaching methods are the same as elsewhere. Those in charge do not understand and are frustrated by this, although there is nothing mysterious about these desertions. Quite simply the companies have lost everything by trying to gain too much. Having invested heavily in the physical premises, their decorations and so on, they have economized on the teaching materials and equipped the laboratories with poor quality tape recorders. They may have acquired equipment from the same price range as those which produce the best performance; they may pride themselves on this in the prospectus. But prospectuses, as everyone knows, are drawn up to beguile. They should have entrusted these purchases to experts, people capable of verifying whether these machines fulfilled the promises made.

In fact, in language laboratories, the use of equipment of the highest quality is an absolute necessity. Every weakness, whether mechanical or electronic, may hinder or even block the learning process. When I say "mechanical," I think first and foremost of the playing of the tape. In this area, the slightest imperfection makes the whole process void, for it introduces parasitic noises and distortions of greater or lesser importance which result in making the original acoustic signal unrecognizable or at least seriously altered. If the student is put in the position of having to correct, minute by minute, the sound message transmitted to him, this extra effort which he is forced to make will (1) jeopardize the pleasure of learning and (2) in the long term cause weariness...and flight! Moreover, there is good reason for the student to give up because in such conditions his goal cannot be attained. A tape recorder whose frequency range is cut off after 3,000 or 4,000 Hertz produces an auditory curve the very opposite of that required. I have even tested machines where everything began to fade after 500 and some even after 300 Hertz. Of course, I know that actual norms allow for a drop after 5,000 Hertz, but in the very important process of learning foreign languages, this is not good enough. A tape recorder should be able to respect, with the utmost rigor, the preferred frequency range, the slope of the envelope curve, and the latency time of the language being studied. This means that in the case of British English, for example, an accurate response range up to 12,000 Hertz must be maintained; if not, the ear may be seriously thwarted.

If the apparatus offers all the desired guarantees, if the student is motivated, and if the teacher properly fulfills the role of "mouthpiece" (the expression should be taken literally), rapid progress is ensured. With the assistance of the Electronic Ear, the learning of a foreign language can be accomplished in a minimum of six months. This seems lengthy compared to what certain laboratories promise, but I am not a salesman. I am satisfied with giving the results of experiments which have actually been conducted under scientific control.

That being said, I too have my secret weapon. Specialists used to agree that after the age of 14, it is no longer possible to bring about a genuine bilingualism in anyone. Now I can declare that with the techniques perfected in the area of audio-psycho-phonology, this limitation has been shattered. The ability to master a foreign language is now open to people of all ages. Appropriate listening training is all that is necessary.

This insight has commercial value, too. I am sure some readers remember those employees of the Hachette publishing house whose spokesman was made to speak in the whole range of languages he knew — *unknown to himself*. They had not come to see me just to witness some kind of theatrics, but rather to consult me on a particular matter. The editor whom they represented had just put together a reading primer which he hoped would sell widely in French-speaking Africa. But the book was not nearly as successful as he had expected. What had gone wrong? For them, it was a guessing game; for me, the reason was apparent as soon as I glanced at the text.

The first phrases for the reader to repeat were as follows: Je dis (I say), Je lis (I read), J'écris (I write). As far as frequency level goes, the phoneme "i" rises above 2,000 Hertz while the letter "j" extends considerably above this frequency. The French-speaking African ear is more attuned to lower frequencies in and around the range of the sounds "bo," "bou," and "dou"; so a glaring incompatibility showed up in the first pages of the book. The book's very first linguistic task demanded too great an effort from the young students for their first lesson in French. As a result, the book was judged to be too demanding and was ultimately abandoned because the auditory challenge was too great. The book's penetration into the African market was nothing more than a flash in the pan. I explained to them that it would have worked quite differently if the reader had first encountered phonemes situated in the lower part of the sound spectrum. In that case, no doubt an auditory adaptation would have gradually occurred.

The interdependence of reading and listening remains to be discussed.

There's nothing remarkable about that, you may say, if we are talking of reading aloud and, therefore, of vocalization. But, surprisingly enough, this interdependence remains valid with silent reading.

I myself worked several years before accepting this idea. The gradually accumulating facts, all pointing in the same direction, compelled me to elaborate this apparently paradoxical thesis: "One reads with one's ear."

From the beginning I noticed that high school students who became good students of spoken English after working with the Electronic Ear also obtained better results *in other subjects.* When parents thanked me for this, one phrase kept recurring: "Now my child reads much better." This comment recurred so systematically that I could no longer believe in simple coincidence. I investigated and observed that the development of audio-phonatory interplay made acquiring the mechanics of reading much easier.

After all, is that so surprising? The written symbol in itself is merely a sound to be reproduced. Is it not revealing that the Latin word "legere" meant "to read" (in the sense which we understand it today) and at the same time "to gather by means of the ear"? In ancient Greek "lexic" meant primarily "saying, speaking," and "dyslectos" (from which our word dyslexic is derived) meant "having difficulty in expressing oneself in speech." Let us consider, too, that in England today a "lecture" is what the French call a "conference." From this point of view, every letter calls for vocal elaboration in tones which can be understood. Writing, therefore, may be considered a recording of sound since it aims to store up sounds. In fact, writing constitutes the first tape recorder in the history of humanity.

If we have forgotten this, it is because silent reading, by means of one's eyes, is a relatively late acquisition. It is probably connected with the widespread distribution of books after the invention of printing. I am sure that if ancient civilizations had known of the tape recorder, they would not have taken the trouble to perfect a writing system. In other words, the written symbol is a sound and only expresses its full value by its restoration to sound. Writing only carries meaning when the reader "hears" the sound of the words in front of him.

Precisely how the ear is involved in silent reading remains to be defined. In fact, the entire body enters this dynamic process. A language well learned is a language well embodied, or well incarnated, one finds ample support for this view in experiments carried out by McGuigan, a specialist in electromyography.[6]

McGuigan studied muscle reactions by recording them on a special electronic machine fastened to the subject by electrodes (as many electrodes as desired

---

[6] See, for example, McGuigan and Winstead (1974) "Discriminative relationship between covert oral behavior and the phonemic system in internal information processing." Journal of Experimental Psychology, 1974, 103, 5, 885-890.

once a computer was employed to do the calculations). He observed the musculatory reactions of a series of people while they were reading aloud. He noted that when dealing with the same person, the pronunciation of the same word or phrase produced the same response at the electronic level. But even more interesting was that these musculatory reactions continued to be produced when the person concerned was asked to read in a low voice or even to murmur. In other words, it was not merely putting actual utterances to work that stimulated responses. This hypothesis was confirmed when McGuigan imposed silent reading on his subjects and registered similar responses. Silent reading, then, brings into play our entire bodily dynamic.

The results of this piece of research did not surprise me. They merely corroborated older observations. About 30 years ago, a researcher at the Sorbonne had the idea of making the mouth, tongue, and pharynx opaque to X-rays by having someone swallow a product that deposited barium on the surfaces of these organs. This ingenious system enabled an observer to follow exactly what was happening within the oral/pharyngeal cavity when a person spoke. One could establish that the tongue executed the same movements at nearly the same amplitude when the person articulated his name, for example, as when he only thought of it.

This is not surprising to anyone who has talked to a person and seen their lips moving in sync with his own. I have often experienced this. It is as if the person listening to me whispers at the same time and in the same rhythm what I am saying to him. In reality, he is satisfied with thinking it, either because he has already heard us saying the same phrases and knows by the next word what we are about to say, or because he is in perfect intellectual harmony with me and would use the same phrase himself. Characteristically these sequences of labial mimicry are always followed by a vigorous acknowledgement.

To speak is to create interplay with another's body. Of course, not all those who agree with us exhibit this mimicry. The type of interlocutor just described does not inhibit muscular movement as others might, or else only partially inhibits it. We engage our whole body in speech, whether this is vocalized or not. In this way the ear becomes involved in reading, improperly described as reading "with the eyes."

When I became thoroughly convinced of the fact that reading was connected to listening, I also asked myself whether reading difficulties (otherwise called dyslexic problems) could be treated by the ear. Such a connection could offer immense hope for those children who are handicapped by these troubles in their schooling and mental development. There are one and a half million of them in France alone. I had no right to neglect this possibility. Problems connected with dyslexia then became one of my vital preoccupations.

I asked McGuigan to take some measurements of dyslexic children. He reported back that the muscular response among this group was always anarchic.

The body did not know how to respond. It was not very difficult to deduce that the dyslexic was a person who had not incorporated speech. If the experiment were to be repeated with a musician and an unmusical person, I am convinced that one would see the same phenomena registered as the result of listening to a given musical phrase. The muscular reaction of the first would have a structure (which would be reproduced at each new application of the stimulus), while that of the second would be variable and haphazard (for the good reason that the notes have hardly any meaning for the unmusical person).

The less one has mastered speech with one's body, the less gifted one is for silent reading. This also means that silent reading is necessarily a late acquisition compared with reading aloud. It is a great mistake to continue teaching silent reading before teaching reading aloud for there is a great risk of blocking all spontaneity and comprehension. Nevertheless, this is precisely what is being done. At the very moment I observed this in 1965, out of ignorance of the laws which govern learning, a Minister of Education demanded that from infant school onwards, children should carry out reading sessions *in silence*.

Of course, this decision was not arrived at in a purely arbitrary manner. It was based on the writings of the philosopher Alain,[7] who claimed this was the way he learned to read. I would like to believe it. But Alain simply had forgotten that if he had not begun by reading aloud like everyone else, he would never have reached this stage.

Similarly, one would not know how to make an outstanding musical conductor out of someone who does not know how to read a note of music. The greatest conductors are able to read a whole page of a score at a glance, even if it is from a work requiring 120 players. Nevertheless, they too had to begin their career by learning the ABCs of music. In verbal reading, as in musical reading, brilliant performance is a matter of absorption. It is necessary to be steeped in an *acoustic* environment for a long time in order to be in a position to exercise such mastery; it is indisputably necessary that a large number of nerve-cell references be evoked and, in some way, imprinted.

A human being is like an enormous jellyfish of which the skull-cap is the brain and the infrastructure is the nervous system. Every stimulus provokes a response at the sensory level and, at the same time, at the muscular level. Thus are established, little by little, neural circuits which just as quickly translate themselves into motor or bodily responses. This may be seen very clearly when a dyslexic child is asked questions, even simple ones. Immediately, he shows what one calls "synkinesis," that is, involuntary movements which accompany the activation of speech, movements which are clearly uncoordinated. He agitates his hands, his arms, his legs, and his feet, and finally, starts speaking. One is tempted to say "like a foot" (very badly). He speaks as his feet move,

---

[7] The pseudonym for Emile Auguste Chartier.

waving about aimlessly, out of control, without ever being able to reach the level of properly expressed thought. This parasitic agitation of the body uses up all the energy that should be employed by the nervous system to organize and verbally express thought. Proper verbal expression is strictly dependent on a certain economy of body movement.

Dyslexia as a research topic is still wide open. I have written more about it later in this book and have devoted another entire book, *Education and Dyslexia,* to its study.

In defense of the practice of reading aloud, as far as children are concerned it constitutes a vital stage in their psychic development. Adults also will find it an excellent and very simple means of establishing audio-phonatory control. It might suffice to recall the rule imposed by St. Benedict on the monks of his order: "Everyone should read in his cell in such a way as not to disturb his neighbor." Here is proof enough that for him all reading should be carried on aloud.

Throughout this period of my life, my attention was focused increasingly on my work; my family life received less and less of my time. I worried about the future of my home life. For one, it needed to be reorganized. It was a bad idea, I thought, not to have made a neater separation between my apartment and my professional practice. My children experienced my absence all the more when they knew I was physically close at hand. I thought it might be a good idea to settle my family in the countryside near Paris. We moved, but it turned out to be a serious mistake. Every evening I lost a ridiculous amount of time traveling home. My work and research were disturbed by the long trek, and I saw my children even less than before. The chasm between my wife and myself grew ever wider.

Our divorce was finalized shortly thereafter.

7

Death Sentence

Though my father never approved of my marriage, he was deeply distressed by my marital problems. Our relationship very nearly turned sour because of them. It was not that he was very religious. In fact, his religious beliefs had grown weaker, and he no longer really believed in either God or the devil. However, he clung to an old-fashioned sense of social proprieties. He discarded a good many old-fashioned ideas but continued to think of divorce as one of those things which is "just not done." Marriages must be saved at any cost. Not only did he decide I was wrong, but he bore me a considerable grudge because he felt that this shameful event would reflect on him and blemish his own position in society.

I knew there was no other reasonable solution. In any case, my wife left. The idea of living together became unbearable for both of us. Besides, all the good and bad reasons given by two separating marriage partners are just so many attempts at rationalization, as psychoanalysts would say. If one goes to the root of the matter, divorces have only one cause, and it is always the same: lack of love. As far as I am concerned, it is from this point of view that I understand the old saying, "What God has created, let no man destroy." For me, I repeat, God is love; God is the one supreme Love, and, in fact, what love has built is indestructible. A couple who love each other, where each partner understands the slightest nuance of the other's personality and moves harmoniously in mutually given joy, is assured of a lasting partnership. Without love, on the other hand, no union works.

It was clear in my case that love had not been invited to my wedding. That being so, my wife and I were unable to operate on the same wavelength. I am not trying to minimize my own responsibility. My professional experience shows me that the major effort in the task of mutual adjustment falls to the husband. I do not deny the deficiency on my part, but how could I manage entirely on my own? My wife needed to meet me part way.

It was no consolation, of course, but I learned much from this failure. Suffering can be a good school, not only for the soul but also for the spirit. Without this heart-breaking experience, it is very likely that today I would not be able to assist couples, as I do, to achieve a balanced relationship. At the same time, I learned all sorts of things about the children of divorced parents, which helped me do my work more successfully.

For example, I observed first hand that for the child it is the mother, and she alone, who counts. This is regardless of whatever efforts the father may make and whatever the mother's failings may have been. For it is the mother whom the child needs to seek out, whether or not she offers herself, whether or not she is capable of giving the child her tenderness. The father's duty (psychologists have never sufficiently insisted on this) is to encourage the child to love his mother and to help the child to do so. This is vital. A child who no longer loves his mother no longer loves life. Naturally, it took me a long time to understand this and, above all, to admit it. I recognized that I had faults, and, not being a saint, I was also acutely aware that my wife was not perfect either.

Divorced fathers who have been granted care and custody of their child or children simply must get it into their heads that these children are *always* crippled by the loss of their mother — *never mind what sort of mother*. All divorce laws, even those enacted with the best intentions, the most respectable humanitarian scruples, and the most punctilious spirit of justice, are null and void when they do not address the psychological problems involved.

Excellent jurists made these laws. I do not dispute that. But, as far as the maternal relationship is concerned, they generally do not know much more than the mass of laymen. And then, the majority of such jurists are men. The legislation does not take enough account of other more secret laws — the laws of love. They tend to forget, for lack of understanding, the imperatives which govern a child's growth. In my opinion, we urgently need to revise all divorce laws in order to submit them to the one great principle which admits of no exception: whatever a man's powers of tenderness and goodwill and whatever his personal merits, he will never succeed in any circumstances in taking the place of his children's mother.

My divorce shook my father badly, and I myself was brought to the verge of total collapse. It was as if all the accumulated fatigue and those repeated refusals to take any rest, leisure time, or holidays began to make themselves felt all at once. I pushed myself too far. I committed excesses in my work as others indulge in excesses of pleasure, and now my body was presenting me with the bill.

It was a stiff one. I, who had never had a particular taste for food, had not ceased putting on weight: I was obese, weighing 122 kilos (268 pounds). My blood pressure crept up alarmingly, and I suffered severe attacks of asthma and eczema. Cardiac troubles appeared, and I had three heart attacks.

Added to the shock brought on by my family drama, I had to deal with the openly disapproving attitude of my father, and the fact that my debts, newly added up, rose to seventy-five million francs (about $140,000 at the time). The time had come for me to draw up a balance sheet, in every sense of the term. I was 35 years old. I calculated that I needed seven years to pay back all I owed, provided I did not go further in debt and I could count on a regular income. In a way, this realization came just at the right moment. For it was exactly in seven years' time, according to my most objective diagnosis, that I was bound to die. In fact, I did not doubt for a single moment that a premature death would be the price of my overspent energies. Moreover, the colleagues whom I consulted, heart specialists and others, let me understand that on this subject they held the same opinion as I did. It only remained for me to set my affairs in order before leaving this earth.

Something unexpected, however, changed this gloomy picture. At the moment when all seemed lost, I at last found real love. Some time before this I had hired a laboratory assistant who gradually proved to be remarkably efficient. This young woman knew how to do everything. I could delegate to her both secretarial and administrative jobs. She was perfectly capable of editing a scientific article. I had never ventured to hope for such an ideal collaborator. My contacts with her were greatly simplified because I was unconsciously categorizing her mentality as "masculine." This was oversimplified and wrong. In our dealings, she always said what she really thought, and she placed our conversations on a strictly asexual basis. Her willing, matter-of-fact, and objective spirit greatly assisted me. This also enabled her to become the representative of the staff around me. She helped sort out conflicts, if necessary, by showing me when I was wrong.

My first feeling for her was admiration. Later on, I learned that this was shared. Now I am convinced that mutual admiration is an excellent starting point for a love affair. I will go even further: Without admiration, it is very difficult for a genuine and lasting love to be born. In any case, an emotional relationship developed between us, one which became closer as the days passed. I dared to think of remarrying and setting up house once more.... but, no. I was only a "dead" man on remission. Well, of course, everyone is. But I knew my reprieve was strictly limited. I was the least desirable prospective bridegroom imaginable!

After we admitted our shared feelings, we had a long conversation about marriage. I explained my situation to her from every point of view: divorced, father of four children, up to my neck in debt, and fated to disappear pretty soon. Should she involve herself with a dying, penniless man with the added burden of four children? She replied calmly that none of that was of the slightest importance and that she was ready to face the situation. Was it really so bad? After all, we loved each other.

This was what saved me. Such a splendid, unshakable proof of love sowed in me a fierce desire to escape my fate, to put a stop to the inexorable, in a word, to live — to live, despite the sentence of death that medical examinations pronounced.

My body was injured and damaged, and I needed to start with a definite achievable goal. I decided to lose weight first, although it had always been impossible before, even when I followed every sort of diet — low calorie and fad — one after the other.

I tried everything. One week I ate without drinking. The next week I drank without eating. Nothing happened. I did not lose so much as a gram, although I was an exceptionally disciplined patient and did not allow myself to deviate at all from each diet.

Growing fatter all the time, I reached 268 pounds. There I managed to settle. My skin could not stretch any further. In contrast, my blood pressure continued to increase and reached 32! I became almost helpless. I could no longer cover 50 yards in my apartment without having to stop and rest. Climbing stairs was out of the question. When I made house calls, I asked patients who lived in buildings without an elevator to be kind enough to come down to the concierge's apartment to be examined.

I finally decided to consult Dr. Maurice Delor. Like Professor Moulonguet, he was an independent man who kept out of the rat race. He was a physician in charge of Internal Medicine at St. Michel Hospital, a remarkable writer, and the originator of the Cénacle (a liberal doctors' organization whose purpose was to defend medicine against those members of the profession who tended to forget that political in-fighting can compromise freedom). Dr. Delor was curious about everything and had even visited me to find out about my work. I regarded him highly as a doctor.

I sat in his consulting room and told him about my case in great detail.

"I know, I know," he said, nodding his head every time I embarked on a new chapter of my troubles. Then each time he added, "And you are going to die!"

I knew that only too well, but there was no way of stopping him from repeating it. "You are going to die!" punctuated our entire hour and a half consultation.

"What if I stop eating entirely?" I finally asked him. "If I undertake a fast, don't you think I might succeed in losing a few kilos?"

"Perhaps," he said simply just before I left.

This "perhaps" reverberated in my mind with the same force as another doctor's comment, that of Dr. Carcopino who, when I was a child, said "I must search." I grabbed onto this "perhaps" and began to transform my whole life.

I had read voraciously about diet, but I had no knowledge about fasting, theoretical or practical. Perhaps I never would have dared to do what I did if I had been better informed. I took advantage of my first real holiday in more than 15 years to submit myself to a draconian regime. I ate absolutely nothing, contenting myself with a glass of water whenever I felt hungry. I passed my days stretched out on a chaise lounge. After a few days, my general state improved slightly, and, since I felt better, I continued. After fasting for ten days I weighed myself at the nearest pharmacy. I was stupefied to find that the needle of the weight scale still pointed to the same figure! Had all my heroic deprivations been for nothing? That did not seem possible, but I simply could not deny the evidence.

This setback might well have ended my efforts, except that Dr. Delor's "perhaps" kept ringing in my head. I persevered, even more enthusiastically because my blood pressure returned to normal and I felt that I was definitely reviving. I was invited to Corsica by friends, composer Henri Tomasi and his painter wife, Odette Camp. While the others spent meal times together, I went for a walk. Seven kilometers at midday, and sometimes seven kilometers in the evening. I continued to take nothing but water and surprisingly felt a real improvement. I waited until I had finished my third week of fasting before I weighed myself: this time I *had* lost a few pounds. It was certainly very little in comparison with what I had hoped, but it was an encouraging start since now I could walk long distances, even though two weeks earlier I could not manage 50 meters without chest pains to stop me.

Intending to accelerate the improvement, I decided not even to drink water any more. Then I had a fainting spell and those around me begged me to eat normally. I compromised by allowing myself one meal a week. I chose the day —— Tuesday. Two months later, I weighed 220 pounds. When I got down to 198 pounds, I modified my regime a little further. In kingly fashion I granted myself two meals a week, on Tuesday and Friday. This time the process of getting thinner was well under way. I was melting away slowly but regularly. I found I felt lightened in many ways: I regained muscle-tone, could breathe more easily, and stabilized my blood pressure. I had no more heart troubles, and my expectation of life was suddenly prolonged. The only person in despair over my transformation was my tailor. My old clothes hung so loosely about me that I began to resemble a tramp! The poor tailor went to great trouble to make the necessary alterations.

"It's not as easy as you think," he lamented. "You've become quite another man now. Look at your trousers!"

In fact you could have put a plough horse in those trousers and still had room to spare! I consoled my tailor by ordering a whole new suit. For three months I held myself to two meals a week. When at last I stopped fasting, I had lost 92 pounds in seven months. I am tempted to add *only* 92 pounds, which is how I looked at it then. I thought that such a starvation diet would surely thin a person into a skeleton or perhaps even kill him long before the seven months had run out. But no, I weighed 176 pounds, which was still a lot for my thin frame, and, far from being dead, I achieved a genuine rebirth.

I gradually allowed myself to eat normally, but soon put on weight. I decided then to submit myself to an ascetic routine. Every year for a month I would fast. And to appease my tailor once and for all, I ordered several suits, each of which corresponded to a stage in the process which from one year to another made me expand and contract like an accordion —— between 176 and 220 pounds. I was satisfied with this regime until I eventually found a way of stabilizing the process through diet.

I remarried in August, 1958 in the little church of Grau d'Agde in the South of France. (My first marriage had not been celebrated in the Catholic church.) Since I was still overweight and still destined for a premature death, the marriage shows just how far my second wife's strength of character extended. It is a quality she continues to possess; from it I draw the greater part of my own vitality and tenacity.

From the first moments of our marriage we established a lasting dialogue between us. Communication was so rich, intense, and profound that "communion" is a more appropriate term. I, who had not opened my mouth for more than 12 years during my previous marriage, now talked without stopping! Every word uttered seemed to bring us closer to one another and to cement what we were in the process of building. We still share this precious feeling today; our two personalities are truly blended into one. It is an easy formula to talk about (and it has even become a cliché), but is difficult to achieve, if I may judge by what I see around me. We know how to listen to each other and enjoy doing so. Nothing falls from the mouth of one of us that the ear of the other is not ready to welcome. Nothing reaches the ear of either that the mouth could not have spoken. Perhaps I might say that together we have brought about an ideal audio-phonatory circuit.

At the same time as what I might call my "resurrection," the dawning of my passion for modern painting occurred. This interest has been one of the greatest joys of my life. I was ignorant of almost all modern art when fortune favored me by sending two or three painters to me who were suffering from hearing troubles. Talking to them made me want to get to know their works. With the benefit of their explanations, and finding myself able to understand each canvas in relation to the man who painted it, I plunged into this new world. My sensibilities were touched. I felt that I had discovered something of vital concern to me.

These painters were the Symbolists. I particularly admired Aujame, the marvelous painter of the forests of the Auvergne where he was born. We met often and he was my principal guide. He introduced me to many other painters, and it was through them that I met one of my dearest friends, Georges Massié, painter and poet and director of Beaux-Arts of the city of Paris. He was a former engineer for the city of Paris and was in charge of maintaining supplies for Paris during the war. He dazzled me with the range of his culture and the extent of his gifts, but even more than these, his human qualities really impressed me. I often thought that just knowing one man like that in a lifetime makes everything worthwhile.

At about the same time I was treating a colleague's wife who published some works on painting that drew a lot of attention. She was a woman of great intelligence and dynamic personality — one of the most brilliant women I have ever met. She, too, helped me get to know many artists: the famous photographer Ingrid Morad, wife of Arthur Miller, and also the fine abstract flower painter, Hartung, his wife Ana Eve Bergman, Pillet, Lacasse, Terry Haass, and others.

Non-figurative painting held no attraction for me for quite some time. I could not identify with it, and contact with it did not awaken my sensibilities. I met abstract painters and argued with them, often impressed with the insight and subtlety of their spirit. But their paintings remained a closed book to me.

One of Pillet's friends had some nasal troubles and I treated him free of charge, as I always did with artists. He thanked me by presenting me with one of his own sculptures, a work he called "A Crucible," but which I was hard pressed to name. His gesture was a touching one, but I hardly appreciated the actual object. My ignorance of abstract art was total. My recent initiation into figurative painting made this ignorance all the stronger.

My first impulse was to hide the crucible in the back of a cupboard somewhere. I could not bear to look at it. Yet, I could not bring myself to think that people who raved about abstract art were completely wrong. I knew too many of them who were neither snobs nor dupes nor lacking in taste or culture. I gradually saw my failure to understand contemporary art as a true deficiency. It was as if I were blind to something others could see, or deaf to a language others could hear.

I took the sculpture out of the cupboard and set it up in my consulting room where it would be right before me. I studied it constantly and with characteristic obstinacy, waiting for illumination to dawn. Astonishingly enough, revelation did take place and in the most abrupt way: all of a sudden, I understood modern art. I do not mean to say that I merely understood the artists' intentions or that I could now tolerate looking at their works. I mean that in the twinkling of an eye, I recognized as my own this world which had remained closed to me until that moment. Without my moving, chaos had rearranged itself before my eyes into a new and rigorous order. Nothing had actually changed. It was I who was now situated *inside* this vision of the world instead of outside.

My "conversion" to abstract art was instantaneous and permanent. I bought other works from Pillet. When I had ten of them he said to me with an honesty I am pleased to stress, since one does not come across it every day, "Now you have enough Pillets. Move on to something else."

He guided me in my choice, and his help was invaluable, for many artists were his friends. He contributed to the magazine *Architecture Today* and used his influence to help young painters become better known, particularly Soto, Cruz-Diez, and Guzman. I gradually enriched my collection with their works. Really, the only thing missing was enough space to display them.

And still I did not stop acquiring new works. I was especially tempted because more and more of my clients were painters. It was not by mere coincidence; they sought me out because I was capable of solving some of their problems.

In fact, I began to perceive —— and I was the first to be surprised at this —— that a certain organic interdependence existed between hearing and the act of painting. When a painter lost the precision of his line or the richness of his palette, he was suffering at the same time from auditory problems of a more or less obvious nature. Problems associated with blues and greens, for example, corresponded to losses in the higher frequency range. Quite a correlation could be predicted between the frequency range of sounds and the spectrum of colors. I was almost tempted to say "One paints with one's ears!" Although I wanted to thoroughly investigate this phenomenon, I was already snowed under with my other research projects.

The problem of taste is one of the headaches of aesthetic philosophy. I certainly do not claim to have solved it, but I noticed a few things which might advance our thoughts on this subject. When I changed my apartment and was able at last to hang my pictures, I discovered a remarkable homogeneity of themes in my collection. Despite the difference in artists and styles, the works harmonized very well together. Blues and greens predominated nearly everywhere. Although the paintings came from different pallets, they were perfectly compatible. So it was within *me* that this harmony existed. It must have been the fruit of some sort of selective perception which interpreted the essence of all sorts of conditions. I am convinced that listening and audio-vocal control actively shape some of these impressions. One could gather valuable information about the psychology and psycho-physiology of aesthetic preferences by studying the auditory curve of art collectors and relating it to the characteristics of the pictures they collected. Our history, geographic origin, cultural base, character, and as will be seen later, the depths of our personality are clearly shown through them.

8

Stutterers

As the '50s rolled on, several subjects captured and held my attention. I tackled intrauterine listening, which is the very complex and fascinating subject of a later chapter. This was to prove the most fundamental of all my investigations. From the moment I embarked upon it, it has not ceased to absorb me completely. I know that it will always fascinate me because it is a subject which the human brain can never exhaust. By posing this problem, without being aware of it, one has posed the problem of Existence itself, neither more nor less. One might also say one has asked the greatest question of all.

Another area in which I made several interesting discoveries and proposed new hypotheses was stuttering. This began when a great actor, Daniel Sorano, consulted me about his lost voice; some singers had given him my address. Since he himself was formerly a singer in Toulouse, I thought of applying the same training to him as I had to other singers. Why not? I had no other solution on hand that might be helpful to him. I knew nothing at that time about problems of speech and language.

After he was given "Caruso's ear" by means of the Electronic Ear, he regained his absolutely magnificent voice. My whole staff enjoyed listening during the audio-vocal training sessions. Sorano took advantage of the treatment to prepare Moliere's *Le Malade Imaginaire* for the Theatre National Populaire. Meanwhile, he finished performances of Berthold Brecht's *War*. We were fascinated to see him develop the part before our eyes, enriching it and gradually introducing more and more subtlety. Sorano was a man of superior intelligence, and he made the text speak with captivating eloquence.

He was so happy to be able to perform on stage once more that he willingly agreed to take part in some experiments. In one of these I blocked off his right ear. Immediately he began to stutter. Interpreting this phenomenon in terms of audio-feedback, I offered the following theory. It was the right ear that controlled speech, and stuttering was bound up with the loss of this controlling ear. I already knew how reconditioned listening could improve vocal utterance. When the ear was able to hear the lost or damaged frequencies correctly, the ability to utter them was immediately and unconsciously restored. From that point I could envisage, so far as my original proposition was acceptable, an approach for treating stutterers using the Electronic Ear.

Nevertheless, I first had to verify this proposition. As I examined more and more stutterers, I became even more convinced that all these patients were suffering from a minor auditory deficiency in the right or *directing* ear. But I needed further confirmation and set out to get it. I researched other current scientific work being done in the field of audition. I certainly needed to rely on colleagues because I myself did not have all the necessary knowledge about the subject. The investigations of two Americans, John Lee and John Black of Georgetown University, caught and held my attention. They had perfected an experimental test called "delayed feedback."

When a person listens through earphones as he speaks into a microphone entering a tape recorder he can hear himself as he speaks, but with a very slight delay which corresponds to the time needed to bring about the *return* of the sound. As early as 1949, Lee and Black set up an experimental apparatus in their laboratory so this feedback time could be shortened or lengthened at will. On their machine the playback head was mobile and could be moved by an operator a precise distance from the recording head. They could thus induce a time-lag between the vocal emission and the auditory feedback which could be varied for experimental purposes.

According to the distance between the recording head and the playback head, if the speed of the tape is known, the time between the utterance and the "feedback" received by the listener may easily be calculated. What interested me most in their experimental reports was that the individual *always* began to stutter when the distance between the recording and its restoration reached a certain threshold. Though this is an artificially-induced stutter, it is evident that a relationship exists between a listening deficiency and the occurrence of stuttering.

Lee and Black pinned high hopes on this discovery. They thought that by increasing their research efforts in this direction they might perhaps reach the point where they would find a solution for stuttering.

An Italian researcher, Azzo Azzi, took advantage of the experiments with delayed feedback to identify workers who were feigning deafness. Some workers exposed to high levels of noise were tempted by the prospect of a disability pension and falsely claimed that their hearing had deteriorated. It is not always easy to expose such malingering or to distinguish it from genuine cases of industrial hearing loss. Azzo Azzi then suggested subjecting these people to delayed feedback. If they really did not hear, they would not be troubled by this delayed listening; on the other hand, if they were only pretending, they would automatically begin to stutter!

Personally, I wanted to make more exact measurements of the phenomena demonstrated by the Americans. Unfortunately, the delayed feedback apparatus they used in their laboratory could not be found in France. I asked the Association of French Language Acousticians (GALF), of which I had been a member for a very long time, if they had any way of obtaining a "delayed" telephone line. But this request involved such complications that I decided to improvise with a simple plastic hose pipe. I bought one which was 340 meters long, after making sure that a voice passed through it satisfactorily. The delay time from one end to the other was one second.

Lee and Black noted that articulation difficulties appeared between one-tenth and two-tenths of a second, so I had more than enough pipe. I refined the experiment by making a series of holes in the pipe at intervals corresponding to delays of one-tenth of a second. I then spoke into a funnel inserted at one end of this interminable flute-like pipe and I listened by means of a stethoscope applied to one hole or another. In this way, I could study all manner of delayed feedback to my heart's content. I established by this means extremely accurate measurements, even more accurate than if I had had the benefit of equipment from an electronic laboratory. My only problem was how to store this picturesque but appallingly cumbersome apparatus in my apartment.

Most of my conclusions confirmed those of the Americans. For example, I determined "stuttering zones" very exactly. But one conclusion made me skeptical about the possibility of my two colleagues ever fulfilling their desire to treat stutterers. In fact, for stutterers to benefit from the delay between the recording and the replay, the replay must *precede* the recording! Why? Because the spoken word is merely the end product of a provisional stage during which the ear, in its own way, already rehearses what is going to be pronounced. It must be obvious that no machine, so far, is able to rehearse something which has not yet been spoken. No machine can make audible what we are going to say before we say it.

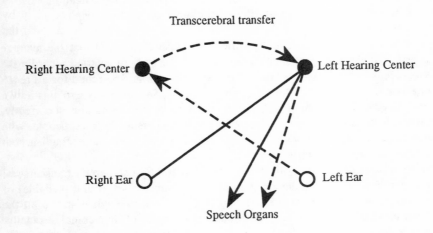

Figure 4. *Straight lines show normal trajectory of nervous impulse when the right ear is dominant. Dotted lines show the trajectory with brain-transfer that a stutterer has (left ear dominant, with general lateralization to the right).*

After observing many of my patients, I thought that those who had not yet established a directing ear for the control of their own speech (auditory lateralization) thereby provoked a sort of physiological delayed feedback.

The difference between a well lateralized audio-phonatory circuit and a poorly lateralized one is explained by my conception of how the various nerve pathways work. Poor lateralization, in contrast with good lateralization, introduces an element of delay caused by an extra step in the transfer of information. Instead of a direct pass from right ear to left brain, information passes from left ear to the auditory center of the right hemisphere and then to the left brain center.

As stated earlier, this transfer of information across the hemispheres may last between .05 seconds and .4 seconds but remains specific for each individual. Stuttering appears when it occurs within .1 seconds and .2 seconds with a peak at .15 seconds. Outside these limits, symptoms vary, which is why someone may lose the "directing" ear and not necessarily begin to stutter. This additional factor must be taken into account when considering our original theory. André le Gall wrote most correctly, in the paper already quoted, the following:

Two conditions are always present when stuttering occurs in a French speaker:

(1) Incompatibility between the directing ear and the general later-alization of the individual, or the absence of a "directing" ear owing to the absence or inadequacy of general lateralization.

(2) A transcerebral delay time of the order of .15 seconds.

Why is a French speaker specified? Because I observed that the average duration of physiological delayed feedback among stutterers varied according to their *language of origin*. Whereas, for example, it was .15 second for a French speaker, it was .2 second for an English speaker. This disparity explains how a multilingual speaker could stammer in one language and speak almost correctly, although without fluency, in another. I have personally met people who expressed themselves without much difficulty in Arabic and English, but stuttered a great deal in French.

It is most illuminating to compare the duration of a stutterer's transcerebral transfer and the average length it takes to pronounce a vocal unit (syllable) of the language in which he is stuttering. In French, as in English and in all the other languages I have investigated, these two lengths of time coincide exactly. The average length of a syllable in French is .15 seconds, that of an English syllable is .2 seconds, and so on. In this way, too, the repetition of syllables, which characterizes the stutter where its symptoms appear, may be better under-stood. It is the outward symptom of "delayed feedback." With these repetitions the subject is in some way attempting to catch up with himself.

It must be emphasized that this attempt is a reflex phenomenon and not a conscious one. In fact, the stutterer is only vaguely aware of what he is doing. If he is asked to stutter voluntarily, he will be quite unable to do so. He will speak like everyone else for the good reason that by fixing his attention on what he is going to say, *he will begin to listen to himself.* In other words, the stutterer is typically a person who makes sounds without listening to them. This is a very important point. One of the cardinal mistakes that can be made in the treatment of a stutterer is to record his stutter and make him listen to the tape. Most people are usually disappointed when they hear themselves on tape because their voice is less rich than they thought it was. But with stutterers, the experience can turn into a sadistic trial. They are brutally confronted with a speech disorder they had no idea they possessed. The dejection which ensues may lead to nervous depression and even suicide.

Recovery from the delay is a phenomenon which is always instructive to observe. When they are at ease, if I may put it this way, stutterers double or triple syllables, but when they are more attentive they introduce other processes, this time in a deliberate way. At the Bichat Hospital, I once treated a friend of my chief of staff, the great actor Louis Jouvet. As everyone knows, Jouvet was a stutterer in his private life (in this, he was like a number of great actors, Roger Blin, for example). In daily life he stumbled over his words often, but never on stage, for he found an excellent way of getting around the obstacle. He overcame his delay by slowing down the tempo of his phrasing in the musical sense of the word. The result was a flow of speech so characteristic of him that it contributed to his celebrity and was the joy of all his imitators. The more he became aware of any time lag, the more he lengthened certain phrases, "Biza-a-a-a-re, my dear cousin-n-n-n? I said biza-a-a-a-re?" In addition, he knew how to use silence by increasing the pauses between phrases and then by firing off salvos of words.

I asked my colleagues to send me all the stutterers they knew in order to make a closer study of all these phenomena. For a whole year, starting in 1950, I saw stutterers on an almost daily basis. There was a total of 70 in all. I was practically living with them, so to speak, and this involved certain problems. To make a long story short, I became quite a stutterer myself; when I subjected myself to the test of delayed feedback on John Black's machine, I continued to stutter for three days!

In every case, the examination of these patients strengthened my basic intuition. They all exhibited a delay of between .1 seconds and .2 seconds so it seemed likely that their troubles were due to the nonintegration of the dominant ear, that is to say, to a lack of auditory lateralization. Let the reader understand clearly that when I say their troubles were "due" to this failing, in no way do I claim to have resolved the whole cause and nature of stuttering. When some psychoanalysts became aware of my research they exclaimed, "But stuttering is only a symptom!" I quite agree. In the majority of cases, the psychological or psychoanalytical causes advanced in order to explain the troubles of rhythm are perfectly well grounded. My only contribution was to identify the physiological mechanism which had taken charge and allowed them to express themselves in body language. On the other hand, I am inclined to think that when confronted by a stutter of purely physiological origin (which also exists), the transfer across the brain hemisphere must have a certain psychological repercussion.

If the loss of the directing ear were indeed the decisive element in the loss of rhythmic control, this could be treated by stimulating the right ear or by blocking the left, and so bringing about the lateralization that is lacking.

A single session of this treatment was enough to cure one of my 70 patients. The others stopped stuttering at the end of several days, several weeks, or several months. One year later, in every case, the success of this group was complete. I really thought I had found the secret.

I might have been satisfied with this if I had not been lucky enough to encounter two further cases of stuttering whose resistance showed me that the problem was not as simple as I had at first imagined. These two stutterers proved to be totally impervious to the treatment process even after a whole year's treatment. I was not disappointed. On the contrary. In the realm of science I have never believed in easy victories. When solutions are found too quickly, there is every reason to suppose one has gone astray. The difficulties which arise are a real blessing; without them we would think we had made definitive discoveries, whereas science really progresses through a constant, never-ending process of self-correction.

These two recalcitrant stutterers compelled me to reconsider my theory. I asked myself all sorts of questions about them. I examined every aspect about them until the day I suddenly realized that they were both blue-eyed blonds, and that those who had been treated most rapidly had dark hair and brown eyes. Perhaps it was only coincidence. But when I established that the relationship between these parameters (color of hair and color of eyes) and the success rate of the treatment was the same for each of the stutterers I treated, I realized that it was not a coincidence at all. The problem of understanding this obvious but nonetheless strange relationship remained. As I pondered the question, I asked myself if it was not perhaps a particular sensitivity that was in play. It was certainly not an auditory sensitivity, for at this level I had not recorded any significant differences between the patients. Perhaps it was a sensitivity of the skin, a possibility that I finally decided to pursue.

I thought, in fact, that the skin ensured continuity between the ear and the rest of the body. As I proceeded along these lines, I soon perceived that the ear was not, as I had first believed, a differentiated piece of skin; on the contrary, *it was the skin which was a differentiated piece of ear.* The further I go, the more I am convinced this formulation is true.[8]

Then I carried out some cutaneous audiograms, a sort of dermogram. I beamed sounds over the skin to obtain reactions by which I might be able to distinguish, first, the various types of cutaneous surfaces, and second, zones of clearly distinct sound sensitivity within the same area of skin. In this way I succeeded in setting up the geography of sensitivity to sounds to which I have already alluded. One of the most sound receptive areas is between the thumb and index finger of the right hand. Another is the part of the forehead between the eyes.

This experimental validation showed that the two stutterers who did not respond to the treatment presented a particularly high degree of skin resistance. Whereas the dark haired patients with black eyes reacted by means of new cutaneous sensitivity to stimulations of about five or six decibels, the other two remained insensitive to stimulations which reached 80 and even 100 decibels.

Let us move quickly to our findings: Cutaneous sensitivity and the quality of phonatory control are in constant relation to one another. I also noted that *the more precise the control is, the more the rhythm is correctly followed, and the more acute the sensitivity of the skin remains*. Almost deprived of their cutaneous control mechanism, my two recalcitrants were unable to receive much information from the verbal flow over their body. The treatment had no effect on them because it was directed only to the ears. Now, if the ear controls not only utterance, but its intensity, duration, and volume, it possesses the power to control the verbal flow only insofar as the cutaneous register can take charge of the corresponding sounds. The control of this acoustic wave emanating from our mouth as we speak reverts for the most part to the skin. If the skin lacks sensitivity, the whole process is endangered; incorporation of the word is no longer possible. Treatment consists of teaching the patient to use his body like a musical instrument. The skin must be able to transform itself into a veritable "cutaneous keyboard" so that the patient may finally be in a position to "play on his body" in order to talk to someone else. Speaking, in the final analysis, is nothing else but this.

This theory led to the development of another apparatus capable of allowing, at one and the same time, an audio-vocal control by the ear and the materialization of the verbal "flow" over the body in such a way that its progress is imprinted on the cutaneous keyboard.

This theory also had an interesting psychological repercussion. My blue-eyed

---

[8] Tomatis expresses this point in a literal sense. He contends in *Vers L'Ecoute Humaine* (1974) that phylogenetic data suggests the ear preceded the nervous system and further that the sensory cells found in the skin (Meissner's, Pacinian, Krause, Merkel's) are differentiated cells of corti. He points to this evolution of the sensory cells of corti towards cutaneous hair cells of the skin as support of his hypothesis.

blondes had fair skin. In a verbal exchange, when they were placed in a difficult position, they quickly began to blush. The reason for this was that they were as vulnerable to sound as albinos are to light. They did not know how to defend themselves against it. The ear and, by extension, the skin obey a sort of "all or nothing" law. In their case, either they heard nothing or they became suddenly aware of sounds from 80 to 100 decibels. They experienced a real "attack." The speech flow pouring over their bodies caused stress. On the other hand, an excellent musician possesses a cutaneous covering of extreme sensitivity. Five to ten decibels are enough to trigger the cutaneous response mechanisms to the sonic information. Such a person can adapt to and defend against sound incomparably better. Between these two types of people exists a difference in skin properties which I think can be measured. I suggest that this sensitivity, great or small, might be determined by a "degree of timidity" (since it corresponds to manifestations of timidity) which, to be strictly accurate, has no relationship to a person's emotional nature. The two sorts of reaction are quite distinct.

In the United States, John Black, whom I have met, continued to find the problem of reversing the recording head and the playback head a baffling one. He sent me one of his students, named Strumsta, who worked with me for a while and with whom I kept in touch after he left.

I believed that it was a malfunction of the ear *as a whole* which prevented a stutterer from hearing himself properly. At the end of his own investigations, Strumsta challenged my theory claiming that it was *uniquely by bone conduction* that a stutterer did not hear himself. He went back over his work several times to improve and correct it. He always came to the same conclusion.

Today, I think he was right.

If a stutterer has poor hearing, it is because he is incapable of auditory awareness at the level of bone conduction. What happens when we speak? We project sounds into the air where higher sounds are thrown out in a straight line and lower sounds spread out everywhere in our environment. (This explains why our recorded voice always seems to us higher than it naturally is.) But at the same time, the skull vibrates and transmits sound information directly to the ear. Great opera singers who have a technical mastery of their art control their voices essentially by bone conduction. But stutterers, on the other hand, lack harmony between the auditory curves for bone conduction and air conduction, in which the latter is always more sensitive.

Based on this observation the idea of a training program to re-establish harmony became clear. For this I needed to perfect the Electronic Ear to improve a person's responsiveness to sound by exerting variable pressure on the stirrup muscle or hammer muscle. I began using a system of electronic gating mechanisms, and at the same time, I arranged to impose a dominant right ear.

Developing right ear dominance is a somewhat delicate procedure in that it has to be effected without the patient being aware of it. If he becomes aware of what is happening, he immediately develops resistance to it. This psychological refusal of treatment may seem abnormal, until one realizes that it is not the prospect of a cure that he is resisting, for he wants nothing more than to speak like everyone else. What he does not want is to grow up.

Let me explain. As far as speech is concerned, the stutterer remains fixated at a stage of development between two and four years of age. His unconscious self finds enough advantages at this level to want to maintain it. When he feels that this status quo is threatened, he fights like the devil to protect it. So it is advisable not to awaken his mistrust.

Regarding this infantile speech fixation, the repetition of syllables characteristic of a stutterer is also a constant in the way little children express themselves (Papa, Mama, pee pee, etc.). From this point of view, a stutter is only childish babbling which has become chronic instead of giving way to properly articulated speech.

When a stutterer is told that he can achieve an excellent elocution, provided he abruptly covers the ground which separates the speech of a two, three, or four year old and his real age, it is rather like offering a young person a pill which will enable him to attain the pinnacle of wisdom, but which will also turn him into an old man. Progress, oh yes! Aging, no! Consciously, he agrees and even desires to speak better, but unconsciously he wants to hold on to his fixation. The result of treatment depends on the result of this conflict.

Besides, therapy for stutterers runs into numerous difficulties. The person who does not hear himself stutter because he refuses to listen to himself will in the same way refuse to hear himself speak well. To treat a stutterer presupposes not only skill and patience on the therapist's part, but also a considerable evenness of temper, for they can be extremely aggressive and have a certain spiritual force. A stutterer, in fact, is the most difficult kind of patient because he is the most susceptible to psychological *transference*.

By this, I mean that he involves the therapist in a relationship very much like the one between the psychoanalyst and the person being analyzed. The patient transfers to the doctor unconscious feelings and desires which originated with another person. With stutterers, the therapist finds himself taking the place of the stutterer's father. Often, it is just this conflict with the father which has provoked, or at least accentuated, the patient's speech problems. At a symbolic level, the refusal to let the right ear be dominant corresponds to the rejection of the father (the person who brings speech) and the rejection of growing up. Unless the therapist is careful (speech therapists and language pathologists are not as well prepared to accept the shock of transference as psychoanalysts are), he will find himself tied up in a dense network of ambivalent relationships, with love and hate inextricably mixed, and he will gradually lose his way. Bogged down in the transference, he will be totally incapable both of helping his patient to overcome his difficulties and also of getting out of them himself.

The danger is all the greater because, as a general rule, stutterers have a very strong personality which easily influences anyone speaking to them. It is only necessary to remember the case of the South African stutterer. When he spoke, everyone present began to reproduce his gesticulations and to stutter themselves.

Although the speech of stutterers reflects an infantile fixation of an emotional type, the fixation does not extend to their intelligence. On the contrary, the majority of stutterers have a high I.Q.

My observation goes against the more accepted, but illusory, impression that includes among stutterers children who cannot master speech because of an intellectual handicap. This inclusion is a most unwarrantable assimilation. Let us not confuse babbling with stuttering or mental retardation with difficulty of speech flow. To think that a stutter depends on lack of thought structure is to make a tragic mistake and really to judge people by appearances, which has never been a very scientific approach.

While a stutter does intervene in the intellectual sphere, the best proof that it originates outside this sphere and keeps an autonomous relationship with the sphere is that it can affect other channels as well as vocal utterance. I have seen stutterers repeat syllables in writing and repeat notes when playing a musical instrument. Should it be said that they do not know how to write or how to play a score? Not at all. The problem clearly has no connection with mental capacity. Rather than lacking something, the person is surrounded by obstacles. This is not the same thing at all.

On the other hand, to stumble in expressing oneself does set up an obstacle to the outflow of thought. In this sense, treatment always causes a certain freeing of the intellect, from the point of view of its most obvious manifestations.

At the Centre Tomatis which I founded in Paris, the training sessions now begin with the help of the Electronic Ear specially adapted to simulate hearing through bone conduction. This has the immense advantage of putting the listener in touch with himself in a much more intense way. At the University of Potchefstroom in South Africa, a center highly specialized in the problems of stutterers has existed for more than ten years. The staff there employs the same procedures and produces excellent results.

Even in the mildest cases, the treatment must be directed towards the underlying cause of the trouble. It must not be limited to a purely physiological realignment. If problems of rhythm appear as a result of a neurotic conflict (which is most frequently the case) merely correcting them physiologically will not by itself free the person from his neurosis. No doubt he will stop stuttering, but perhaps begin to suffer from asthma or an outbreak of eczema. To obtain more than superficial results, mere mechanical re-education must be accompanied by psychosensory steps (with the help of intrauterine sounds, in particular, and sonic births, which will be dealt with in a later chapter) which allow the patient to make what I call his own self-analysis of his neurotic state. By this, I am suggesting that for a true cure he has to free himself from Oedipal attachments in order to take charge of himself and bring about, in a sort of way, a self-transference. Instead of trying to attach himself to another person, he must welcome and cultivate quite a different desire: to have a true encounter with himself and others through mature verbal communication.

Oddly enough, it is by this indirect route that he comes to make an effort to listen to himself. He is not going to do so for pleasure, for that might trigger off a narcissistic condition. Rather he will do it simply to be better understood by the person to whom he is speaking, by means of his own proper listening. If he speaks badly, it is because he does not make any effort to speak, to apply audio-vocal control. If he makes no effort, it is because he does not think anyone else is important enough. He is blocked in communication in the same way that a car driver is blocked in the midst of a bottleneck because he will not let anyone else pass him at any price. In a way, it is courtesy and a willingness to oblige that are lacking in him.

This is so true that when a stutterer feels that his stumblings are embarrassing the person to whom he is speaking, he generally tends to multiply their number and to accentuate their importance. Nothing makes him happier than to see the other person stutter in turn. To return once again to the comparison with the bottleneck, he is just like the driver who does not at all mind not being able to proceed provided that someone else is also prevented from doing so. This presents a clearer picture of what I refer to as the aggressiveness of stutterers.

Objectively and without moral judgment entering this analysis, the psychology of the stutterer is rooted in duality or, in fact, in duplicity. From this view, stuttering can be grasped as an unconscious effort to camouflage one's real thoughts. The unconscious hides things and prevents their escape by setting up barriers in the form of speech difficulties.

The duplicity of the stutterer becomes more clear when considering how he uses his stutter. I often observed a client's rhythmic difficulties get worse from the moment he entered a discussion with a third person. Through these tactics, the stutterer first disappoints and puts off the person to whom he speaks. Secondly, he succeeds in making the listener swallow almost any story, which is very useful in matters of business. A number of stutterers are found in the business world where they generally have successful careers.

When the stutterer finds himself in difficulties in a business discussion, his unconscious discharges a profusion of stuttering, just as an octopus discharges ink. Like the octopus, he succeeds simultaneously in concealing his difficulty and creating a diversion. He may succeed in this so well that the psychology of the other person begins to change. Seeing the stutterer struggling with speech, the person contradicting him feels physically uncomfortable (he suffers with the speaker) and feels the need to help him. But by helping him, he loses the thread of his own argument, and it is at this moment that the stutterer, who is waiting for this very thing to happen, wins the game. To sum up, his stutter is an *unconscious* secret weapon which enables him to triumph over the other person by taking advantage of the charitable spirit that emerges. This is a kind of duplicity, even if the Machiavellianism coming from the unconscious is not a deliberate one.

I am not one who thinks that the Oedipus Complex, as defined by Freud, is a universal reality. Before going any further, perhaps I should define my connection with psychoanalysis more precisely. It has often been said that I am anti-Freudian because many details in my theory are opposed to that of the Viennese master. I feel my position ought to be more clearly defined, so that no misunderstanding persists.

I have always held the greatest respect for the work of Sigmund Freud. His originality, power, and genius have enabled him to develop a prodigious synthesis of somewhat disparate cultural elements which then constituted the universe of specialists in psychism, scientific disciplines, and metaphysical tendencies. His advanced neurological knowledge enabled him to demonstrate in a remarkable way man's behavioral mechanisms, from the starting point of this famous "unconscious" which has so liberally — and so dangerously, one might add — invaded the twentieth century world. Additionally, from his knowledge of Jewish esoteric matters, the "father of psychoanalysis" knew how to apply to medicine the enormous insights afforded him by the Jewish tradition, for example, the interpretation of dreams so admirably presented in the Cabala.

Freud was himself the child of several systems, and he was able as no one before him to dominate them, combine them, and go beyond them. More than that, he knew enough to avoid becoming the hostage of his own discoveries. He never stopped evolving, and in the end no one could oppose Freud except Freud himself! It is probable, in the light of his last writings, that if he had lived 20 years longer, the whole of psychoanalysis might have been transformed.

The mistake made by a large number of his disciples who operate on the basis of strict obedience is to maintain a more reverent attitude about his theories than he did himself. Finally, it is they who, by desiring to be more Freudian than Freud, are the real anti-Freudians. The trouble is that they are not aware of this and mask their intellectual rigidity behind a sort of terrorism: "Freud said...." Bow down before Freud or be damned!

Anyone who enters the psychological profession today is called upon to meet Freud, whether he wishes to or not. There is no reason to sanctify all the theories put forward by the master, which he himself did not want to do as he followed the thread like a journey. He undertook a vast research that involved groping, temporarily losing direction, and acknowledging matters that simply led to further questions.

Personally, I part company with Freud's ideas on several points, and the most important one is this: I do not believe that the elucidation of "complexes" is enough to trigger or bring about therapeutic action. In other words, I do not believe that the power of elucidating unconscious conflicts constitutes in itself a healing power.

I think that a genuine healing involves not simply bringing something to a conscious level, but also to a conscious grasp, which is not entirely the same thing. This conscious grasp causes problems because it has nothing like an automatic mechanism, and it demands of the subject altogether exceptional abilities.

Let me explain. In the course of psychoanalysis one is gradually led to a quasi-microscopic vision of one's own deep personality. This vision brings to light the cause of emotional fixation and, in particular, the negative influence of one's parents, which appears considerably magnified as a result of this experience. In a manner of speaking, psychoanalysis leads to "killing" both father and mother. Actually, it is a question of putting to death a certain image or symbolic dimension of Father and Mother. The essence of this is defined by the cultural background and the family relationships within it. It is not a question of severing, entirely and finally, all the ties which attach a person to his parents. The only question here is, how many people are there who possess enough subtlety and skill to draw a dividing line for themselves between the "good" and "bad" parental images? How many people can separate what constitutes a shackle among these ties we have just evoked from what, on the contrary, helps them to find an anchorage in life?

It is risky to deprive someone of his relationship with the Mother, the universal life-giver, and with the Father, the universal life-implanter, and also the solar source, which enables the seed of life to grow. To "kill" this Mother and Father because of their participation in constricting complexes from which we wish to be free is also to kill the aliveness and growth in one's own self. The penalty for such acts is immediate, and it is brutal as well as cruel. It leads to fathomless despair and collapse as soon as the gates of growth are shut in one's face; it brings the terrible threat of suicide. The being with no ties —— without Father or Mother, without God or Devil —— floats in space, drifting between the branches to which it can no longer attach as if it were a poor distressed monkey.

It is well to remember, however, that it is not always complexes (in the psychoanalytic sense of the term) which intervene in problems of rhythm. In 1958, a well-known actor was referred to me by a French movie director, Jacques Clouzot. This actor was starring in a very important film when shooting had to be interrupted because he suddenly began to stutter. Though he saw several doctors, he continued to stutter. His anxiety grew from day to day until it finally brought about a genuine psychological trauma. He had to be hospitalized for depression. The film, which seemed assured of success, never saw the light of day. The actor was in a desperate state when he discovered that the weeks of forced rest had in no way improved his elocution. Much later he consulted me. I solved his problem in just a few minutes by simply removing a wax plug which was blocking his right ear. In this case, I was in the presence of a purely mechanical stutter.

I noted before that a certain number of stage actors were notorious stutterers. A closer look shows that this is not entirely a matter of coincidence. In fact, many stutterers find that taking to the stage is an excellent way of asserting themselves, fulfilling themselves, and thereby even overcoming those complexes within their psychic nature that make them stutter, among other things. The psychological profile of a stutterer gives him good prospects of being able to express himself on the stage.

The temptation to act is all the stronger because, on the stage, the stutter disappears for several reasons. When they sense they are running into difficulty, some stutterers employ subterfuges like Jouvet. Many do not even need that and are sustained by knowing that what they are saying is a text "learned by heart."

In this way, stutterers do not need to control the content of what they say, and they can apply all their attention to intensity and voice modulation to immediately ensure proper rhythm. Command of utterance takes place without the necessity of auditory control. In particular, having to foresee the next word (that silent word which occurs before the word itself is uttered, and so can interfere with speech being effectively delivered) no longer interferes in the process once the subject no longer has to think of what he is going to say.

Even so, I have met stubborn stutterers incapable of reciting without stumbling over a text learned by heart. They are influenced by skin sensitivity, having insufficient dermal control. They do not succeed in speaking to others no matter what the conditions, because they do not succeed in speaking to themselves. If a stutterer in our first category is isolated and is asked to speak aloud in a room where there are microphones (unknown to him so as to remove all inhibitions), he can be heard to speak like everyone else. Compelled to speak to himself, he is also compelled to listen. I recorded the results during just such an experiment.

"He uses a clear, steady voice, often sonorous; he follows the flow of his thought admirably in his speech and sticks to it closely." However, I also observed, "All this wonderful arrangement collapses as soon as the spell of being alone is broken. The rhythm no longer has anything in common with that which characterized the flow at the beginning, and (an essential fact, very noticeable in recorded analysis) the voice tone changes: it becomes monotone, without quality or resonance." When he is placed in the same experimental conditions, a stutterer of the second category performs almost the same as he habitually does. He continues to stumble, even when he is left alone because he does not succeed in reaching the only possible listener in those circumstances, namely himself.

One last detail on the latent abilities of stutterers. While many are able to become actors, others win fame as singers. In performing, the control attained is that which is exercised when learning by heart. The intensity allows for better listening, and, finally, the latency time of each syllable is long enough for repetition to be avoided.

Stuttering is certainly one of the most difficult problems to analyze in the whole realm of audio-psycho-phonology, and I make no claim to any definitive solution. Developments so far are scarcely more than the beginning of a system which remains to be perfected, or at least constructed. At least they cause some doubt to be cast on the multifarious accepted notions which impede us in our approach to the actual phenomenon itself. The professional literature puts forth an incredible tangle of definitions and theories, among which it is almost impossible to find one's bearings. This is certainly a sign that stuttering is an exceptionally difficult clinical entity. Explanations about it are of a stupefying diversity, ranging from reflections of scientific investigations to the results of researchers' personal obsessions. They lead us from one end to the other of the etiological spectrum, from genetic deficiency to psychoanalytic conflict.

One thing, however, remains certain: whatever the primary cause may be, concrete symptoms result from a certain difficulty in listening. This difficulty, whether it is manifested by distortions more pronounced on one side than the other or by lack of symmetry of a different kind, represents anomalies caused by a lack of auditory laterality. This is true whether the difficulty is caused by rejection of the paternal image or by a simple blockage of wax. What a stutterer lacks is the ability to *aim or direct sounds*.

As far as the stutterer is concerned, the control circuit is disturbed. The idea of a *feedback loop* came to me early in the 1950s as a result of observing stutterers. Even the formulation of the idea is bound to make one think of cybernetics. However, at that time Norbert Wiener's theories had not yet spread in France, and I was ignorant of them. When I heard that this talented mathematician had laid the foundations in 1949 of a science dedicated to "The Study of Control and Communication in Animals and Machines," I recognized immediately that I was dabbling in cybernetics without having realized it. I was neither the first nor the only one.

The term "cybernetic" was coined from the Greek word "kubernesis" which means "the action of governing or directing." Even before it was used by Ampére to designate the art of government, the term appeared in the writings of Plato. Certainly the Greek philosophers gave no thought to modern cybernetic theories such as remote control and automation. Yet the original idea on which these theories are founded was already present in the thought of the ancients. As soon as the notion of a feedback loop appeared in a theoretical system, a cybernetic concept was being called into play. This particular rapprochement was a fruitful one for me. I gained great insight, not only into problems of rhythm, but also into all the manifestations of listening and speech, both normal and pathological.

I continued to study stuttering and discovered many exciting insights, one of which has always impressed me. From the moment I began to read sacred books, I realized that such study was very enriching, both spiritually and intellectually. I knew well the parable in St. Mark where a stutterer is cured by Christ, who takes him "away from the crowd," wets his own finger with saliva, and places it first on the stutterer's tongue, then into his ears, and says, "Be opened!" The text adds, "The ear was opened and the tongue was untied." What interested me in this parable was that Christ made the correction of the stutter depend on the opening of the ear and, therefore, on the power of listening. This confirms my original idea. As for the symbolic gesture of untying the tongue, there is no need of further explanation. However, I was puzzled for a long time by the detail about "the tip of the tongue." Why was this so precisely worded? I only understood this much later when I became aware that when stutterers speak, *they use essentially the back part of the tongue.*

The tongue is a complex organ of 35 muscles (17 on each side and one in the middle) which in the act of phonation divides the air found in the oral cavity into two parts: the front part extends as far as the teeth; the back part as far as the pharynx. One becomes aware of a hypothetical barrier when pronouncing a hard "g" or a hard "q." When most people go to utter a phoneme like this, they do not know whether to *place* it in front of or behind the barrier. With stutterers, it is systematically placed *behind*, as virtually all other phonemes are. When the stutterer wishes to speak, a blockage occurs at the level of this barrier, and the phoneme is thrown back to the rear. When he tries at the same time to utter the sound and to produce vocal quality, there is an obstacle because the two operations are incompatible.

The tongue is, at the outset, essentially a digestive organ. It can only become a fluent speech organ by means of its most mobile part, the tip. Everyone who speaks with the back of the tongue has considerable difficulty, whereas those who use the tip of the tongue do not. Moreover, if you ask someone to speak with the tip of his tongue, you will hear his voice take on increased tonal quality, and you will see his face become more expressive.

An observant person will notice something more. The two halves of the face lack symmetry. The right side is more active than the left because the right side of the mouth, when one speaks with the tip of the tongue, is more involved than the left. On the other hand, when the back of the tongue is being used the asymmetry favors the left side.

It is enough to experiment on oneself to establish that these observations are well founded. According to whether one speaks "to the front" or "to the rear," it is the right side of the mouth or the left side which engages more.

The use of the right side of the mouth defines the "right" voice, which is the ideal one for eloquence, or even simply for free expression and fluent utterance. Everyone who speaks well, speaks on the right. This does not mean that the left side of the mouth makes no contribution. In fact, it works equally well and synchronizes with the right. It simply makes movements which are smaller in scope.

If an electromyograph is taken of a stutterer, by placing electrodes on his lips and at the corners of the mouth, it will show that in his case the movements of the right and left sides of the mouth do not synchronize. This lack of control helps to explain the repetition of syllables. It is almost as if the two halves of his mouth pronounced each syllable in turn rather than simultaneously.

Mastery of speech greatly depends on lateralization to the right of the audio-phonatory circuit. If human beings wish to realize all their potentialities, they must be much more right-eared and right-mouthed than left.

9

Sonic Birth

A knock on the door prompted me to call out, "Come in!" It was my two anesthetists. At this time, I was still operating so much that one anesthetist alone was not enough to help me. Although these two colleagues worked closely with me each day, they knew very little about my research activities. They had heard certain rumors, however, and wanted to know more.

"Now Dr. Tomatis, we have come to find you because, well, it appears you have constructed a sort of machine?"

"A machine? Yes, I have. So?"

"A machine that really works?"

"A machine that I find very useful, it's true, in certain circumstances."

"For the treatment of singers, isn't it? Forgive our persistence, but what we heard excited us very much. Could you explain it to us?"

"Certainly." I succinctly described the principles of audio-vocal re-education and of the apparatus itself. "But of course," I said by way of conclusion, "it is only an experimental machine."

They looked at one another.

"Experimental?" asked one of them.

"But haven't you taken out a patent?" asked the other.

"In fact, yes, I have taken out a patent."

They looked at one another once more.

"Listen. Would it interest you to distribute these machines? The machine deserves a wider circulation, doesn't it?"

I was not expecting this. "I assure you, I have many other problems on my mind."

"All the same, this is important."

"Everything depends on what one's priorities are. As far as I am concerned, I haven't the time to spend in this business. All I can say to you is that if anyone wants these patents, I'll give them to him."

They seized them with eagerness, then quickly sold them again to a group with whom I found myself tangling for years. I had a tough struggle to recover my own patents!

This incident was only the first step in my unpleasant dealings with the business and commercial world. I was a poor businessman and salesman because I signed anything put in front of me. My attention is fixed on interests other than the power of money. It is impossible to pursue every passion, and research is a sufficiently exacting mistress for me.

The consequences of this casualness in business were unpleasant, including a reputation among certain people of being a grocer, a sort of society doctor, more intent on making money than obtaining cures. It was my fault, I admit. All I needed to do was pay more attention. Occupied night and day with my work (consultations, operations, re-education sessions, lectures, and theoretical studies), and convinced for a long time that I only had a few years to live, I paid too little attention to what was happening around me and going on behind my back. But I was the only one who did not notice. Soon all sorts of ill-natured gossip arose. Exaggerations and fabrications made me a picturesque legend. The flashiness alarmed some of my colleagues. They were afraid that these reports, whether genuine or not, might be prejudicial to them. Meanwhile, a singer whom I had treated, who was well-known for his gift of gab, went all around Paris singing my praises. He did this so enthusiastically that everyone assumed he had been paid for his words. This singer had many friends, and soon my name appeared in the press. Suddenly the Medical Faculty was roused: I was accused of violating the sacrosanct rules against advertising.

This was the first time that an experience of this sort happened to me. Alas, it was not to be the last, so an explanation is necessary at this point. If I have sometimes offended by omission or through negligence, others have deliberately misrepresented the truth about me. However, the situation did not get out of hand because I had an eminent man to defend me.

Doctor Huet came to my rescue. It was his practice, even his vocation, to help the young. He will be remembered by many as a staunch and skillful defender of medicine against the efforts of people to bring it under the influence of privilege or ideology. It is my pleasure to hail him as a champion of liberty. When I heard that he had been appointed secretary general of the free hospitals, I said to myself that here was a man in exactly the right position, and that no one could be a better standard-bearer for a post which was more in accord with his own ideas.

I had never met Dr. Huet before. Mutual friends told him of my work, and, without ever letting me know, he followed my progress sympathetically. He stood up for me when he found out why I was being criticized. I was told about his intervention by an old schoolmate from the Neuilly Lycée. As was only proper, I went to thank Dr. Huet personally for coming to my defence.

"You don't have to thank me," he said. "I know what you are doing, and I know who you are. The least one can do for a young fellow committed to his work is to help him in this kind of vexatious situation. It is an opportunity for me to make myself useful —— an opportunity, I assure you." Dr. Huet never failed to grasp such opportunities, and defended many young doctors.

I remained in touch with him. His conversation was always marvelously enlightening. He was a man of great helpfulness. For example, one day he telephoned me to say, "I have a friend, G.B., whom you really must meet. I know what material difficulties you are encountering in your research projects, so see him for my sake. He is a remarkably forceful and enterprising fellow. I have already talked to him about you. He is very much interested in your work, and particularly in what you are doing in the domain of foreign languages. Perhaps he will be able to help you. I don't know, but call him anyway."

A few days later I had a meeting with this G.B.

"Huet talked to me about your machine," he told me. "I am sure you can get me out of my difficulties in language teaching."

He wasted no time in empty talk, yet was a remarkable diplomat when necessary. He tirelessly shaped all sorts of projects, great and small. He was boiling over with ideas. He was at one and the same time a *creative* person, a catalyst of the first rank, a coordinator without equal, and an exceptionally gifted public relations man. He used to meet people in all disciplines and then arrange meetings between them. He was without equal in making people investigate and resolve particular problems, the solutions to which also benefitted him.

When I agreed to work not *for* him but in partnership with him, he launched me in 100 different directions. Some of them could not and, in fact, did not lead anywhere. Some, on the other hand, enabled me to make great progress. I was caught up in a whirlwind of activity. All that I had known so far was nothing compared to it!

"I will make you known," he assured me.

He had few scruples over how he did this. Time and again I wondered whether I was an investigator specializing in audio-phonology or the star of a circus ring, recruited by a new Barnum.

He was only eager to promote me insofar as he thought it would serve his own interests, which was fair enough. Though my ideas did become well-known because of him, they were tainted with commercialism in the eyes of many people. Some wondered if my Electronic Ear was more of a slot machine than an apparatus for re-education!

I understood how people might have thought that. If I had been outside the situation and had to judge by appearances, I would probably have considered myself a huckster. In any case, my reputation suffered because of it. At first I took no notice. When at last I woke up, it was too late. Those who considered me a charlatan had gone too far. They would have had to expose themselves to ridicule if they had retracted their stories of me. So, instead, they became even more hostile.

I had to bear this while my *protector* stood passively by; yet I am aware of all that I owe him. Every coin has its reverse side, but in the same way every reverse has its obverse side. He demanded so much of me that I felt compelled to refine my thought, make it even more precise, and push my extrapolations even further. I thank him for driving me on during all those years. He urged me to give lectures, which allowed me to gain both an overall view and a sharper awareness of my discoveries. By being compelled to formulate them, I perceived more clearly their strengths, weaknesses, and interesting possibilities. This chance to put things into perspective offered the best means for forging ahead.

Through this same person I also rubbed shoulders at summit meetings with important international scientists. Even limited association with them was of great benefit to me. I had access to such intellectual highflyers as Huxley and Oppenheimer. G.B.'s obsession was to bring learned men together. One day he decided to establish an important scientific center whose purpose was to attract some of the leading lights of contemporary science. The project was ambitious but, so far as I knew, perfectly valid. Unfortunately, it coincided with a speculative operation in real estate, which caused the project to run aground. At the start, the problem was to put a magnificent idea into concrete form. At the finish, the whole affair came down to selling some villas and apartments. G.B. had not known how to successfully bring together the two halves of the enterprise, the scientific and the commercial. Money, no doubt, proved to be too great an attraction for him. Things turned out very badly. In the end, G.B. was in serious trouble and had to withdraw from the business world for a long time.

I was completely content to be on my own again. However, I was not yet through with businessmen. Soon afterwards, a member of the Rockefeller Foundation suggested to me that I abandon all my research projects in France to work in a laboratory at Georgetown University in the United States.

"What is your future here?" he asked me. "The same as it is for all French researchers — no credit, no consideration. You will be much better off with us. We know how to be generous. Believe me, this will be the best way of putting an end to all your debts and detractors."

"Listen to me," I objected. "You forget something which for me is essential. I am not merely a laboratory worker. I am also a therapist. I don't want to turn my back on medicine."

"Come now, you have a duty to your research. All these consultations are just a waste of time and energy."

"You are quite wrong there! I have always learned from facts, and it's in my practice that I encounter facts," I protested.

"But you have amassed enough facts already. What will you learn from the examination and treatment of ten, twenty, a hundred or a thousand more patients?" he asked.

"You are mistaken. In science, progress only occurs if there are new problems to be solved. At least that is what I believe in the depths of my being. Neither examination nor treatment ever goes without a hitch. Unexpected difficulties arise. Accepted knowledge or practice must be thrown open to question again. Repeated corrections bring me gradually nearer to a truth which remains a distant one. Progress is slow, yet without this resistance provoked by facts, I might travel faster, but in the wrong direction. Contact with patients stimulates me, keeps me from extrapolations that are too pure and too abstract, forces me to focus on what is real. It acts as a safety railing, you might say."

"By working in a laboratory, you will find other safety measures. You won't be the first scientist to carry out his research in these conditions. You're not going to tell me that all the others are wrong."

"By no means," I said. "But what I am telling you holds true for me. What I need to deal with are human beings, patients, not pieces of paper. In any case, I have just recovered a freedom which I do not wish to lose ever again."

"Wait until you've thought this over. You may change your mind," he cautioned me.

I was sure I would not, but he refused to give up. He got in touch with me again a few days later.

"Doctor Tomatis, I am still convinced that it is to our common interest that you settle in the United States. Be reasonable. I can offer you 50 percent more than the amount I mentioned last time. What do you say to that?"

"Nothing more. I need to keep my freedom because I must have direct contact with my patients," I answered.

He misjudged my sincerity and believed that I was merely trying to raise my price. As a result, the price kept rising. Every day the amount increased. I had the impression that I was the stake in a sort of auction sale.

News of the matter spread. A Council Member from the Medical Association wrote me a letter which said essentially the following: "I hear that you are in the process of selling yourself to the Americans for four hundred million francs — it is an enormous sum, but you cannot do that to French medicine." It was truly an enormous sum but it was not just 400 million francs, it was a billion and a half! My only reply to this correspondent who was so concerned with the interests of French medicine was to tell him that he had no cause for uneasiness. I was not, never had been, and never would be a man who put himself up for sale.

I was advised to think the offer over, but I did not. I had already given it my full consideration. In fact, I did not lose another moment's sleep over this proposition. However, many of the people around me did. The magnitude of the sum involved sent them into a veritable trance. They were shocked that I turned the American offer down, especially those who thought that some crumbs might find their way into their own pockets if I accepted. One of them refused to consider the matter closed. He left for the United States to market me for his own profit: thirty-six million for me, all the rest for him. But he had no luck, for though I usually sign blindly, this time I refused.

I congratulated myself every day for not giving in. I am convinced that my work would have been less fruitful in the United States than in France. To be sure, the most perfect and up-to-date equipment would have been put at my disposal. But a fine apparatus never enabled anyone to dispense with ideas. Ideas are born as a result of difficulties, because difficulties make ideas necessary, even vital. Of course, I lost certain material advantages by not embarking on this adventure, but whatever they were, I would not have known what to do with them once my debts were paid. I did, however, preserve something beyond price — the chance to fight, to face stubborn dissenting facts, to find the way through a narrow gate and along a path strewn with traps.

Moreover, I feel that if I had gone to the United States, I certainly would have lost the opportunity to tackle all sorts of problems with an open mind, that is to say, according to the fine Cartesian formula of avoiding "with great care violent hurry and prejudice." I would have been hostage to my own hypotheses, instead of acting as a kind of permanent devil's advocate. I would have focused through the distorting lens of my role as licensed investigator, instead of allowing the facts to surface while juggling ideas as my experiments progressed. In France, as a sort of sniper whose discoveries were suspect, I continued my investigations as a traveler with no baggage to weigh me down, mistrusting *a priori* reasoning, always ready to make subtle variations of approach, and challenging my own ideas when fresh facts compelled me to do so. I am a scientific adventurer, advancing into unknown territory without consulting any guides, encountering difficulties and acquiring experience in the field. I enjoy being astonished by what I see; I enjoy being put in an awkward position by concrete facts. Above all, I am suspicious of a point of view that shows greater loyalty to oneself (and whatever system one is setting up) than to observed phenomena. One must let oneself be challenged by facts if one is to have any chance of understanding them. Only something that does not involve a predetermined course of explanation can be explained really well.

When G.B. had to leave us, I still felt the need to delegate my power of administration. Once again, I made a mistake and gave the keys of the safe and the authority to sign to a plausible swindler. In the course of ten years of collaboration, this man ruined the reputation of our Language Centre and drained the bank account.

He was an ex-patient who soon commingled the funds of the center with his own and drew on them heavily. By the time he left us in 1974, we were destitute. We did not recover financially for many years.

As a result of his misappropriation of funds, some fundamental research projects could not be pursued, and hundreds of patients who might have benefitted received no effective treatment.

There was also a moral stigma involved. Our administrator — unknown to us, but nevertheless with full powers as our representative — gave the appearance of a flourishing shark and presented an unreal picture of the Centre and myself to the world around us. Consequently, and here lies the bitter irony of the situation, at the very moment when I was ruined and utterly crushed by

124 • THE CONSCIOUS EAR

the effects of this betrayal, I was being described as a merry millionaire with no scruples!

When I was told about other discreditable actions which our hero committed during his life, I was able to recognize what mankind can offer in the way of mean and shabby deeds. It is a painful sight, but not a useless one. The important thing, when faced with such realities, is never to forget that this only represents one aspect of things, and not the whole truth. The horror of some details should never obscure the great beauty of the overall picture. In spite of this disagreeable experience, I remain an incorrigible optimist.

The further I go in telling my story, the more I realize how likely I am to disappoint those readers of biography who are looking for spicy details, remarkable events, and fantastic adventures. Yes, I have lived through amazing experiences, but always within the context of my laboratory or consulting room. Yes, I have traveled a great deal to give lectures, direct conferences, and give advice in every corner of the world; still my finest journeys have been made in the laboratory or in my examination room helping a child in difficulty or seeking a solution for an adult's painful problem. In the course of these experiences, I have visited unexplored regions and discovered unknown territory. I have worked hard and so have not had the chance to rub shoulders with "society" people, nor have I been able to frequent fashionable places. This has not prevented me, however, from meeting many exciting people, whether celebrated or not. So my life, viewed from the outside, could be considered commonplace by some. However, it reflects exactly who I am.

My story is above all one of groping in the dark, of trials and errors — the daily bread of a researcher. This is not a story of the Wild West adventure, and it has none of the suspense of Papillon's[9] story. But for me it is just as thrilling, just as moving as the most fantastic adventure. I can understand very well the fascination of such mysteries as the Nazi war treasures or the colossal statues of Easter Island, but what fascinates me more than anything is a human being's acquisition of language.

What a prodigious universe is that of human speech! The fantastic side of it only escapes us because we are steeped in it from the moment we are born, and even, as we shall see, from the moment we existed as an embryo. To step back a little and look at the phenomenon of language is to become conscious of what is wonderful about it, in the strongest sense of the word.

Let us begin, for example, by asking ourselves how a person is able to produce articulate sounds. Too often, people casually sweep aside this important question by sheltering it under so-called "evidence" that our body is supposedly endowed with an apparatus whose purpose is to fulfill this function. This is a

---

[9] A well-known novel by Carriére on which a movie of the same name was based.

perfect example of an unexamined and meaningless commonplace belief. In fact, the answer to this question does not lie in this direction at all, for nothing is less physiological than the act of speaking. Contrary to what the majority of people imagine, no organ of utterance exists in the way that digestive and respiratory organs exist. We speak using elements in our body that were not originally intended for this purpose. Oral language is the result of a combination of two complex structures built to fulfill other functions. These two structures are composed of the organs belonging to the digestive apparatus (lips, mouth, soft palate, tongue, teeth) and those belonging to the respiratory apparatus (nasal passages, larynx, diaphragm, lungs, thoracic cage).

Simultaneously, ear and larynx are diverted from their original functions. The larynx is put into the service of speech; the ear takes on the role of analyzing acoustic information, whereas its original function was to maintain balance and to provide the brain with energy.[10] Listening and speaking are interdependent insofar as an organic link exists between the ear and the larynx, a link that is confirmed by every anatomical and neuro-physiological study. If it is true that one speaks with one's ear, it is also true that it is sound that fashions the ear. Briefly, a person speaks insofar as he or she hears and tunes in to spoken sounds as a matter of choice.

What is the origin of this need to speak? Other animals are capable of producing mere sounds, more or less articulate, and yet true language is not within their power. Language is what characterizes man and makes him different from other creatures. In other words, language brings people together as a group. Some accept this simplistic explanation of why language exists — it is nothing more than the desire to communicate with other people. This desire is founded on two needs, to enrich others with one's own impressions, feelings, and pieces of knowledge and to benefit from the learning and information collected by others.

I remain convinced, however, that the correct answer is situated on an entirely different plane. By his very structure, man is a kind of receiving antenna of a self-expressive universe which reveals its real presence. Man is plunged into an apparently limitless environment, the true manifestation of an unfathomable presence which everything reveals, which everything registers as its phenomenological answer. In short, and also to provoke reflection, I prefer to say that it is only God who speaks, and man exists to translate this message — very awkwardly, it is true — into human language.

Going more deeply into the question posed above, whence comes the need

---

[10] In his theory (1974) Tomatis speaks of the charging effect of sound, especially high-frequency sound, on the brain. Through their action on the corti cells of the inner ear, the great majority of which are responsive to the higher frequencies, these sounds increase the electrical potential of the brain.

to maintain permanent contact with other people?

While looking for an answer to this, I remembered a phrase I had read when I was studying ENT (Ear, Nose, and Throat). I was studying *The Mechanisms of the Larynx* by Negus, an English scholar and world renowned specialist on this subject. He wrote a vast tome, which had all the attractions of a dictionary including an extraordinary collection of original observations and valuable viewpoints. One observation in particular struck me: "If the eggs of singing birds were hatched by non-singing birds, there was a risk that the little birds when they came into the world would turn out to be non-singing birds." A little later he said, "If the eggs were hatched by birds which sang in a different way from their real parents, the newly-born would risk singing the wrong sort of song when they were born."

After making some headway in my own work, I formed a hypothesis to explain this phenomenon. Surely it was an audio-phonatory conditioning process that caused the little birds to reproduce the vocal behavior pattern of those who had sat on the eggs. This was not impossible. But if such were the case, it had to be admitted that the conditioning process began at the egg stage, *in ovo*. Obviously, this was a very bold speculation. But if it were true, I must be on the track of one of the great secrets of the desire to communicate.

I would have liked to have repeated these experiments myself, but for want of time, money, and eggs I had to give up the idea. Nevertheless, the problem remained in the back of my mind, and fortunately I soon found my opinion confirmed by some experiments carried out by Konrad Lorenz, the great ethologist and Nobel Prize winner (1973).[11]

Lorenz established that after he spoke regularly to certain eggs, the ducklings born from those eggs turned their heads towards him and rushed headlong in his direction as soon as he uttered a word. It was as if genuine spoken communication existed between them and him. In the same way as butterflies are attracted by light, these ducklings were attracted by Lorenz's voice.

If a tropism of this kind exists for some species, might it exist among human beings, too? But there again it was very difficult for me to verify this by my own means.

Luckily I came across the works of André Thomas (summarized in his book *Neurologie de Nourisant*), who was carrying out very exciting investigations on babies at the breast. My attention was riveted by what he called "the Christian-name sign."

The experiment could not be simpler to carry out. During the ten days following birth, when the baby possesses great muscular tonicity, a group of adults, including the parents, pronounces the child's Christian name, each in

---

[11] K. Lorenz, The Companion in the Bird's World, Auk, 1937 54, 245-273.

turn. No reaction on the baby's part is observed until the mother speaks. At this moment, the infant's body leans over and falls in her direction.

It seems to me that this is exactly the same behavior as that of Lorenz' ducklings. The newborn reacts to the sound of a particular voice, *the only voice of which he or she was aware while still in the fetal stage.*

It must be inferred from this that the fetus is capable of hearing, which was certainly not a generally accepted idea at the time. Studies of normal hearing, which I carried out in order to get a better understanding and appreciation of the hearing problems of dyslexics, led me to discover step by step how the baby at the breast hears. But I had to stop there, very dissatisfied because I felt that it was my particular vocation to study phenomena within the womb. My own experience as a premature baby often stirred up and guided my *libido sciendi,* my desire to know. I was more aware of these problems than other people. For example, what comes to mind is my experience in the cabin of the aircraft, which was reminiscent of the prenatal conditions which caused my premature birth.

I persisted in my investigations of what an embryo could hear with a desperate eagerness which scientific curiosity alone could not explain. I was more and more convinced that communication of sound is the most important link between a mother and the child within her. Once she has given it a nest within herself, she nourishes it in every way, *especially with sounds.* She reveals herself to the fetus by all the organic and visceral noises she makes and, above all, by her voice. The infant is steeped in this environment of sound. It draws all its emotional material from its mother's voice. This voice also lays the foundations of its mother tongue, but let us not jump ahead.

Thus it is that primitive audio-vocal communication is founded. When the circuit is properly established, the embryo draws a feeling of security from this permanent dialogue which guarantees it will have a harmonious blossoming.

In 1953, I finally devised a system which enabled me to get an idea of intrauterine listening. Besides microphones and loud-speakers, it utilized large sheets of India rubber, by means of which I avoided as much as possible the effects of air pockets, which were capable of compromising the whole experiment. Unfortunately, I did not have microphones and transmitters at my disposal which could work under water. In spite of everything, I succeeded in producing a reasonably sophisticated setup. I was now in a position to study the acoustic impressions of the fetus.

The fetus hears a whole range of sounds, most of which contain low frequencies. Due to the way the human ear is constructed, it acts as a filter. When the ear is filled with water, it carries out a selection of these frequencies. The universe of sound in which the embryo is submerged is remarkably rich in sound qualities of every kind. The fetus experiences internal rumblings, the movement of chyle at the time of digestion, and cardiac rhythms at a sort of gallop. It perceives rhythmic breathing like a distant ebb and flow. And then its mother's voice asserts itself in this context, a little noise superimposed on all the other sounds, a noise in the form of a coded message of exceptional quality.

Starting with this elementary apparatus, I set up experimental situations to record music and other sound combinations the fetus could hear. On each occasion, I found myself in the presence of a fantastic reality which was most delightful to experience. The acoustic ambiance resembled, slightly, that of the African bush at twilight (at least as we imagine it and as fictional films present it to us). I heard distant calls, echoes, stealthy rustlings, and the lapping of waves.

I was genuinely fascinated by all this and continued to make similar experiments. After some time it was no longer enough for me alone to hear the recordings. I had to make other people aware of them, too. When I invited one man to listen to these sounds, it resulted in a significant discovery.

He was a patient whom I knew very well because he had come to consult me several times, although it had nothing to do with intrauterine listening. First of all, this man had a voice of poor quality, which I improved by means of treatment under the Electronic Ear. But he also needed to consult me regarding a very particular linguistic problem. When I first met him, this patient was an engineer in an oil company. He was a very easy-going and pleasant person and a doctor's son, clearly familiar with medicine. He was also a man with a great generosity of spirit, which made him sensitive to the social needs of others. He wanted to explain to the workers under his command certain advantages they would gain by a modification of the working conditions proposed by the management. Unfortunately, every time he tried to explain this, his audience quickly and obviously showed signs of boredom, even of going to sleep. He believed so thoroughly in what he wanted to tell them, and he thought it was so important to circulate this information, that this setback, repeated at every attempt, was a cruel blow to him.

The improvement in his voice hardly changed his situation. The problems arose from an aspect of verbal communication about which he knew nothing. To *speak well* (in perfect French and with an excellent voice) is not enough to gain a hearing. In fact, people will not hear if the speaker addressing them uses a frequency range to which a listener has become *deaf by choice*.

That was precisely the case with these workers, whose ears were constantly assailed by intense noise. The factory's business was to refill butane gas containers, and the handling of these from morning till night caused a great racket. The majority of these workers suffered from an industrial hearing loss which noticeably distorted their auditory curve, with particular impact on the higher frequencies. In practice, they experienced the greatest difficulty in hearing sibilant sounds and, therefore, in following any discourse whose length demanded an accumulation of terms containing sibilants. The ear, in fact, is obliged to restore the missing sound qualities in order to analyze the message. The effort can be sustained for a certain time, but eventually a moment comes when the ear becomes tired. From then on, the meaning of the discourse becomes incoherent.

I asked my patient to record for me some of what he wanted to say to the work force. The sound analyses showed that the vital part of his message was in the exact frequency range in which his audience could not grasp it. When he spoke, these workers found themselves confronted by a language almost unintelligible to them, although it was the most polished French.

After I helped him understand the problem, my whole treatment consisted of helping him speak in another frequency range. In particular, I made him aware that the same things could be said using words with fewer high frequency sibilant sounds. This technique is common practice among many radio and television announcers who instinctively apply it to reach the average media audience. The speech of the man in the street is often full of low frequencies and devoid of high frequencies.

By merely modifying his choice of words our engineer finally succeeded in making himself heard. He was so successful that the management asked him to carry on his public relations efforts in all their other factories.

Do not think we were dealing with an isolated case. I have faced the same problem several times, in particular with Reverend M., one of the best known members of a Protestant church.

Reverend M. came to the aid of representatives of the Algerian Liberation Movement after some troubles arose in Alsace and was then considered by the Lausanne synod to be particularly suitable to promote the scriptures in the industrial suburbs of Paris. The evangelical mission, however, ran into difficulties, which he confided to me one day. He knew about some of my work with speech and language and wondered if I could help him surmount the obstacle.

This turned out very well since many workers from the Cachan region to whom he wished to speak worked in the Air Force arsenals, and I already knew their hearing problems and the failings involved in them. Once again, the speaker was in the paradoxical situation of being incomprehensible just because his speech was of too high a quality. It was not that he spoke too "well" in the sense of using very elaborate or specialized terminology. If the hearing of his audience had been perfectly intact, they would have had no trouble understanding what he had to say. With their hearing impaired, as they were victims of industrial hearing loss, they were in no state to make sense of Reverend M.'s clear and simple message. As the result of this dialogue of the deaf, both sides developed a weariness and confusion which depressed Reverend M. very much. By means of sound filters, I allowed him to hear how the workers in question were hearing his statements. Impressed by this, and indeed convinced, he revised his vocabulary and way of expressing himself and ultimately obtained excellent results. Others were encouraged to follow his example, and he became more and more prominent in the service of his church. At the same time we became friends.

Great orators know instinctively how to adapt their speech and their choice of words in one direction or another to the characteristics of their audience's understanding. These characteristics are quickly grasped on the basis of certain responses. According to their audience, their voice focuses on the higher or lower frequency bands, or one that is more or less spread out. Moreover, the form of discourse changes, according to whether they address people of a high or low sociocultural level. This observation and the situation just described emphasize the important influence of the psychological dimension on the neurophysiological instrument in human communication.

But let us return to my patient, the engineer. At his request, I also helped him to speak English. A little later, I treated his little girl, who was having difficulty in adjusting to school, and then his wife. As in the case of the Reverend M., our relationship became closer and closer. His scientific training and his nostalgia for the world of medicine stimulated him to find out more about my laboratory work.

One day I suggested he listen to the acoustic impressions of the fetus, as far as I had been able to recreate them. He enthusiastically accepted my offer. I asked his wife to have her voice recorded, then told my patient I was ready to begin his initiation into the matter of filtered sounds.

He came, accompanied by his little girl, whom I sat down in a corner of the laboratory while I explained to her father how I went about obtaining the strange sounds he was about to hear. I told him too that I had put a loud speaker in water surrounded by a rubber diaphragm. By playing a tape recorder, I injected the recorded voice via the immersed loud speaker into the water medium. I then registered the resulting sounds via a microphone also plunged in the water and similarly protected.

I gave my friend a demonstration. He was thrilled, and asked me to begin again and provide him with a full explanation. We played around for quite a long time listening to these marvelously fluid noises, like the sounds of a fairyland, which corresponded to the acoustic information perceived by a human fetus. Then I decided to reveal to him what I believed to be the sonic birth. Suddenly another voice was raised in the room. It was the little girl, nine-years-old at the time, whose presence we had completely forgotten. Now she became the center of our attention.

"I am in a tunnel," she said. "I see two angels at the end of it, two angels in white clothes!"

She continued outlining a kind of fantastic waking dream. Her father and I were dumbfounded. However, my experience as a surgeon enabled me to recover my composure quickly. I had lost none of the words uttered by the little girl, and my brain was working at full speed. Abruptly, the explanation forced itself upon me. The child was in the process of visualizing her own birth! It was as if she were in the birth canal (the tunnel) and could see the doctor and the midwife at the other end in their white coats (the two angels).

Her father, meanwhile, showed all the signs of profound agony. Only the reassuring presence of a doctor prevented him from collapsing. I could see by his distorted face that in the course of this experiment, I was in the process of touching something very profound. I knew very little about the psychoanalytic dimension of the human personality at that time, and I had no desire to play the sorcerer's apprentice. All the same, I felt the experiment should not yet be stopped.

The child continued to tell us about the long and complicated journey she was making. After a few minutes, which seemed to us like years, she cried out:

"Now I see mommy!"

Doubt was no longer possible.

Her father's eyes popped out of his head.

"You see mommy! You see mommy! And how do you see mommy?" he blurted out, frightened and overexcited at the same time.

"Like this," said the child. Carried away by automatic gestures, she fell back and took up a gynecological birthing position until the tape came to an end.

Then she left the laboratory and spent the rest of the time playing, as if nothing had happened.

There was really nothing mysterious about what happened. By playing around with the experimental apparatus, I had just recreated for the child the conditions of her birth. I was to define it later as a *sonic birth*, that is to say, the progress from liquid hearing (the way the fetus listens) to aerial hearing (listening as the baby does at the breast).

That the fetus hears is a fact, but not in the same way that the baby does after being thrust into the world. After birth, the auditory function evolves and the ear is gradually opened.

To begin with, the ear has to be able to function in a liquid environment. Acoustically speaking, the external, middle, and internal parts of the ear are adapted before birth to perceive frequencies transmitted by water. Among these the frequencies which transmit speech reside in the high range. After birth, it is only the inner ear that retains its aquatic milieu, whereas the outer and middle ear have to adapt themselves to the impedance of the air around them.

During the days that immediately follow birth, the baby remains in a transitional state as far as acoustic experience is concerned. For ten days the middle ear (and the Eustachian tube in particular) retains some amniotic liquid and so remains attuned to the frequencies of a liquid environment. When the middle ear empties itself of this fluid, the infant loses his perception of high frequencies. He even enters into a period of *sonic shadows* during which he hardly hears any longer. The muscular tension associated with listening to high frequencies during fetal life diminishes and the infant settles down and sleeps. Now he must concentrate all his energy on increasing his power of aural adaptation. This learning period lasts for weeks until contact with his mother's voice is reestablished, this time via the surrounding air instead of through the liquids of the uterine world.

Little by little, the auditory diaphragm gradually opens to the world of sound, around an axis situated between 300 and 800 Hertz.

The infant gradually rediscovers the tympanic tension necessary to reexperience the perceptions registered during fetal life and, in particular, can come to recognize the voice that supported him and made him feel secure during the long uterine night. This voice has changed, of course, but not from the point of view of rhythm or inflections. When the infant rediscovers this, he makes no mistake. He will aim his ear in his mother's direction in the hope of reexperiencing that nirvana-within-the-womb associated with her.

This vocal nourishment that the mother provides to her child is just as important to the child's development as her milk. The infant awaits the mother's voice just as much as he awaits its next drink at the breast. The eagerness with which a premature baby placed in an incubator *devours* his mother's voice offers a most palpable proof of this. That is why I persist in stating that every facility for premature babies should be equipped with an apparatus capable of injecting the mother's voice into the incubators, a voice which is just as vital as the food being brought to nourish them.

My friend's daughter experienced an artificial sonic birth, which seemed to have simulated for her the conditions of her birth. It was possible to consider then that one might be able to bring about reactions which touch the depths of the psyche simply by using acoustic information of a certain kind. In other words, one could envisage a method of regulating (or at least of exercising a direct, guided action upon) those bits of acoustic data capable of producing well-defined psychological effects. Perhaps it would be possible to make use of the ear to relieve certain psycho-pathological disturbances.

I did not have the training required to answer these questions myself. I had a hunch that I had put my finger on something important, but first I had to look at it more clearly, and collect some authoritative opinions.

So I took up my pilgrim's staff and went to visit colleagues in the field of neuropsychiatry, especially those with psychoanalytic training.

The majority of them showed interest, particularly those associated with René Laforgue, a Freudian psychoanalyst. However, they were all snowed under with work and, therefore, could afford to be more generous with advice than with concrete help. I sat in my laboratory waiting in vain for something to happen.

I was at a standstill in my investigations when I became acquainted with Dr. Bernard This, a young psychoanalyst and a follower of Françoise Dolto, who was a student of Laforgue. Dr. This brought me one of the most extraordinary patients, a child of about 12, a great fat baby of astounding vitality. He screamed so piercingly that he emptied my waiting room. Every five or six seconds he jumped so high in the air that he could kick himself in the back with both feet, a performance I have never seen from anyone else. He did not speak, but his face was always alive with an extremely vivid mimicry. He looked as if he were sucking something without stopping. His mother accompanied him, but he repelled her as if they were two electromagnets of the same polarity!

I was flabbergasted. I had never seen nor even heard about anything like it. At this moment a woman I did not know entered my consulting room, a woman of admirable style, remarkable moreover for the richness of her vocabulary and her power of expression. It was Françoise Dolto.

After we introduced ourselves, I begged her to throw some light on the nature of the young patient who was continuing to cry out, mimic, and gesticulate.

"He's a schizophrenic," she told me.

"I have heard about this psychosis," I said. "But can you explain to me what it consists of?"

Dolto replied, "To tell you the truth, we do not know very well what it is. All I can tell you is that children like that are, psychologically speaking, not yet born."

"Not yet born?" I said. "You intrigue me. At this very moment I am carrying out an investigation into intrauterine life and birth."

"Yes, I know. Bernard told me. That's why I am here with this child. I think you may be able to help him. May we try?"

As I was happy to agree, we made an appointment and also arranged for the boy's mother to record her voice in my laboratory for the experiment. She made a recording of about 20 minutes.

On the appointed day, Françoise Dolto, Bernard This, the patient, his mother, and I met in my laboratory which I had set up in the office of the apartment and adapted to the needs of the investigation.

The mother was sitting in front of one wall while the child was lying flat against the opposite partition on which he was scribbling with a piece of chalk he had grabbed. The two psychoanalysts took their places beside the mother. I was near the door, in a good position to operate the equipment.

I set the process in motion.

I did not want to bring about sonic birth at this first session. I simply wanted to make the child listen to filtered sounds that resemble the acoustic impressions the fetus receives in the womb and, in particular, the mother's voice, which comes across like a fantastic rustling. I had eliminated all low notes in order to simulate intrauterine hearing. All that remained were the high notes that corresponded to this rustling. Since the high notes were propagated in a straight line, it was easy for me to "touch" the child's body by means of a directional loud speaker suited for just such a purpose. I aimed the sound waves in the direction of his head.

Immediately he became still and stopped scribbling. Then he flung himself towards me and hit the switch to turn out the light. In the twinkling of an eye we were plunged into darkness. This gesture took my breath away — not that it was difficult for me to understand. On the contrary, it was perfectly clear that the child was only trying to recreate the lighting conditions of his fetal life. But I was puzzled because that presupposed some latent intelligence in the psychotic boy. In fact, he had instantaneously located a switch which was not easy to find, even for an adult in full possession of his faculties.

At the same time, I felt myself overcome by a certain anxiety. Knowing what prodigious leaps he could make, I was very much afraid he might wreak all sorts of havoc in the room. Nevertheless, I restrained myself from switching the light back on. Instead I followed his movements by the feeble glimmer of the pilot lights on the electronic apparatus.

While the tape continued to run, I saw him gradually leave his place and move towards his mother. I followed his movements as well as I could with my sonic beam. Finally, he sat on his mother's knees, took her arms, and put them around him. The next second he began to suck his thumb. He remained in this position for as long as the tape recording lasted. It was almost as if he were back inside his mother. What he did was all the more remarkable because for the last ten years or so he had not seemed to know her — that is, when he was not looking upon her as an openly hostile character.

When the tape finished, he got up and switched the light back on.

"Very interesting," Françoise Dolto said to me. "Could one perhaps go a little further?"

"Let's all meet again in a week," I suggested. "Then we will try to bring about a sonic birth."

The psychoanalysts and the boy's mother agreed, and we arranged a second meeting.

A week later, when we were once more together in my laboratory, the mother told us that her child had made definite progress. On several occasions, he had moved toward her. He had even caressed her face, which was not at all the sort of thing he usually did. In brief, the outline of a reconciliation had visibly taken form. For us doctors, this development was very encouraging. We thought there was no longer any reason to hesitate. The sonic birth would doubtless merely hurry matters on in the right direction. It would enable the child, we firmly hoped, to reach a really new stage.

The setting for the second session was in every way the same as the first, at least at the beginning. The child was scribbling when I made the sound emerge. He stopped at once, ran to the switch, plunged the room into darkness, went to sit on his mother's knees in the fetal position, and put his thumb in his mouth.

But when I produced the change in the acoustic impressions from those received in the fluid environment *within* the womb to those received in the aerial environment *outside* the womb, I obtained a new reaction. Suddenly he began to babble.

Such chatter was in itself a form of expression. We had awakened in him the desire to communicate with his mother, a desire which had remained dormant until that moment. The child began to produce sound effects of all kinds, making us understand that we were witnessing a genuine birth of language.

At the end of the session he stood up on his own, just as he had done the previous time, switched on the light once more, and returned to his mother's side to button her coat, which she had kept over her shoulders.

"That's it," Françoise Dolto said to me. "He's finally been born."

His behavior in fact was very symbolic, something which could not escape the eye of such an experienced psychoanalyst. It was as if he had closed behind him the door of a room, one that he had decided to leave forever. He had left the womb, never to return.

We were in the process of discussing all this when we realized that the child had disappeared. I immediately questioned my fellow workers, but no one had seen him leave. This was not surprising, for the apartment in which I lived was full of immense, winding corridors. We looked for the boy everywhere without success. At first the mother succumbed to panic, then she sped like an arrow through the front door as if a rope were drawing her outside, or as if someone were calling her.

In fact, maternal instinct had come into play. Her son was calmly waiting for her on the sidewalk in front of the house. She brought him back to us a moment later.

The strangest thing about it was that he somehow had gone out without being seen. We finally determined that he had used the service staircase. There again, what powers of observation this child had! The door that opened onto this staircase was hidden from view by a bookcase which I had to put there because there was no other place for it. Most of my staff had no idea up until then of the existence of this exit. Our schizophrenic, however, had found it right away and used it. None of us would have thought him capable of figuring this out.

As a result of this adventure, Françoise Dolto drew conclusions that seemed to me then, and even now, to be highly apt.

"You will notice," she said. "Not only has he left his mother's womb and fastened the door behind him, but, more than that, he took a totally different route out of this house. In this way, he is showing that he wants to separate himself from his mother in order to assume his own individuality and exist outside her."

I thought we were going to repeat the session the following week, but this did not take place. The psychoanalysts were against it. They wanted to make a more rigorous study of the material they already had. Moreover, they were somewhat apprehensive of the eventual outcome of the experiment. I do not blame them for this. "I never thought things would move so fast," Françoise Dolto whispered to me, after the child had rebuttoned his mother's coat. Even I thought that perhaps I had gone too fast.

It turned out that I had. A little later the schizophrenic child showed disturbing signs of self-destruction. I learned from Françoise Dolto that he had tried to scratch his own face, and that he again had turned against his mother. Did this mean that the sonic birth did not have therapeutic possibilities after all? I did not think so and the future was to prove me right. Our setback had come about solely from having gone too fast. It was not the Method that was faulty, but the inexperienced way in which we used it.

Françoise Dolto preferred to leave it at that, but I did not give up. Setbacks have always stimulated me. A new direction was opening before me. The present problem was to find the means of profiting from the advantages of the sonic birth without its attendant drawbacks. I advanced with the greatest precautions, and this carried me a long way, this time without mishap.

The results obtained were as remarkable as the process was slow. Today the passage from listening in an aquatic environment to that of listening in an aerial one is only brought about after long preparation, every stage of which is precisely defined and controlled. To pass from one level to another, the operator waits until the subject himself asks for the change, although, of course, we are talking about an unconscious request, one which is not explicitly put into words. Current ideas of depth psychology are a great help to us now since they enable us to recognize the unconscious entreaty of the infant. Besides, we now collaborate on a daily basis with psychiatrists, psychologists, and psychoanalysts since we are convinced that many fertile ideas are born from a common approach. This, in turn, gives rise to further possible lines of investigation.

The application of this therapy has given me a better understanding of this *need to communicate* which, in my view, lies at the very root of language. Above all, it is born from the desire not to break off (or renew at a later stage) the sonic relationship experienced with the mother during prenatal life. A human being wants either to keep or rediscover a way of being in touch with the outside world and with another person, a way which gave him the greatest satisfaction when he was still in the embryonic state. From this point of view, we are all of us, as one of my commentators wrote, "homesick for the womb."

The cry with which the infant greets his entry into the world is a cry of distress. Already it weeps for the lost paradise which was being experienced just a few moments earlier in his mother's womb.

I know by heart the objections usually raised against this theory. Isn't the contact of the fetus with the mother essentially a physical one? Isn't it going too far in this context to bring up a relationship of a psychological nature? I answer these objections with an argument the reader already knows: Language, too, possesses a physical dimension. By causing vibrations in the surrounding air, language becomes a sort of invisible arm by which we can "touch" the person listening to us in every sense of the term.

If the word did not have such negative connotations, I would say that the desire to communicate is "regressive" since it is a maintaining or a restoration of a symbolic umbilical cord. Indeed, the person returns to the memory of life in the womb. It is *not* a regression in the sense of being a handicap since this symbolic return to the fetal stage actually represents an extraordinary opportunity for the person who accomplishes it. It is as if by being plunged into one's own past, one were being offered a better way of mastering the future. By bringing the ear back to its earliest influences, the filtered sound treatment enables it in this roundabout way to achieve the most advanced stage of its evolution, that of "human listening." A particular state of attention and tension of its components produces this, and filtered sound restores it.

The verbal exchange, thus readjusted, prolongs and perfects the "dialogue of the flesh" between the human embryo and that first "other person," the mother. It fulfills the desire to maintain a fleshy contact with another in the most physiological sense of the term. We have just seen how this is so. To be born is to pass from an environment limited by the walls of the womb to an environment whose limits are moved back indefinitely. In other words, whoever is brought into the world achieves an awareness that the womb has burst open to become the universe. In a way, one never leaves one's mother's womb; the maternal environment is merely given further dimensions. The walls of the womb grow into the sides of the cradle, then of the room, then of the family, then of one's native country, then of the whole earth, and finally of the cosmos.

My work with filtered sounds and the sonic birth has considerably extended my intellectual horizons and, in a more general way, my outlook as a human being. The fact that I have been able to be present "live" at the birth of language has led me to a fundamental study of communication problems, personality disturbances, and, as a result, psychopathology. This cleared the way for me into psychology, which in turn opened the gates of philosophy. In this way, I branched out far more widely than ever before from my original specializations, ENT and surgery.

I evolved because necessity drove me. It was fine to gain access to all these psychic phenomena "through the ear hole," but I realized that my training had become insufficient —— both to understand the phenomena myself and, above all, to make others understand them. I found myself confronted by a language difficulty. I quickly became aware that the vocabulary and working concepts of a laboratory technician well trained in electronics were not at all suitable for my new investigations.

I went back to school. In my case, *school* took the form of St. Anne's Hospital, a psychiatric facility in the south part of Paris, where I attended psychiatric consultations of inestimable value.

This initiation enabled me to get to know many psychiatrists and psychoanalysts whose company soon proved to be of great benefit. But I also experienced a misadventure which is worth relating.

One of my colleagues, a doctor in the psychiatric hospital service, was attracted to my field of auditory education through a group which worked with psychotics. Through him I had the opportunity to carry out a research project within the hospital service. I obtained permission to conduct some investigations in an establishment in the north of France.

Of the 230 hospitalized children, I estimated that it was possible to improve the condition of about 180. Hospitalized? I wonder if that is the right word. I was dumbfounded to find in this hospital, in 1961-1963, children shut up in beds which were like cages, surrounded by bars, even on the upper part. Others remained confined all day in straight jackets. It was an hallucinatory universe, atrocious, worse than Kafka-esque, where *the mad* seemed to be the victims of some horrible relic of the obscurantism of the Middle Ages. And yet, the hospital doctors were open-minded people. Otherwise, they certainly would not have had anything to do with me.

I used my own equipment to begin treatment on those children who appeared to me capable of recovery. At the same time, the other members of the team, which was a remarkably dynamic one, undertook a more purely psychological treatment, based on such techniques as psychotherapy and psychodrama.

Quite quickly, the children moved toward normalization and began to need some sort of elementary academic education. One morning we had the satisfaction of seeing them line up to go to the village school. The villagers were deeply moved by this, but not in the way one might have expected. The villagers were indignant, or terrified, to see these *crazy* kids walking in the streets and attending the same school as their own precious children. Complaints poured in. The deputy-mayor of this out-of-the-way place, who was also a government minister, joined the outcry and demanded an immediate end to this "deplorable scandal." The lack of understanding was total. They would not even consider our point of view. The mad were the mad and were condemned to remain so for the rest of their lives; they should not be allowed to "disturb normal people."

Under pressure from certain families whose interest lay in keeping their child confined, and by the direct intervention of the minister, order was restored in the country. I was ordered to pack up my machines and clear out. The colleague who had made it possible for me to conduct the experiment was passed over for promotion and ultimately transferred. He was refused any appeal by the hospital service, although he was certainly entitled to one. As for the children, they were put back in their cages.

Thus I had been, unwillingly, one of the chief actors in a pitiful social drama. Once again I had been naive enough to believe that routine could be disturbed with impunity, that entrenched habits of thought could be challenged, and that a priori reasoning could be overcome because it was manifestly absurd. An established structure must never be disturbed. To do so is very bad, and one is not forgiven. I suffered deep and lasting injury as a result of this sad business. What pained me most was to learn of the part certain of my colleagues played in the matter. Such lack of understanding on the part of others in my profession was very hard to bear. Too many of them, alas, are more willing to serve a venerable institution than to serve the truth. They forget that there is no spectacle more heart-rending than little children suffering, abandoned by all, while the heirs of Hippocrates tear one another to pieces.

10

Laterality — It Must Be Right

The painful adventure I just related was a severe blow to my morale. However, it only strengthened my determination to come to the aid of psychotic children. While continuing my experimental work, I increased my therapeutic endeavors. "I saw children in my consulting room who were sometimes impaired at a very deep level. Nevertheless, I made it a rule to respond to every appeal and always attempt some treatment, however unfavorable the prognosis. I never said "No" to parents who begged me to help their children."

For this, too, others criticized me. I have been accused of being a universal dabbler, with no doubts about anything. Despite these criticisms I remain unruffled. If I have any doubts about my approach, I reassure myself by recalling Dr. Carcopino's words: "In medicine, when one doesn't understand something, one searches for the answer." Similarly, when one does not know what to do to relieve a patient's suffering, one searches for a solution. One cannot escape the problem by proclaiming "Nothing can be done." No doctor has the right to give up. It is not a proper reaction for a doctor to avoid getting involved — indeed, it is exactly the opposite. Everything must be attempted to bring about even an iota of improvement. How can one be sure an effort will be useless if one first has not made it?

I absolutely disagree with those doctors who make the diagnosis "incurable" and then wash their hands of the matter. Moreover, I am convinced that in this field no effort is made wholly in vain. *Something can always be done* if only to give the family love and help them to better understand what is happening. It is unworthy of a doctor to leave them in their agony, in total darkness, under the shadow of a terrible sentence with no appeal.

Even if the treatment undertaken has no effect on the patient, dealing with the parents can bring them some comfort. Though it may be only slight comfort, it is always appreciated. It is extremely important to make the mother and father understand, for example, that they are not personally responsible for what is happening to their child (very often, they believe they are); that the child's problems have caused a crystallization of an illness within the family constellation (we shall see presently that three generations are needed to make an autistic child); and that if the family is sick, ultimately it is because society itself is not in a good state.

It is a humanitarian duty to give people these facts, not only to comfort them, but to make their burden a little less crushing by relieving them of unwarranted guilt. Unfortunately, some doctors deliver diagnoses to parents brutally. The door is cruelly slammed shut and all hope is lost when the doctor pronounces, "Things must be faced squarely" or "The situation must be accepted as it is."

One thing is certain: this kind of final verdict falling like a guillotine on the heads of unfortunate parents puts an end to investigations and attempts at treatment which, if pursued, might have brought about some positive improvements in the child's state. A doctor worthy of the name has no right to neglect such a possibility, however remote.

Is it wise to use staff and materials in "desperate" cases to achieve a purely hypothetical improvement, when there is already so much work to be done for children classified as good candidates for treatment? I asked myself this question at the start of my career and, after mature consideration, my answer is "Yes." Something in me cries out, "These children must not be abandoned." If this were a scientific argument, and I had only the weight of my convictions, I would not be taken seriously. Once again, I would be treated as a visionary, a sort of Don Quixote. But my special plea is also based on results actually obtained, results which are tangible. Experience has fully proved to me — and I keep a record of all the proofs — that there is no case so desperate that one cannot bring at least the beginning of relief. Stubbornly refusing to follow what good sense dictates while aiming for the impossible has brought me some of the greatest satisfactions of my professional life. By proving *something can always be done*, I experienced delight that words are inadequate to express. It was not the pleasure of being right that brought me this reward, but simply the pleasure of having done my job and helped somebody to experience a better life.

The slightest improvement can bring great appreciation. It is often enough to show a family that one is tackling their problem with all the seriousness and energy it requires for a sense of relief to appear, a relief which by transforming certain psychological conditions may perhaps help to make a treatment work (to some slight extent) that otherwise would never have worked at all. Every specialist in these problems knows well what a simple change of ambiance can do.

Today it is considered proper and desirable to treat autistic children and the poor, desolate, disinherited outcasts who suffer from major speech and language disorders. It is now recognized that some of their deficiencies can and should be improved by treatment. So much the better.

Right at the start I asked myself the question, "Is it really worth treating autistic children?" To do so means bringing them into a world which, to say the least, is not easy to live in. Perhaps their craziness provides them an opportunity to escape the aggression of the real world and its attendant agonies. When I thought about these children, who are so convulsive and dynamic, so seemingly unaware of the difficulty of existing in this world, I wondered if I had the right to bring about a significant improvement in their condition and, while doing so, plunge them into a hostile environment. To what sort of normality would they be normalized?

After prolonged wrestling with my doubts, I decided that their treatment and reeducation must be attempted. Their sickness might be a shelter for them, but fundamentally, they were existing only in a very crude protective mechanism or *animal* state.

Every time I brought up this dimension of "animal nature," those around me winced, psychoanalysts in particular. So I must explain myself. In my opinion, there exists a close relationship between *animal nature* and *spirit* (*anima* in Latin). The animal nature of autistic children does not prevent them from having feelings. Quite the contrary. It is their sorrow taken to extremes which imprisons them in such a remote darkness. It removes them from the world of human beings into their own *dead* universe. Yet just a glimmer of awareness could reanimate and revive them.

As proof of this there is a certain reaction which I have often noticed. In the course of treatment leading to normalization, the autistic child starts by appearing quite indifferent to everything taking place. The child is remote, and hardly capable of emotional reactions like our own. Yet, at the stage where he comes to accept his mother's voice, he bursts into a flood of tears. It is impossible to stem this torrent. The child appears inconsolable and gives every sign of intense despair. This child, whom one has hastily judged from his looks as incapable of moral suffering, has now for the first time suffered a moral wound, or mortal wound? Do not let anyone speak of the insensitivity of autistic children. It is just a myth based on misleading appearances.

Why do these children experience this distress? They insert themselves into a body occupied by an unconscious power that seems to have shut the doors against them. They feel excluded from the nucleus of their own being. When they first attain self-awareness it only serves to emphasize this exclusion, this deprivation.

Happily, this is only a passing stage. A phase of increasing freedom follows this suffering phase, in the course of which various manifestations appear (particularly vocal manifestations, such as cooings and other noises). In order to cause passage from the first phase to the second, the mother plays a specific and important part. Her involvement in this process is a very positive element, and it may be a virtual necessity. Often the success of the whole treatment depends on the mother's intervention. This necessity was not immediately apparent to me when I began working with autistic children. It only became apparent as part of a long-term process.

Using the mother in her child's treatment causes extremely delicate problems. On the surface, the idea of asking a mother's help in treating her child might seem a perfectly natural request, unlikely to raise any particular difficulties. In fact, it is much easier to request the help than it is to attain it.

The mothers of autistic children may themselves suffer from disturbed psychological and emotional states. This type of child is often brought into the world by women who repress their own anxieties, whose whole personality may combine elements which cause their children's problems.

Clearly then, if action is to be taken with reference to the direct cause of the psychosis, the mother may also need treatment. An excellent way of getting her to come to her own aid lies in involving her in her child's treatment. One connects her, as it were, to the same wavelength as her child. She is made to hear sounds of the same pitch and quality. The effect is startling — the mother's anguish gradually disappears, but above all, the child makes notable progress at the same time.

Seeing the effect of the parallel treatment just described removed my last doubts of the importance of family influence. Moreover, as I have already said, it is the entire family that is sick. For if the mother herself encounters difficulties on the psychoaffective plane, it may be because her own mother had to contend with abnormally intense anxiety. As I suggested earlier, *at least* three generations are required to produce an autistic child.

"Soon then," someone sarcastically remarked, "I suppose you are going to summon grandmothers to your treatment sessions." Why not? I would certainly do so if I had the means of persuading them to come! In fact, I cherish the hope of succeeding in this one day. Once I had the greatest difficulty in getting mothers to accept the idea of a collaboration. Now they agree. Why shouldn't I succeed, with plenty of patience, in getting grandmothers to agree, too? I believe that, in this area at least, one must strive for the impossible, and I am convinced that one day doctors will be able to treat the family group as a whole.

This will not come about tomorrow, nor the day after tomorrow. Very strong family resistance will have to be overcome, resistance bound up with lack of understanding on the part of the individuals concerned (that same lack of understanding which explains why a meeting between mother and child did not occur in the first place). But since the public now is more informed about these problems, I have high hopes. The popularization of modern ideas in the fields of psychopathology and psychotherapy by the media will at least have the advantage of making people sensitive to and aware of certain phenomena. Years ago when I first tackled these subjects, it seemed I was preaching in the desert. Today people do listen to me and accept what I have to say much more easily.

It is no longer shocking, except to a few limited and reactionary minds, to affirm that the family is responsible (I do not use the word "culpable") for certain disappointments that children experience. To make a child is easy. One only has to pass a few agreeable minutes. On the other hand, to humanize that child to develop a whole human being, that task is no sinecure! It demands attention, permanent care, and availability which is put entirely at the service of the baby, then of the child. It is only natural to make mistakes. Freud said to parents, "Whatever you do is wrong!" Without taking this declaration too seriously, we recognize and accept that mistakes will be made in bringing up a child and then use all possible means to repair them when they occur.

My method of sonic birth has been much criticized, and the theories that lie behind it have been attacked even more fiercely. If I had an appetite for controversy, I could have spent my entire life in intellectual jousting. I continue to have some rough adversaries who oppose me in every respect. According to them, my ideas contain not the slightest particle of truth.

This opposition began with my theory of listening in the womb. As soon as my colleagues learned of my opinion that the human embryo could hear, an armed revolt occurred.

"What a joke!" they said. "This scatterbrained idea of Tomatis' shows such ignorance. He does not even know that the ear of the fetus is not completely formed. How can this poor fetus hear when the junctions between the nerve cells capable of sending the message to the brain (the synapses) are not yet made? At least our dear colleague is not lacking in imagination. A renowned fantasist in his own way; he ought to write science fiction! He's really missed his vocation!"

This was not the first time that I found myself the butt of witty fellows. By this time I was an old enough crocodile not to have my skin seriously pierced by these barbs. I let my detractors sing their little song. The positive results were sufficiently rewarding, enough so that I did not let these pinpricks hold me up.

I adopted this attitude because my thesis was confirmed even before I took the trouble to cross swords with anyone in its defense. In 1962, the investigations of the American researcher Dr. Lee Salk[12] proved decisively that the fetus was aware of the mother's heartbeats. The prestige attached to research projects carried out in the U.S.A. was such that Salk's conclusions were generally accepted. Abruptly people admitted that, in fact, the fetus could hear these sounds. But for all that, they still did not agree with me. The fetus could hear heartbeats —— so what? What did that prove? Well, at least that proved that it was capable of hearing! And if it could hear those sounds, in spite of the unfinished condition of the ear and non-establishment of the synapses, it might well be able to hear other things, too!

A little later, work in embryology revealed that the ear of the fetus was able to function fully from four and a half months after conception. Better still, Norwegian experts proved this with audiograms as support.[13] They constructed

---

[12] L. Salk, "Mother's heartbeat as an imprinting stimulus," Transactions of the New York Academy of Science, 1962, 24, 753-763.

[13] F.H. Hon, E.J. Quilligan and P.J. Disain, "Auditory-evoked potential in the human foetus: a preliminary report," Acta Otolaryngologia 57, 188, Stockholm 1967.

these audiograms to estimate the damage caused to the fetus by certain maternal maladies, for example rubella (German measles) which is capable of injuring the auditory nerve. To obtain these audiograms, sounds are sent in the direction of the uterus by means of vaginal probes. The fetal heartbeat sound is monitored in response to the sound being sent. According to the cardiac reactions, an exact idea may be obtained of acoustic sensitivity. It is a question of determining what the listening powers of the embryo may be by means of the counterreactions provoked at the neurovegetative level.

I myself am sure that hearing within the womb starts even earlier. Many phenomena which occur immediately after the fertilization of the ovum escape our notice. When we learn to recognize them better, we will realize that the embryo is sensitive to sound much earlier than people are now willing to admit.

Not long ago, I treated a child of four and a half years who was brought to me with a total verbal block. The little girl responded quickly to treatment and soon began to speak. She came to treatment sessions with her mother, as I asked, and also with her father who drove the family car.

This father was a merchant seaman and not often at home. I was lucky that he was on land at the particular stage of treatment where I often needed the father's cooperation. It was better luck still that this father did not show any great resistance, unlike many fathers, to what was happening. He was very interested in the proceedings, asked questions, talked to me about what was happening, and, in general, willingly accepted his part in the treatment.

The child had already begun to speak when her father said to me, "Listen, Doctor, I don't know what is happening but there is something that seems to me extraordinary. My wife and I have four children, which makes it difficult for us to find privacy in our apartment and say things they ought not to hear. Well, we've solved the problem. When we need to communicate this sort of thing to each other we use English, which we both speak fluently. Now the child you are treating gives the impression of understanding English even better than French! But she has never had a single English lesson in her life."

"Then surely," I retorted, "your wife spoke English during her pregnancy."

"During her pregnancy? Oh no, not at all!"

How puzzling. We were going to have to find another explanation. Since I was overwhelmed with work, I did not give it another thought until a week later when the child returned for another treatment. As soon as he saw me, her father said, "I owe you an apology."

"An apology?" I asked.

"Yes, I made a mistake last week. I made a categorical statement, but when I went to verify it, I found I was wrong. I questioned my wife and she reminded me that when she was pregnant with the child she worked as an English translator in an import/export business."

"May I ask you at what stage of pregnancy?"

"Only for the first three months," he said.

I suspect this anecdote will only serve to prolong theoretical argument. Yet the incident is in no way an isolated one. I run into unsolicited examples of this sort every week, if not every day. I only related this one because it is one of the most recent and so more immediately memorable.

The development of listening takes place in the deepest darkness of the womb. I place its beginning in the first days after conception. That is early enough; I do not embrace the theory of a previous life, as some people do.

Plenty of questions remained. For example, what phenomena occurred when a child whose mother was unbalanced psychoemotionally was born autistic? How did the transmission take place? To what system or process must one refer? Should one indict, as some people do, the whole package of genetic factors? I myself lean more towards a strictly psychological formulation.

Thus the process in question had to be determined. For that purpose, I carefully studied the case histories of patients and of their mothers. I interviewed the mothers in depth. As a result, I soon established a positive correlation between the begetting of an autistic child and rejection by its mother who had not wanted the child (no doubt because she herself lacked the desire for life), had borne her pregnancy with difficulty, had sought an abortion, etc.

The refusal or rejection of a child is what makes it autistic. Even at the embryonic stage it is going to be aware of this negative reaction on the mother's part. The intuitive "registering" of this more or less manifest hostility brings about, on the fringes of the growing child's awareness, a sense of being cut off from the external world, as opposed to the sense of bonding or belonging which occurs in normal children.

However, the repercussions of a mother's rejection are not the same for all children. Most happily, not all children who are unwanted are born autistic. What makes the difference is the system's ability to bend in one way or another by virtue of one's inborn temperament.

Characterization assists us in this matter. We classify the most fragile types as emotional, intuitive, or spiritual. Degree of vulnerability is proportional to degree of emotiveness. Those who become autistic attain the level of a paroxysm. They cannot bear any cutting off of contact with the mother. When the mother introjects the idea into the embryo that it is rejected, she triggers a crisis which is going to weigh heavily on the whole future of the child.

Even before birth the child feels itself cut off from the world, so it will protect itself from this hostile environment by developing a refusal to live, a determination to "not exist" in the most basic sense. Rather than consent to be "human" in the full sense of the word, it will become after its birth an animal of purely vegetative nature, and yet one endowed with colossal energy.

If such children do not integrate language, it must be emphasized that their ears are nevertheless perfectly normal. In fact, they could not be so dynamic if they were unable to hear. It is not the picking up of sounds that is in question. It is the symbolic realization of thought by means of the word that does not take place. It does not take place because the child's relationship with its surroundings, already disappointed at the embryonic stage, is no longer welcomed. What useful purpose could spoken language serve?

One of the characteristics of autistic children is that they do not have any desire within themselves to communicate with the environment. They do not experience that longing to go back to the womb, common among children who have been aware of their mother's love even at the earliest stage. Once born, the autistic child has no lost paradise to regain.

A human being's journey to maturity begins with a dialogue between the embryo and the womb. It finally achieves its goal when the individual becomes part of the social framework. An ideal sonic pathway exists which must be followed in order to reach maturity. When the fetus and mother establish communication, the fetus desires to pursue this further. After birth, the infant wants to extend this communication, first with the mother, then with the father, and then with society in general.

This ideal sonic route determines, at one and the same time, one's way of listening, speaking, and reading. Accidents during different stages cause specific types of problems. The path leading from the fleshy communication of the fetus with the womb to the most subtle and complex verbal exchanges is strewn with traps.

However, the "ideal" path is only an ideal which exists on the horizontal of the real and which reality only succeeds, at best, in approaching. A little something always exists, a grain of sand, a frog's hair, as Professor Leipp[14] likes to say, to throw one off the perfect path. As indicated earlier, as far as a child's education and upbringing are concerned, no program can be guaranteed to bring success. It is useless for parents to hope that no mistakes will be made, that no accident or untoward happening will occur. A wide range of problems exist between a benign speech problem, which often corrects itself, and the absence of any desire to speak which is peculiar to the autistic child. All blunders, all unlucky chances are not accompanied by such serious failings! In the vast majority of cases, listening and language finally establish themselves in a satisfactory way, even if enormous difficulties have to be overcome to achieve this. Sometimes, the process of readjustment comes about by itself. In other circumstances, with problems such as stuttering, dyslexia, or a certain type of deafness, outside help is necessary.

Up to this point, I have used the word treatment to describe such help. I

---

[14] A well-known University of Paris Professor, Director of Psychoacoustic Laboratory who died in 1987.

would like to make it clear that this is solely for reasons of convenience. "Training" seems to me a much more suitable term. Isn't it a question of coming to the aid of someone imprisoned in his own immaturity? I do not *treat* the children who are brought to me; I *awaken* them. For the same reason, the term "re-education" should not be used. To awaken potentialities that have not yet been expressed should not be called "*re*-education" but just "education." After all, existence can be considered a permanent process of education.

I recommend a method that is simple in principle: by means of a conditioning process, make the client follow the ideal sonic path from which, for various reasons, he strayed too far.

After establishing the most appropriate acoustic program to enable the personality to blossom, I use the Electronic Ear and some other special electronic connections to make this a living reality for the patient. I recreate the five main stages comprising the ideal journey.

We have given the stages names, whose only value lies in the use made of them by those who use the Electronic Ear. They are:

(1)   Sonic Return
(2)   Filtered Sounds
(3)   Sonic Birth
(4)   Prelinguistic Stage
(5)   Language Integration

The Sonic Return

Over time we have learned how people react to filtered sounds and what potential value results from them so that now we can prepare the individual by guiding and educating him, step-by-step, towards this quite exceptional and difficult-to-encounter intrauterine listening. The term "sonic return" conveys this preparation process. This journey is undertaken by means of a musical theme, usually Mozart's music which, in itself, is easy to take in. The time allowed for this sonic return process varies according to the discrepancy or distance (which sometimes seems astronomical) between the individual's auditory mode and the ideal listening posture. In fact, the time is rarely long, and after a few sessions, the filtered sounds are easily perceived through the earphones. These filtered sounds are the ones which reveal what is perceived in the womb other than purely visceral noises.

This return to fetal life can sometimes be accomplished in a single half-hour session. It is remarkable to witness the extraordinary power which the ear possesses during such an adaptation. In taking this step, we acknowledge something that is true in every human process: everything is possible. It is only necessary to find the correct form and manner of accomplishing it. This is as true for a child as it is for an adult, and particularly so for mothers. When mothers are asked to participate in listening sessions at the same time as their child, they often show a certain reluctance — not to say hostility — in the face of this suggestion. They do not understand the request since they feel that they are not personally affected. Also, to impose filtered sounds upon them without any preparatory phase is liable to produce a refusal, based on the impossibility, in their present state of enduring what seem to them to be such heavy, grating, even painful sounds. Thought must be given to guiding them, without rushing them, toward that universe of sound which they themselves have at some time refused during their own fetal life. A program has to be devised, based on music filtered somewhat differently. This procedure is more humane because it is more gradual. It ensures a more confident beginning and increases the chances of ultimate success. It is only when a child, or an adult, has been gently and slowly prepared for this ascent to intrauterine listening that we may consider proposing a journey by means of filtered sounds.

Filtered Sounds

In intrauterine listening the embryo is immersed in amniotic fluid. This state can be artificially imposed on an individual by means of a system of electronic filters that treat sound in such a way that only certain high frequencies remain on the track. Filtered in this way, the sounds take the patient back into conditions simulating his prenatal existence. This method of perception should rekindle his desire for a relationship with his mother, the most ancient and fundamental of human relationships.

One should not be surprised that filtered sounds are brought about on the basis of the mother's voice. This is both sensible and indispensable. The whole "secret" of one's relationship with the environment is contained in this, for this voice comprises a true "law of love." Our clinical experience proves that we do not obtain the desired results when we use another woman's voice.

This may present problems. For example, what can be done when the mother is no longer available, because she is dead or because adoption is involved? Actually, adoptions are not the most troublesome cases. We have sometimes brought about a certain re-creation of intrauterine sounds by using recordings of the adoptive mother's voice. I emphasize that this procedure is only possible when we work with a *loving* adoptive mother, one capable of loving her adopted child for its own sake instead of to fulfill her own needs.

Consider adoption to be something that provides a deep, unselfish, emotional support rather than mere material support mingled with the satisfaction on the part of the adoptive parents of handing down their name or compensating for something they lack. Many adoptive mothers agree to bring up and nurture a child to satisfy what they call their *maternal instinct*. But this instinct is not the same as a pseudo-devotion which often hides a desire to possess. Even bearing a child cannot induce a material instinct in the heart of those so-called *sterile* women or women who are not carriers of life.

The first task is to give the children back the sense of life that their own mothers did not know how to pass on to them. Several times, in Europe and particularly in South Africa, I was able to procure for a couple the joy of having a child while treating one or the other of the pair with filtered sounds, starting with the voice of their own mother. The desire to communicate, and so to share, to transmit life, appeared as a result of these treatments. It was then possible for these couples, who had been so crippled, to contemplate starting a family.

Here again the value of filtered sounds, connected with the idea of intrauterine listening, deserves further discussion. What does the dialogue with life represent during the fetal journey within the womb of a mother full of love, a mother who is preparing her child not for herself but for humanity? I explore this question at length in *La Libération d'Oedipe* (1972). This *ideal mother* exists in every woman, but is masked by her own mother's personality, a personality largely formed by a grandmother's ego that did not know how to free her child at the most appropriate time.

Listening to the adoptive mother's voice through the Electronic Ear may have positive effects on the development of the emotional relationship between the child and the adoptive mother. These relationships, as we all know, are often troubled by tensions and obstacles caused by the adopted child's frustrations of which he bears indelible marks. He will never forgive the woman who took him to her home for wanting to take his mother's place. He will never forgive the man who gave him his name for trying to play the role of his father.

We find ourselves at quite a disadvantage when a divorce or death deprives a patient of his mother. Then we have to turn to a different source of sonic material, starting with a chosen musical theme. But this new approach requires a very delicate touch. On the one hand, the technical laboratory work is very difficult, and on the other, the choice of music poses considerable problems since different musical themes do not bring about the same reactions. The musical themes which are the richest in high notes are the most effective, since they reach the area of the cortex where the cells that are intended for cortical recharge are most concentrated. One of the functions of the ear is to stimulate the cortex to give it the means of animating the body and the spirit for which it is responsible. High frequency sounds, transmitted harmoniously, help do this. Among the hundreds of pieces of music tested over 25 years, we selected and retained works by Mozart and Gregorian chants, owing to the good results they have enabled us to obtain. Much remains to be done in this area, particularly in the choice of modulations capable of being filtered.

The cooperation of the mother, moreover, does not resolve every difficulty. In certain cases, so much time elapsed and so many events took place between the pregnancy and the moment when the patient is brought before us that the mother's voice has appreciably changed. Then our first task is to make it sound young again in the laboratory in such a way as to restore the higher harmonics in the voice so that it meets the criteria necessary for proper filtering. Thus the ear to be educated does not have to play guessing games in order to be immersed in the recall of embryonic life.

In order to prepare filtered sounds of mothers' voices, we must get them to talk, something which is easier said than done when one is dealing with the mother of an autistic child. When such mothers are asked to speak into a microphone, after the process and the reasons for it have been clearly explained to them, often they can find nothing to say. Often, too, they flatly refuse to say anything whatsoever. Those who finally agree to do so, but without the slightest enthusiasm, end up saying some breathtaking things. A few moments of listening are enough to reveal just what extent they are implanting not love and life but hatred and death in their manner of speaking to their child. In these circumstances the emotional and psychological block experienced by the little boy or little girl is not at all surprising.

To overcome this difficulty, we changed our approach and asked these mothers to read a passage from a text of their own choosing. This amounted to taking a step back in order to produce a better start. All the same, the passages these women tended to select were frightening and confusing. In most cases, they consisted of comfort for themselves, who had never wanted to give life, in their position of refusal. While the majority of them no doubt believed their choice had been a haphazard one, their unconscious really dictated the selection. To give an example, not at all the worst, I pass on the words of a mother who recently recorded her voice at the Tomatis Centre in Paris, a recording which of course we remade after suggesting different content for the dialogue. Having left her glasses at home, this mother agreed to speak into the microphone and to offer, as instructed by the lady in charge, some gentle, pleasant words directed towards her child, a young girl of fifteen, who was suffering a deep personality disturbance. This is what she gave us:

"I do not know what to say to you. Yes, I know that you asked me to come here. Very well, here I am. I will do everything I can to make you happy and to bring about your good health. Of course, I have suffered terribly in my life because your father was so jealous. When I was pregnant with you, there was no difficulty with your father; on the contrary he would have done anything, as much for you as for me. He wanted a little girl; I have told you that I once lost a little girl called Aline, and at any cost I wanted another girl. At the beginning I only wanted boys, not girls, and when Aline died, I became pregnant straight away and had Richard. Although I was happy to have this boy, it was Aline I wanted. Then I said to your father, all right, now we must try again so that I can have a girl. So you were to be called Aline, after the dead girl, and you came and were named Aline. I was happy; papa was happy, too. In you we had a little girl who had been lost and found again. You were not at all like her because the other little girl had blue eyes, and yours are brown, like papa's. I do not know what has happened to you —— you say it is my fault and papa's fault that you are like that. I know that since you grew up, we have not been happy. Unless this could be the little one I lost, I do not know.... (silence). If you need help, I will do anything, no matter what it is. It is difficult. I do not know what to say any more. That is stupid. I hope that things will work out. I love you very much. I am happy to have you."

All this was spoken, in a monotonous voice, without any voice quality, any life, or any conviction.

So we were forced to choose another text from the passage ourselves, a delicate task insofar as these passages have to be free of all potentially aggressive impact on the child. The ideal text would clearly be one which had no psychoanalytic loading of any kind. Unfortunately, laying hands on such a passage is about as easy as finding a squared circle! Language, as soon as it occurs, carries an underlying meaning; as soon as human "nature" intervenes, a psychoanalytic dimension begins to appear. Since there is no technical possibility of getting our young patients to listen to music from heaven, we are obliged to be content with approximations. In fact, we have to satisfy ourselves with the most neutral material possible, knowing full well that it cannot be altogether so. If possible, we try to use text that has a positive effect on the child.

How can one assess the likely effect of a given text? Very simply, by observing the reactions it excites in the patient when transmitted to him in the form of filtered sounds, that is to say in a form that seems indecipherable when first heard, but which the child knows very well how to decode. If the passage is pleasant for him, he blossoms, gives signs of joy, becomes radiant. If it is not, he breaks down, begins to cry, and leaves the listening booth in despair. We have experimented with many texts. One of those which is better accepted and most likely to produce a state of well-being is Saint-Exupery's *The Little Prince*. It pleases both the mother who reads it and the child who listens to it. This text has never been refused by any mother or child.

Every mother records about a 30-minute tape. In order that the higher frequencies may be maintained for good filtering, recording apparatus of first class quality is required. The tape recorder should work perfectly up to 15,000 Hertz, and the tape must respond perfectly. Furthermore, the recording takes place using the Electronic Ear to ensure that the voice has maximum tone.

The filtering process carries the mother's voice just as it sounded across the liquid layers within the womb. This reproduction is made possible by modifying the acoustic impedance.

The number of half-hour sessions of filtered sound is increased or decreased according to the case being treated. Preferably, they are administered in intensive sessions at the rate of four to six sessions a day in order to as rapidly as possible set in motion the processes, which we shall speak about shortly. Dramatic changes are sometimes obtained after only ten to twenty hours of auditory training. An average length program for a case of dyslexia generally requires 50 to 80 hours. Of course, more severe language and communication disorders, such as autism, require many more sessions.

It seems that progress beyond the first stage does not occur as long as the patient has neither accepted the idea of communication nor begun to derive any pleasure from it. The aim here is to get him by means of a deconditioning process to rediscover the desire to live and to reveal himself outwardly. Moreover, the patient is not restricted to perceiving filtered sounds; we wait and watch in order to weaken his most personal resistances by inviting him to play. We suggest to him that he paint and draw, do jigsaw puzzles, and play games.

Such distractions are not always successful in deceiving the unconscious. In certain cases, the unconscious presents such aggression that it is cannot be put to sleep so easily. The patient may reject the filtered voice of his mother and demand to be delivered from this infuriating noise, which is making him so ill at ease. "It is like a bee right near my ear," a child said to me one day. "It is going to sting me!"

Such reactions are very significant. If one persists in a sufficiently subtle way (for example, by alternating the sessions comprising the mother's voice with those of filtered music), an acceptance of intrauterine sounds is finally accomplished. A desire to listen becomes apparent which is a prelude to the desire for dialogue. The "registering" of embryonic life of which we have spoken enables the child to reconnect with a past distant enough to be still untouched by any negative experience. It is a little as if all the obstacles which locked him in a painful situation and made our help necessary finally were removed.

Sonic Birth

Having overcome this first hurdle, we can move on to what we call the *sonic birth* (SB), the passage which leads from liquid to aerial listening. Several sessions are needed to accomplish this transition. However, we proceed very gradually when we foresee very lively reactions at the time of the sonic birth. In fact, there are some children who do not want to be born, so they must be invited to this experience with the utmost tact. In these cases, we start by working with sonic births brought out by music (SBM), and we defilter the sound program little by little in the course of several sessions. It is only after this *descent into the underworld* by means of music that we tackle a sonic birth brought about with the use of the mother's voice. This is carried out in an equally gradual manner until the child joyfully rediscovers his mother's now unfiltered voice.

However, it is not as if every problem is settled by waving a magic wand — far from it! To get a child to distinguish his mother's voice when he hears it is one thing; to bring about a new adaptation in this child's ear is quite another. When the sonic birth is brought about, we are not finished. On the contrary, everything is ready to begin. Now that the child is equipped for a new means of sonic communication, he must be prepared step by step to use this means to encounter *the other person*. He is not dragged roughly from the handicapped state (where, for various reasons, he took refuge) to a satisfactory auditory state. Artificial sonic birth must pay due regard to the successive stages that take place in natural sonic birth.

In other words, the patient will not immediately begin to hear *properly*. What he will perceive at first is scarcely more than a sonic blur — just like the one experienced by the newborn child when the middle ear is emptied of amniotic liquid and filled with air. So the sonic birth should not be imagined as triggering a reaction all at once. Rather, its action is comparable to the slow and gradual opening of a diaphragm, by means of which the child will rediscover the mother's voice only after a certain period of time. In order to renew the relationship of deep intimacy which he had with this voice during the last months of life in the womb, he will be plunged into a foggy chaos of sound which will only clear up little by little, until at last the first clear gleam of recognizable sound presents itself.

By means of his relationship with his mother (particularly his acoustic relationship), the child has the chance of finding his place in the universe just as comfortably as he found one in the womb. A happy relationship could give a human being, in the depths of himself, the awareness that he is a molecule in the cosmos, not by any means hurled there by chance, but placed in the unthinkable plan of transcendent creativity. It is *unthinkable* because it is far beyond the bounds of human thought. To accept this awareness is what may properly be termed "being born into the world." Everyone, unfortunately, does not move spontaneously toward this end.

Many events or accidents in one's personal history may throw obstacles in the way: for example, the lack or prolonged absence of a mother, emotional indifference or inadequacy on her part, the hospitalization of the baby-at-the-breast, or the isolation of a premature baby who is put in an incubator. A certain number of children experience an imperfect and traumatic natural childbirth. In such cases, the idea is to make the child relive it after previously ensuring more favorable conditions for this *rebirth* than for those which prevailed at his *birth*.

For many others, the rediscovery of the mother's voice has not taken place because the initial meeting never was accomplished. The problem at this point is no longer to make them relive the crucial moment of becoming part of the universe, but just to get them to live at all, since this essential step was never taken.

This constitutes an urgent challenge, for insofar as one has not lived this desire to be in the world, one is not in the world with the desire to live.

Prelinguistic Stage

After the sonic birth, the active phase, properly speaking, begins. It is active in a double sense. First, it corresponds to a frontal attack on the difficulties from which the patient suffers. Second, the patient is about to abandon the passive role to which he has been confined up to this point in order to play a part in his own liberation. Step by step, the child achieves a greater and greater mastery of language. But this progress can only take place if he is, in the fullest sense, the active power, or at least one of them.

The relationship with the mother which prevailed up to this phase was, in a sense, unique. It will now break off because the child desires to get in touch with the environment, to build up a dialogue with it, and thus begin a process of socialization. From this point of view, the phase appears like a preliminary education towards socialization.

By this means the child prepares himself to meet *the other person*. Has he not done so already by meeting his mother? No. At the deepest level a clear distinction can never be made between the child and the one who carried him for a long time within her before sending him into the world. Dialogue with the mother is more of a "monologue for two people." Of course, exchanges occur between mother and child: fleshy exchanges before birth and then verbal exchanges afterward. Though at first "infant" (originally meaning speechless), the baby-at-the-breast soon makes his voice heard. If the mutual encounters with the mother have been easy and happy, he is going to become an enthusiastic user of his voice. The babblings of a satisfied baby —— more correctly, the stutterings —— constitute in fact a chattering. Something like "areu...areu" is the first talk addressed to the mother, and it is already rich in meaning. Next will come "mama," "papa," "popo," "dodo," more complex words at which the parents marvel because they seem to convey such obvious meaning, but which actually at first are only simple soundplay.

I was intrigued that these "words" were formed by the repetition of a single syllable. To understand this phenomenon, we must remember that the two branches of the pneumogastric nerve (or vagus, the tenth cranial nerve), which link the brain to the speech organs, both reach the larynx, but by different routes. The distance to be covered is not the same on the left side of the body as it is on the right. This involves a time difference in the nerve impulses, depending on which route they follow. Therefore, it is probable that the repetition of syllables is linked to the displacement between the responses of the two sides of the larynx (the right and the left) to the stimuli which come, each from one of the cerebral hemispheres.

The simple sound modulation "areu ... areu" maintains physical communication between the baby and its mother. If it is eliminated, then "maman" or "mama" and "papa" certainly are the first words in the human vocabulary, as is popularly believed. But at the risk of disappointing many parents, I must make it clear that these two words originally do not indicate the mother and father. Their appearance is a purely mechanical phenomenon, related to the first breath, the very breath of our life. A child's first cry is contained within this breath as a potentiality awaiting only the desire to be expressed. As soon as the mouth wants to open, a cry bursts forth. The cry is bound up with automatic physiological processes. What indeed happens when the jaws and the lips move apart? The tongue and the soft palate move further from one another. When the mouth shuts again, they come closer together. The sound produced, a sort of musical coloring of the breathing, is cut off by the shutting of the mouth, but it is not interrupted. As soon as the mouth reopens (to the rhythm of a sucking motion of the lips, which is the most animal of all our automatic movements), it carries on afresh. Thus it is that the first "ma-ma-ma-ma" is launched into space. The parents, by means of a phonetic coincidence, then project a meaning into the sounds which is not really there.

Does this explanation put an end to a beautiful myth? I do not think so. Of course, this evidence of the existence of such a mechanism removes some of the charm of a baby's first words. But if we look more closely, the structural beauty of human language is in no way affected.

In fact, illusions often create something good. For example, when parents mistakenly fasten significance on a meaningless "mama" sound, they behave in a particular way, with smiles and caresses. This reaction is exactly what stimulates the child's awareness of the speech function. He understands that this "ma-ma-ma" which he emits as he breathes (and because he breathes) can serve a purpose — to attract the gift of tenderness and to make his mother appear when he wants her. I have often said that this is the way a young human serves an apprenticeship to the spoken word; it is how he perceives the power of the spoken word and its informative value. By this process man reaches the human level.

The whole of language is built on this foundation. Isn't the reality of its birth as wonderful as fiction? I have already written: *Truly, it is only the first word that counts.* It counts, yet it costs nothing since it is life itself, the presence of life in a human body. The rest is only a game. The individual amuses himself by making new verbal constructions by using his body, which is his instrument. So he plays scales with language. For example, when the gesture of sucking ceases, the lips retract and the sound "pa-pa-pa" takes the place of "ma-ma-ma."

Because of their usefulness for calling and making demands, these primitive words (or, more accurately, spoken sequences) quickly *become* charged with meaning, a meaning as universal as a baby's lip movements which modify the original cry. It is not at all astonishing, despite the differences of languages and dialects, that mothers are addressed in the same way ("ma-ma" or something like it) in all four corners of the world, for it is the mother who appears when this sound "ma-ma" soars into space. She is the one who suckles the child, just as this same "ma-ma" is rightly associated with a sucking movement.

The sound "pa-pa" is directed naturally to "the other" (a person *other* than the mother, that is to say, the father). Unlike the mother, from whom the infant does not ever entirely separate himself, the father is immediately looked upon as a third party. He might be called the closest of strangers. I like to define him as a constellation, near and at the same time distant, a constellation which more often than not appears threatening to the infant. At the father's touch, he feels crushed; he is afraid of approaching the paternal image. His great, visceral terror is of getting burnt there, for it is a constellation which glitters but which also sets ablaze.

The paternal mythology explains why the desire to communicate with the outside world (the mother still forms part of the inner world) and so to communicate with the father is governed by ambivalent feelings. The infant simultaneously welcomes the desire and mistrusts it, advances and recoils before it. This is what makes the development of the social stage of language so difficult and the introduction of the father's message into the child's life such a delicate, yet necessary, undertaking.

At the start of our experiments we made the child listen to the father's voice right after the sonic birth, but we had to give this up immediately because of the violent negative reactions the Method aroused. This is because the passage from specific language (that of and spoken to the mother) to the language of *the other* and others is not such an easy one. The infant finds that he needs this mode of expression at a certain point in his development, not in order to have dialogue with his surroundings, but to improve in some way his communication with his mother. In a confused way, he resents the fact that he can only attain a more sophisticated level of verbal exchange if he makes the other instrument of communication his own —— the instrument of the other person. So he is going to have to let the third party, that burning, crushing constellation, penetrate the soft, protected, closed world which the orb of the mother has set up. He has to do it, and yet it is difficult to accept. Some children resent this penetration as unbearable. It seems neither more nor less than rape.

The father's voice, which makes itself heard among the filtered sounds, is the horned devil breaking into the world of maternal sweetness, the intrusion of the legendary ogre, or of the beast from grandmother's tales. In this beast, the son encounters the undesirable, the enemy. So he reacts with the utmost violence: he flies into a temper, bursts out sobbing, seizes the earphones, and sends them flying to the other end of the room. The therapist and his aides have great difficulty calming the child. By prematurely injecting the father's voice, a real emotional explosion may be provoked. From a strictly scientific point of view, this type of shock is exciting because it furnishes rich and abundant material for observation. As usual, I learned a lot from my mistakes. The child's reactions to the father's voice, however unbridled they may be, are not without value. They reveal most spectacularly the image the child has of his father. It is significant that such reactions are particularly strong in a left-handed child, the one who specifically turns his back on the father and the father's symbolic equivalents, the right side and the word.

However, the father's language, which is that of society, constitutes an irreplaceable link with the environment, and the child is well aware of it. He is aware, too, that opening up this mode of communication will free him and release his own being from his mother's. But it is precisely this liberation that he does not want. He gets caught in the original confusion of his own ego with his mother's, even while he knows intuitively that this union is doomed.

It serves no purpose to try to defy this infantile refusal, to master it, or to treat it as if it does not exist. It is absolutely essential to remain patient and wait until the child himself solicits the father's approach, for he needs recourse to it to deepen his relationship with the mother. Slowly and unwillingly, the infant will finally approach the father's language of his own accord. This happens after assimilation and embodiment of the first systems of speech, which are set up by contact with the mother. Specifically, his nervous system must be prepared to encode and stabilize the structures and rhythms on which the future social language will take root.

The prelinguistic phase brings about the most rapid, effective, and complete integration of these phenomena from the earlier language system. In short, it constitutes the foundation of the father's intervention. Its goal is to guide the infant's hearing toward a way of listening to language that will be controlled by the directing ear, preferably the right one.

Gradually, we induce an auditory lateralization until the right ear dominates the audio-vocal control. At the same time we have the child listen to musical or vocal filtered or unfiltered sounds, counting rhymes without words, and later with them, and Gregorian chants. Little by little the neural tracts are established which constitute the rails and the vehicle on which the structures of social language will be built. (When we work with an adult, the short stories are replaced by vocal exercises taken from "sacred" songs.) After that, we continue with the structuring of language, which is destined to lay permanent psycholinguistic foundations. These experiences put the child on that path to verbal expression which is so necessary for a mature relationship with the environment.

Language Integration

This new phase begins with listening through the Electronic Ear to phonemes rich in high frequencies, which we call "filtered sibilants." Speech is actually much more complicated than simply a more mature perception of high frequencies and heightened harmonics. To attain this maturity, it is necessary to *open the ear* to these frequencies. The injection of filtered sibilants through the Electronic Ear contributes to this end. By this means, the individual's auditory ability is drawn towards previously unexplored areas. This operation takes place in gradual stages, 500 Hertz at a time, from 500 Hertz to the peaks of perceiving heightened harmonics: 6,000, 8,000, 10,000 Hertz, and beyond.

However, the easy notion of a formula should not deceive us: this is not in any way a passive process, since the individual's conscious involvement in the training is indispensable. This phase demands active participation from child and adult alike. Yet the scope for initiative is limited, since the individual is restricted to repeating what he hears during the spaces left empty of sound. Clinical evidence shows that this is enough to release the audio-phonatory reactions that provide us with a barometer of his progress. When the person perfects the repeating process, the proof will be at hand that he knows how to listen like his model (whoever recorded the tape). From the moment when a dyslexic, for example, listens like someone who is a complete master of reading skills, he is on the threshold of having his dyslexia disappear. A successful treatment from this view consists merely of integrating the auditory posture of one who hears well with the person who has succeeded in setting up an adapted relational system.

Alternated with sessions of filtered sibilants are sessions of filtered music, which relax tensions. The sound bath in which we plunge the child washes away his anxieties. This prepares him in the most efficient way possible for an acoustic encounter with the father, that father who is the carrier of the word of socialized discourse. Even if not perfectly serene, much of the emotional content of the discourse has been removed.

When the problem is to replace an absent mother, Mozart's music is the most appropriate, just as in the filtered sound phase. Why Mozart and why not Beethoven, Ravel, Bartok, or Louis Armstrong?

Perhaps it is Wolfgang Amadeus' precocity that provides the answer. He began to compose excellent works at the age of four and a half. He was born into an extremely favorable environment, where music reigned as absolute monarch. Even before his birth, Mozart was saturated with music. I have no doubt that such a situation prepared his nervous system to listen and to live only in music. Even while still in his mother's womb, he created neuronic musical "engrams" and adjusted his listening postures accordingly. It is not inappropriate to say that musical expression was the true mother tongue which enabled Mozart to communicate with the entire universe.

In a certain way, Mozart came into the world entirely *shaped* by music; as a result of the greatest possible sensitivity to music, he "encoded" his own nervous system and prepared all his neurovegetative responses. His pulse always beat faster than a normal one, a fact which may also explain why he used up his life so quickly. These inner rhythms are reflected in the particular cadences which characterize the whole body of his work.

The diffusion of Mozart's works through the Electronic Ear provides a desirable architecture for the neural foundations of listening (and more generally of perception), and so of the individual's relationship with the surrounding world. Under the repeated massages of this music, which the listener perceives in the guise of filtered sounds (reproducing intrauterine hearing), a whole succession of waves is created and organized. Later this succession of waves will be able to bear a message of semantic value, but at first it simply programs the body to become an instrument for all sound integration, and by means of this, the instrument of speech.

From the universal beginning of the Mozartian message-massage, a gradual differentiation begins to operate in such a way that the underlying pattern of each particular language may be built up. At this stage, the program will not be exactly the same for an Englishman, German, Spaniard, Chinese, Frenchman, and so on, because the way the body is programmed in each of these cases will have its own particular features.

A day comes when the child becomes aware that in order to make his relationship with his mother still closer and deeper, he himself must move towards the sources of the meanings of words, and *so toward semantics, and so to the seed itself.* Only then will he move of his own accord and allow himself to develop social language which the father's image represents (a move for which the prelinguistic phase more or less successfully prepared him).

I write "more or less successfully" because one must not expect too much from this approach. It broadly clears the ground of problems, gets rid of as much anxiety as possible, but it cannot altogether eliminate the ambivalence and intrapsychic conflicts which issue from it. Apart from exceptional cases, the transition to mature language is *always* difficult, even painful. The child is afraid of being overwhelmed by this universe of language which looms before him; he is frightened of being separated from his mother if he steps into this new realm.

Consequently, his reluctance to assimilate the clearly spoken message easily may be imagined. The contents of the message are not separable from its form, and this form itself is not separable from the personality of the father (represented by social language) as it appears to the child.

In any case, the father can never obliterate the image of the mother, even if the mother is absent. If the child is compared to a seed in the process of germinating, the mother might be said to be the soil which receives and nourishes it, while the father is the sun which makes it shoot forth. In a different way, the father is just as necessary to the child's development as the mother. The mother is involved in the emotional aspects, the father in the linguistic aspects.

Since the father represents the semantic realm, he is also what the semantic represents. This equivalence is such that it is not as vital at this stage of the program to engage the child in the universe of language as it was to use the mother's voice at the period of filtered sound. The child's movement towards "the word" may be brought about by following other routes which possess the same power and the same structural characteristics. So it is no longer under the guise of an actual being that the child encounters the father, but under the guise of semantics.

If, in very exceptional cases, the father is brought in to record the tape himself, it is best to filter his voice in a certain way in order to draw off from it what makes it unique and then not to re-echo it immediately in the unshakable originality of its real being. To play back this voice as recorded, in a way that wholly respects the tones and inflections that compose it, is like playing with fire. At the beginning of our experiments, we made this mistake with catastrophic results, such that the intrusion of the father's symbol has the impact of rape. If the problems that arise were limited to a violent but passing crisis, there would be little cause for anxiety. Unfortunately, this shock leaves deep scars; indeed, the damage may be irreversible. The child then would be deprived of proper language forever. His terror is so great that, faced with the word, he develops a reaction of shutting it out, which afterwards he may be unable to overcome.

It is essential for us therapists, when we prepare the tapes, to know how to strip off those elements endowed with too great an impact on a deep emotional level and to eliminate them in order to let nothing emerge but purely semantic substance. This is why it may be said in the form of an epigram that "The father is only heard when he is dead."

It goes without saying that the father must have all this clearly explained to him. He must have an exact idea of the place he occupies in the family constellation. At least in France, many parents ignore all problems of relationship; these remain a matter for specialists who are only consulted when the parents are confused by a treatment program that questions the very structure of the family, though it also lies at the root of the problem.

Besides, the majority of fathers have little or no sensitivity to the idea that a genuine dialogue with their child is vital to establish the linguistic bridge that will enable him to make progress in life. Unless the father's attitude towards his children is open and attentive and he is willing to make himself available to them and unless he makes a lasting attempt to understand what is happening in his child's psyche, the effectiveness of both psychotherapy and the Electronic Ear will visibly diminish.

In brief, the father should participate in the upbringing of the child just as much as the mother. The trouble arises when the father resists serving in this capacity, running away from our suggestions, and opposing them with all the power of inertia of which he is capable. This attitude, of course, has some justification. Unconsciously and very often rightly, the father feels he is personally involved in his child's difficulties, particularly in the area of language problems. At this unconscious level he knows very well that in the family triangle, he is the one entrusted with the word. Nothing related to the word then will be strange to him. In a confused way, he has an inkling that he is shouldering a responsibility that he would perhaps prefer not to assume. In fact, language troubles are often caused by the father's inadequacy, either because he does not want to or is not able to "give" language for a variety of reasons. One of these may be the mother's unwillingness to abandon the power that she exercises over the child and to pass it on to the father. More often, the father withdraws when we ask his help because he is in an obscure way jealous of his child and has no intention of bolstering his rival's strength by supporting the treatment of his weaknesses.

What diplomacy we have to employ to attract fathers within our walls! Some of them agree to cooperate when we make them feel that we absolutely cannot do without them, that their contribution is absolutely indispensable to us at this exact moment of the educational process. Some, however, still resist. We make them understand that if they refuse to cooperate, the treatment will last much longer, and the financial burden on the family will be a much heavier one. This is a solid argument, one which very few of them are able to resist!

As we know in advance the objections they will make, we have plenty of time to prepare our answers. For those who take refuge behind their professional duties, we offer Saturday and even Sunday meetings.

But when a father finally decides to cooperate with us, wholeheartedly rather than just obliging us, astonishingly rapid progress is made. Moreover, the risks of a setback are considerably reduced. There is one kind of case where the results are particularly spectacular — that is when the child's difficulties are the direct consequence of the father's problems. The child is treated by taking care of the father. In our field one must never neglect empathic phenomena. What happens around the family dinner table when the father is troubled and shuts down all communication? No one can get him to open up. An anxious person sows anxiety all around him. How could a child gain any sense of balance if he lives with people who have no equilibrium themselves?

I knew a couple who had four children. The father and mother were of superior intelligence and got on well together. However, all four children were brought to me because they suffered from speech and language problems in spite of obvious talents. One was afflicted with a serious stutter. Another was so blocked in verbal expression that he passed for a mental defective. I am not likely to forget them because in the course of several years I experienced the greatest difficulty in re-educating them. The treatment process was punctuated by regrettable misadventures. At the very moment I set this process in motion, one of them suffered an acute respiratory illness, severe enough to necessitate six months hospitalization in a sanatorium. I had to intervene regularly in order to maintain the good results obtained during the program. I might still be intervening if I had not taken the father himself into therapy.

Besides this man's very remarkable qualities, he also had what I call a *left-sided* voice, that is to say, a badly placed voice. As a role model for his children, he made them all *left-oriented*! From this arose all the problems for which I was being consulted. The children only suffered from one thing in relation to listening and speech: they were not *right-oriented* as they should be. At that point, I educated the father by teaching him to speak on the right, that is to say to express himself in a warm, well-controlled, sonorous voice. Thereafter, his impact on the whole family was remarkable. I had the pleasure a few months later of establishing that the children's case histories had rapidly passed into the archives. Since then I have regularly received satisfactory reports from his family, who from that moment were reunited around the father's voice.

From a more technical consideration, during this period of building language structures, we place great emphasis on the system of audio-vocal control. Using a second electronic gating mechanism, we can initiate a self-listening process at the moment the person repeats what he just heard or, eventually, replies to a question. Without even knowing it, the young dyslexic is led to hear his voice in the same way as a normal child hears his. He establishes a conscious grasp of this little by little and develops greater and greater precision of vocal control. The result is more and more perfect mastery of the self, of both physical ego and verbal ego. At the same time, the idea of "the other person" starts to develop.

The educator, to maintain his role effectively, must be very alert and at the same time keep a very low profile. Too much guidance here is not desirable since the effectiveness of psycho-sensory education is intimately connected with the "spontaneous" establishment of the mechanisms which comprise its foundations. On the other hand, one must be receptive to the child's slightest reactions, come to his aid as soon as he needs it, throw light for him on the process which is unfolding, and make him aware of the progress he is making. As far as this last point is concerned, we take regular soundings and draw up a regular balance sheet of his attainments. When the client's auditory skills have been normalized, that is to say, when he is ready to apprehend another person's speech correctly, then that relationship with a third party (society, the environment) has at last been accepted. From this moment on, nothing more stands in the way of establishing communication worthy of the name, a process which includes people other than the mother.

Once this stage passes the problem is to enable the child or adult to discover and accept himself. In short, after he achieves a relationship with another person, we use the Electronic Ear to bring about an encounter with himself.

This transfer runs parallel with a simultaneous reinforcement of audio-vocal control and the client's own conscious awareness of these mechanisms. In fact, the child will actually discover himself when he attains an absolute mastery of the spoken word, including the various techniques and modes of putting his thoughts into words. This discovery compels an individual to simultaneously adapt to reality, to conditions imposed on him by his surroundings, and also to his own purposes.

The ear is "a royal road" not only for speech but also for all the processes of man's adaptation to self and environment. To triumph over the parasitic power of the unconscious in order to attain a full relationship with "the other person" and then with oneself (both are relationships of objective reality) restores to the ear its true function, while the ear restores the person to his true function. The two operations are interdependent.

The ear fully rediscovers its role as an instrument of communication when distortions of the listening curve, which occur in the course of the infant's development, are suppressed. These distortions are one of the chief results of the interference brought about by deep emotional experience, which is the explanation of every blockage. In this listening curve, the unconscious cuts off one or another frequency band that it does not want to hear. Since each frequency band has corresponding physical features, the damage caused is not apparent merely in the ear, and since the psyche is not separable from the soma and our body sustains a rich and complex mental imagery, psychic problems almost inevitably ensue. For example, the autistic child is someone whose ear is closed to speech, although it is wide open to other sounds, which explains the exceptional dynamism of this type of child. The perception of sound can in fact provide a store of energy, the ear being a sort of generator that charges the cortex with electric power. Moreover, movement, through the excitation of the vestibule, also contributes to this charging effect, from which arises the energy required to maintain our verticality.

The listening training during this stage of the program assumes even more active cooperation from the client. The dyslexic will be asked to read aloud under the Electronic Ear in order to reinforce his audio-vocal control. I would like to translate *read aloud* as *read to oneself* because it seems to me that this better describes the Method's final goal and the interdependence of listening with the core of one's being. The person will still be encouraged to listen to an alternating series of tapes prepared in our laboratory. Some have texts recorded to excite his interest and hold his attention; these will also help motivate him to continue the program. Other tapes carry music, either filtered music to provide a secure and serene atmosphere or Gregorian chant to improve voice inflection.

As the program progresses, the handling of written language takes place with greater and greater ease. There is no obstacle to the child's becoming a real virtuoso in the subject once we have awakened his most subtle powers of listening and self-listening. Everything becomes possible from the moment dialogue is established, and the individual reaches this point when he considers himself to be a distinct element and yet inseparable from the whole human environment. Having reached this point, it is up to the school to carry on the process. The school often finds that the child who returns to it has become a pupil who desires and delights in learning. After a long dark, or semi-dark period, his understanding of letters seems like a liberation, bringing with it a sense of euphoria. In short, what we are creating are minds ready to learn. It is up to the teacher to form and expand them, without fear that the teaching may not be understood or may be distorted.

We advise the child when he leaves us to continue reading at home every day, in a loud, clear voice. I mentioned earlier the importance I attach to this exercise. It is not only those who suffer, or have suffered, from dyslexia who should do this, but the entire population, adults as well as children, those able to juggle with words as much as those who are intimidated by words. Reading aloud half an hour daily seems to me the minimum to be prescribed. Besides its deep though not always visible benefits, this method offers an advantage that may be immediately appreciated: it ensures a most effective storage of information. I often repeat to my clients that what has been learned in this way is never forgotten. Everyone must become convinced of this: educators more than anyone else should ponder the question and then reconsider certain a priori pedagogic assumptions. Which system is superior: to learn more or to learn better?

A child who learns his lessons by repeating them aloud assimilates them — more slowly, yes, but also much more securely and lastingly. The benefit will be still greater if he takes care — and this is what we ask our young clients to do — to speak towards the right hand and particularly the area of the skin between the thumb and the index finger. In this way, lateralization is strengthened, and this is always favorable to self-affirmation and self-realization. When involved in a discussion or debate, I always arrange my own seating as far as possible on the left of my principal interlocutor if we are side by side, or on his right if we are on different sides of the table. This little trick enables me to avoid ever losing my line of thought or having difficulty in finding words to express them. Try the same thing yourself; after several experiments you will be amazed at the ease you have acquired at such small expense.

The results obtained from the audio-phonatory system reach other areas as well as speech and listening. In particular, they concern the person's behavior, his natural gifts, and his reactions within his environment. The child who emerges from a program under the Electronic Ear is noticeably better balanced. His moods are less capricious, he has lost much of his hostility towards people and things, and he is more ready to enter into group activities. His joy in living lights up his face and expresses itself in appropriate reactions to events. His appetite becomes more regular and his sleep serene. He falls asleep more quickly and deeply, and nightmares become rare.

All these improvements promote better academic results which, in turn, lead to still further improvements such as a greater flexibility of attention span and memory. Increased powers of concentration result from awareness and mastery of audio-vocal control.

Progress at school is not restricted to stronger and more fluent reading, but is made in every subject. Since good reasoning is above all intelligent reading, supported by a complete understanding of the text, every improvement in reading reveals a greater familiarity with the language process itself. This improvement is generally accompanied by progress in spelling along with a more subtle grasp and more discerning application of the rules of grammar and syntax.

In its turn, assimilation of the correct ways of producing the written word brings about greater facility in composition. Also, the interdependence between hearing and speaking and between intellect and self-expression explain why very creditable marks are usually obtained for recitation.

Of course, the child finds a greater facility in learning foreign languages. And he may, as well, show greater aptitude for history and geography, since reading and memory play an important part in these subjects as taught in French schools. Very often the child obtains good results in physics and natural science; and mathematics offers him the chance to make the most spectacular progress. There is no need to be astonished by this: lateralization to the right involves a greater mastery of the notions of time and space, which is very useful for solving problems in arithmetic and geometry.

The child — and this is very important — is not the only one to benefit from the treatment. Indirectly, the family will also profit from these benefits in a general way. The anxiety of family members will diminish, and they in turn will show signs of euphoria. The child who is handicapped in his means of communication and expression involves the family with his own frustrations. If this is admitted, it may also be affirmed that the steps taken by the individual under the Electronic Ear enable the entire group to recover its health, due to the equilibrium regained by the client. Tensions disappear and bonds become more closely knit between various elements of the family constellation. The home becomes peaceful and, with this, personalities blossom as each person's desire for dialogue with the others takes shape. Each feels himself come alive insofar as he opens his own being in the presence of another.

The family gains even more advantages from the child's program when family members closely follow it and actively join in. Of course, not every form of intervention is a good one. For the parents' cooperation to be relevant, they must have clear and precise information. In particular, they must be warned that during the first several months of the child's program, he is going to show unusual reactions which may perhaps be disagreeable to them. If we were to remain silent on this subject, the parents quickly would become distressed, and, once again, their own anxiety would be transmitted to the child. We encourage them to be patient, and, if possible, serene. We also urge them not to become disappointed by focusing on school results alone, as parents of dyslexics often do. The difficulties met at school are only symptoms, the exterior signs of a lack of balance (to be more precise, an absence of harmony) that lies much deeper. It is by working at this deeper level that one will gradually succeed in eliminating spelling faults, reading inadequacies, and obtuseness in grammar and mathematics.

Do parents all agree and cooperate? Unfortunately, no. At least not from the start. There again we have to struggle step by step. Of course, they do not deliberately refuse to understand our work and cooperate with it, but they do develop a number of unconscious resistances.

We became aware of these by analyzing the resistances of the children themselves, which were manifested among some of them by difficult behavior over food: either the client devoured everything put in front of him, or he violently refused to eat anything at all. At first, we thought the hostility behind these aggressive reactions came from the child himself. But by looking at it more closely, we quickly perceived that these reactions were merely a response to a much more secret and underhanded hostility coming from the parents. The whole family was resisting, not just the child.

Even the best-natured of mothers and fathers will find their situation difficult if either of them has an unsuitable attitude to the situation. In this perspective, it is essential to brief teachers as well as to brief families. Unfortunately, it is difficult for us to initiate meetings with teachers in order to explain to them what we are doing; the family has to invite us. When the family understands the necessity of such a meeting, we are very careful not to refuse the invitation for such contacts, besides the fact that they are always fruitful for us by allowing for greater insights into the child's development. Once we have revealed to the teachers the changes in behavior they may expect, we usually must overcome numerous objections. This is particularly true when they understand that they will temporarily have to treat the child with a certain indulgence. In the case of a left-hander, in particular, the period of adaptation which corresponds to lateralization towards the right is sometimes difficult to live through for both pupil and teacher. In fact, before regaining his balance and making noticeable progress, the child may see his weakness increased and multiplied. For example, he will write more slowly than the others and will have more trouble in understanding how to form his letters correctly, which may hold back the rest of the class. However, this will be only a passing phase. Patience is all that is required.

The reception we get from teachers is nearly always an excellent one. Today, especially, it is very rare for teachers to be unaware of the problems of dyslexia. It must be said that such a handicap has epidemic proportions. As I have noted, there are over 1,500,000 dyslexics in France, and this figure increases every day. To come to their aid is a task of the utmost urgency.

Why this proliferation of dyslexics? The reasons are too numerous and complicated to describe in detail, but one of the most important seems to be modern life itself, particularly in big cities, and what it imposes on the relationship between child and parents, especially between child and father. Meetings between fathers and children are becoming less and less frequent. In the Paris region, it is not uncommon for the head of the family to leave home before his young children wake up and to return either after they go to bed or just a few moments before to wish them goodnight. In addition, the increased number of working women weighs more and more heavily on the time which mother and child can spend together. The problem is also one of quality of relationship. Very often when the mother returns home, she has to fulfill all sorts of domestic duties which leave her little or no leisure time with her family. In a growing number of cases, the child is entrusted to a third party from the very first months of his life. This can have regrettable results if he feels himself abandoned. It is a common error to believe that the infant is not aware of his mother's absence as soon as he has someone else to look after him.

To change one's life is of prime importance, but it is the whole of society and its institutions, indeed civilization itself, which is being challenged. At the teacher and therapist level, where one often feels condemned to mending broken fences, the prevention of evils may seem just a wistful dream. But at least one may work at identifying difficulties at the earliest possible stage. This early screening would allow a vast program of action for teachers from nursery school onwards. A preschool dyslexic is easier to realign than a child who has already reached the secondary level. The younger the child, the more powerful the effect of our method of training.

Teachers could readily be shown how to carry out early screening. A few simple tests would enable them to verify and pinpoint what close observation already revealed. Children who do not speak, who express themselves with difficulty, who are inattentive and incapable of concentrating, who are poorly lateralized, and who are emotionally unstable or immature are all likely candidates for dyslexia.

There is no reason why the remedy for such deficiencies could not be carried out within the school itself by qualified teachers. That would indeed be very desirable. In every location where such experimental programs have been set up, in France and abroad, the results have spoken eloquently for their success. Sometimes a few months were enough for the teachers to overcome a handicap that could affect not only a child's scholastic future but also his psychological and emotional development.

No doubt someone will ask, "What about the cost?" Surely to humanize a little child and make him into a man is something beyond price! Also, in terms of expense, the actual re-education of a dyslexic child by traditional methods costs the state far more than the installation of a joint program of diagnosis and rehabilitation using the new methods of listening integration.

11

Listening Specialist

1963 — I am 43 years old, and I am not dead! It has been proven that I can live and, better still, live happily. My wife, Léna, is always an ideal companion and manages everything. When I fancy launching a new idea, starting a piece of research, or undertaking a course of action, everything is sorted out as if by magic and straight away. She even goes so far as to lead me to believe — although I am not deceived by this, or am only half-deceived — that I do everything myself. That is the art of being a true partner. I let myself be led with a certain unexpressed consent, and I benefit greatly from the organization of such a partnership with this woman.

Our union was further sealed by the birth of our daughter, Emmanuelle. She was premature, like me, and we had to use every possible means to prevent her from following my example to be born at six and a half months, on Christmas Eve. With a thousand precautions, she was born on St. Valentine's Day, - February 14. In 1963, she was four years old. She provided both a blessing and a problem for our partnership. Once more I had to choose between my work and my family. In spite of my strong views of the importance to a young child of her father and mother, it was my research (I should say *our* research, because her mother was fully involved) which took first place. We made sure that Emmanuelle had the best possible second-best. My parents-in-law, admirable characters each in their own way, happily fulfilled the foster parents role.

My mother-in-law's greatness lay in her simplicity and gentle firmness. As the daughter of a naval officer, still thoroughly permeated with her Breton origin and as wild as the coast and the neighboring moorland where she played as a child, she had the uncomplaining character of a sailor's wife and daughter. She was humble in every respect, as if aware of the vast horizon, where the secret sea met the mysterious sky. The years had bowed her, and her face was withered and wrinkled, as if engraved by the slow assault of time which erodes and hollows out.

She was an incomparable mother-in-law. I understood her without any need for words. Our silent communion was boundlessly rich and of a never ending quality. She raised Emmanuelle just as she had brought up Léna. Understanding the laws of real motherhood, she never attempted to take her daughter's place. She disappeared when we arrived leaving us alone with our child to have a direct and unambiguous emotional relationship during our moments of meeting. When we had to leave again, my mother-in-law immediately returned, her firm and gentle presence generating a sensation of well-being.

Even though the choice was made, we still found it difficult to live apart from our daughter, and Emmanuelle, too, must have missed us. We tried to make up for this lack, to some extent, by settling Emmanuelle and my parents-in-law at a distance not too far from us so we might visit as often as possible. We found an ideal house, surrounded by a magnificent garden, at Limours near Paris.

My father-in-law was a plump fellow, always jovial, and as roughhewn as my mother-in-law was delicate, but beaming and full of sunshine. He laughed aloud and played with Emmanuelle all day long, hour after hour. He was an excellent teacher, and enjoyed everything that nature brought him. He was equally happy in rain or fine weather; he sang from the time he got up in the morning, until he went back to bed in the evening. He was struck with wonder at plants growing, delighted with flowers opening, and thrilled with bird songs, but he declared war against cats when they disturbed nature's peaceful festival around him.

Near the end of the '60s, certain number of things changed in my life, particularly in the organization of my professional work. I remained an exceptionally active surgeon, operating locally on 50 patients a week. However, in parallel with my doctor's practice, I was carrying out more and more activities in the fields of education, re-education, and psychotherapy. It seemed the meaning of the "Medical Office" sign on my door had become both too narrow and too approximate. So I changed it for a more relevant one, "Language Center."

This was not simply a matter of semantics. This change was one of the great turning points of my life. Before 1960, I was an ear, nose, and throat specialist carrying out research in the field of *listening* (not merely hearing), and I applied the results as needed. After 1960, I considered myself more and more to be a specialist in listening who also had some experience in ENT. Since I was overloaded with work, I had to make a choice. Without hesitation, I embarked on the path of audio-psycho-phonological education. This term seems a little uncouth in its complexity, and I know that it disturbs some people, yet it has the advantage of stating clearly what it covers.

A specialist in audio-psycho-phonology is what I am and what I call myself to those who come to consult me. Over the years, clients have requested more and more my services as *educator of the ear* and less and less services as specialist in ear, nose, and throat ailments. At the beginning only a few candidates for re-education entered my waiting room. Then, gradually, the trend was reversed until almost my entire clientele consisted of such candidates.

Devoted to my profession of surgeon and its practice, I believed that with reasonable good fortune I would be able to continue operating until I was 50 years old, although less and less frequently. I always said that I would lay down my lancet at that age. Very few people believed me, except for my wife. I maintained, and I still maintain, that a surgeon ought to stop practicing while he still possesses full mastery of his instruments, not when he is beginning to lose it. On the first day of January, 1970, I stopped practicing surgery.

Ten years earlier I had abandoned my activities in the Air Force arsenals because of administrative and working condition changes. The enthusiasm many researchers felt when they started had become noticeably blunted, and they resented the constraints imposed by the administrative apparatus, among other vexatious interferences. In the framework of industrial medicine our activities seemed to have less and less of the spice of pioneering and more and more the insipid taste of routine.

Perhaps I might have stuck it out for a few more years in spite of everything if other circumstances had not intervened. My arsenal visits were divided between half a dozen places scattered all around Paris. Back in 1955, I could complete my rounds in one working day. By 1960, with the increasingly formidable traffic problem, I needed one whole morning to get to just one of these suburban workshops and back again. That meant devoting half my time to my Air Force activities, something which I could no longer afford to do. It was a difficult decision to make, but, after much consideration, I submitted my resignation.

Becoming a full-time specialist in audio-psycho-phonology meant distancing myself from official medicine. As I made progress, I became more and more aware of just how inescapable such a rupture was. It is a break that today has been finally and fully accomplished. The development of medicine in the last quarter century has not pleased me. The most essential element, the human relationship between doctor and patient, has gradually eroded in favor of an extremely impersonal type of service, one which makes the patient an anonymous recipient and the doctor simply a machine for providing prescriptions. Medicine today is in the process of transforming those who practice it into computers. I have always tried to work in the exact opposite manner. This is one of my deepest convictions. I would no longer consider myself part of the medical profession if I had to be today's kind of doctor. In the name of my vocation to help and care for *people*, I refuse to be assimilated.

In the center which I direct in Paris, and also in our other centers worldwide, medical treatment in the accepted sense of the word does not generally take place, except in very specific cases which are to be found in certain psychiatric hospitals. In our work we assume a much more educational role. We teach people to "listen," and by now the reader knows all that this word covers. Poor hearing, poor reading, poor writing, poor speaking, poor singing, poor communication, physical distress, psychological illness, emotional disturbance, neuroses, psychoses — all these troubles are in a certain way the expression of poor listening, of the closure of the ear to the speech of other people. It is remarkable that in numerous cases purely medical treatment is made much easier, sometimes even totally unnecessary, by the success of the educational process.

Thirty years ago when I spoke of audio-phonology, many people laughed derisively. Time has passed and I notice that it is now an accepted idea and sometimes even taught at a university. Some of its chief proponents now come from the ranks of those who sneered at me in the past, which does not stop them from continuing to treat me as a charlatan. For many of them the vital element in the term "audio-phonology" is the hyphen which they employ as a symbol of separation! Such a system, as they see it, includes both hearing and speech, but keeps them at a respectful distance from one another. This is so true that in one American university, the best equipped in the world in this field, the laboratories concerned with research on the ear have been built several kilometers away from those devoted to research on voice and speech. This is not merely an anecdotal detail; it is a symptom which, in fact, illustrates the narrow-minded attitudes of those responsible.

This conception is indeed a faulty one. By arbitrarily dismantling the unity of the system, we are condemned to misunderstand its dynamism. It is important we do just the opposite and draw the words "hearing" and "speech" still more closely together by means of an integration represented by psychology. From the moment when I myself introduced this dimension, I grasped the deep and unfailing unity of the two words together. It was also from that moment that I understood that my true goal was in fact "language," in all its types and manifestations, whence came the name "Language Centre"[15] first given to our headquarters in Paris, then to certain French and foreign institutions working more or less closely with us.

I must say a few words about these "branches," which, for lack of sufficient information, have not always been understood in the right way by those who heard about them.

The reader will surely recollect the strong smell of commercialism which accompanied the original promotion of the Electronic Ear, although I had no hand in that matter. Similarly, at one time, without consulting me or even fore-warning me, various people (whose motives were sometimes more and sometimes less good) set up establishments in France and Belgium where they presented, as if it were a panacea for all ills, a machine that resembled mine as closely as a twin sister. Nearly always they had wanted "to improve it." The result? They went bankrupt in record time.

I do not say that the Electronic Ear cannot be improved; it has already developed considerably since my first experiments. But to succeed in this, it is

---

[15] Now called The Centre Tomatis

essential to have an exact knowledge of the physiology of the human ear.[16] Outside that knowledge there is no salvation! All the fittings one may bring to it, however spectacular they may be, are like so many obstacles to the proper progress of the training. The machine might become more impressive to look at, but it loses its effectiveness in the process.

In any case, one cannot hope to undertake a process of teaching someone simply by pressing buttons on a machine, regardless of how sophisticated the apparatus may be. In a therapeutic relationship, nothing replaces human contact.

Despite being well aware of the failure of these establishments, people have sometimes believed — or "chosen" to believe — that I was responsible for them and, in fact, that I was organizing everything behind the scenes, pulling the strings and drawing the dividends. Various people, even including members of my own staff, pretended to serve my interests while aiming to line their own pockets. They involved my name in dubious transactions. When I finally realized this, I began to exercise stricter control over everything which bears the trademark "Tomatis" or "Electronic Ear." It is still necessary for me to be informed of the existence in one or another part of the world of people claiming to be associated with my techniques so that I can intervene.

That being said, many centers have opened with my full agreement, even my collaboration. Financially, administratively, and organizationally, these centers are independent of the one in Paris. I am not their director, and I have no means of putting legal pressure upon them, although I may withdraw the apparatus in the case of faulty employment of the Method. The Tomatis Method is protected by a professional contract, which makes it impossible for certain practices that depart from the Method to be carried out. These centers are in no way branches of the Centre Tomatis on the Boulevard de Courcelles. This center is only one center among many.

Of course, all these establishments have a certain number of things in common, if only their reference to my ideas. When a center is created outside Paris, I am asked to give it the necessary impetus so that it starts in the right direction.

In order to meet our scientific and moral standards, these people must take certain educational courses at our headquarters. They may set up their center in their own way, but only after having satisfied this requirement.

Despite each center's autonomy, the Paris center fulfills a special function in relation to the others. Besides its educational role, it is devoted to scientific research and to the training of future "educators of the ear."

The trainees must take part in several sessions spread over about a year. Even before they undertake this course we try to get a clear picture not only of

---

[16] I have given an account of this in *Vers L'Ecoute Humaine* (Towards Human Listening), 1974, a book not yet translated into English.

their professional ability, but also of their moral integrity and their ability to love others, especially children, and to communicate with them.

Near the end of the training period, the candidates are reviewed by members of the training staff who make up a board of approval. This group may award a Certificate of Agreement to the candidate, who successfully completes the training and applies to use the Method in his or her area of specialty.

I spend a great deal of time organizing different training stages. My co-workers and I run courses, give conferences, make the trainees do practical work, and carry out interviews with them. These tasks are not always easy, for during the transmission of our know-how we are obliged to rid the trainees of pre-conceived ideas. Is this because what we are teaching is so difficult to absorb? Not at all. But the ideas being propounded are so unusual, even sometimes bluntly contradicting accepted ideas, that we can only get them into people's heads by submitting them to genuine deconditioning. The further advanced a trainee is in his own studies, the less receptive he may be to theories which go against what he has been taught already. All the same, now that certain universities are beginning to offer courses in audio-psycho-phonology similar to those we ourselves are giving, it is likely we shall have fewer and fewer obstacles of this kind to surmount.

We do not demand too exclusive a specialty from our candidates. Their formal education varies from the baccalaureate to the most glittering university degrees. Those with bachelor's or master's degrees in Psychology, Linguistics, Speech Therapy, or Education regularly take our training course in Audio-Psycho-Phonology (APP). In fact, we are sometimes highly suspicious of those loaded with diplomas, *because that may be all they have to offer*. Too often we have had the unhappy experience of people coming to us who are good at academic learning and keen to sharpen their skills and yet they are without the slightest human impulse to move close to the children. That is why we are distinctly more demanding of the qualities which concern the heart, altruism and self-giving, than of so-called intellectual qualities. Without doubt, as Péguy[17] wrote, qualities of character do not enable one to do without those of the intellect, and one cannot make a good teacher out of fine feelings. But, whereas the mind may always be educated, cultivated, moved, it is difficult to improve the heart by any external efforts made within the framework of a training course! A succession of disappointments has given us more insight. Today we are better equipped to distinguish the motives of applicants and so to reject those who are simply looking for a job or those who want to compensate for or resolve their own personal problems.

Candidates who are at the baccalaureate level can improve their knowledge and refine their education after having begun work in a center. In fact, they

---

[17] Charles Péguy was a well-known poet who was killed during the First World War.

often retake their studies as they prepare for a diploma in psychology or to obtain a teaching certificate. Those who have a university education clearly find it easier to gain access to positions of responsibility.

As I said earlier, those with a university education arrive at the center from very different disciplines: psychologists, sociologists, musicologists, linguists, speech therapists, teachers, doctors, in fact, every specialty which audio-psycho-phonology includes. The student directs his efforts to discover and learn about the dimensions which complement his own knowledge. For example, the linguist studies the ear and its relationship to psycho-affective reality, while the psychologist attends to the spoken word and to hearing.

Since we use an apparatus christened the "Electronic Ear," even electronic specialists sometimes apply to join our courses. At first what interests them most is the relationship between the machine and the human ear, but gradually they are caught up and want to know how language is born and how it works, what part psychology plays in the process, what are the conditions under which communication takes place, and so on. This intellectual curiosity together with the capacity to love is the trump card of the trainee. As a result of the free play of such curiosity, everyone's cultural baggage ends up the same, whatever his or her original field of specialization.

More and more doctors come to see us. Very few are ear, nose, and throat specialists (two in 15 years!), but an appreciable number are psychiatrists. This is easily explained because psychiatrists receive a more eclectic training than their colleagues and therefore often have more open minds. Many of them possess, in the highest degree, this intellectual curiosity to which I just paid my respects. They come to the center not because they are already convinced that our methods are valid and our theories correct, but to test both these assumptions. They come "to see," as so many say.

They also admit freely that their visit has an element of self interest in it. They are perhaps in a blind alley in their work and looking for the way out. The powers of medication, contrary to what they had hoped, remain limited. Even psychoanalysis fails to live up to its promises any better than drug therapy. Both medication and psychoanalysis, no doubt, have enabled psychopathological therapy to make enormous strides, but now they show their ultimate inadequacy. In numerous cases, psychoanalytic treatment reveals the essential knot of the disease without actually enabling the knot to be cut. Medication that works well in emergencies is much less effective in the long term.

At our center, the qualification for these psychiatrists is the same as for every trainee, regardless of discipline: first of all, to love other people. After having been brought up to date with what we are doing and shown the how and the why of our actions, those whom we have convinced go their separate ways to psychiatric hospitals or establishments for psycho-therapeutic supervision (such as medical teaching institutes), and when those in charge give them permission and provide the means, they begin to treat their patients with sounds.

Of all the cultural deconditioning processes we have to carry out, that involving doctors is certainly the hardest, for every doctor has a tendency to consider himself by reason of his vocation as one who is in command of knowledge. We, of course, suffer some setbacks, but they are compensated for by victories achieved in a battle royal with colleagues whom we never thought would accept our ideas.

The art of persuading a psychiatrist demands extensive patience! One of them, who had seen the Electronic Ear in a psychiatric hospital and had been intrigued by it, tested us out for five years before finally undertaking his first treatments using filtered sounds.

Many of the doctors who visit us wish to gain information about our methods rather than acquire practical experience. Year after year, the demand has become so considerable that we have had to set up special courses for just this purpose. As I have said, I have never seen any French ENT specialists in these courses. By contrast, foreign colleagues have and continue to sign up in great numbers. Men of great merit and sometimes of great prestige have come from North America, Latin America, England, and elsewhere. We have had people attending our conferences who are universally respected. Yet they make themselves as inconspicuous as possible. Some have even wrapped themselves in cloaks camouflaged to the color of my walls, for fear of being caught *in the act* by their French counterparts, who thunder so furiously against me!

This influx of visitors has compelled me to add more and more staff, at the risk of enlarging the Paris centre to monstrous dimensions. These co-workers, I want to emphasize, are nearly all ex-patients. Aware of the profound effects their sessions under the Electronic Ear have had upon them, they want to know more of the physiological and psychological processes the treatment sets in motion. In the course of this journey we have given them the means to undertake, revise, or improve their studies (psychology, education, medicine). Their interest in the world of audio-psycho-phonology has only grown as a result. They keep demanding more and more accurate information, and we have provided it. After a certain time they themselves become fit to enlighten others. We are extremely cautious about turning away young people who show a desire to work with us and to help others as they themselves have been helped. Time has proved us right again and again, as most of them have become excellent assistants.

When an ex-client asks us to introduce him to the theory and clinical practice of audio-psycho-phonology, we take him into the center with us. If he is accepted by the rest of the staff, we begin to entrust him with small tasks, while at the same time providing for his education. If he is still interested at the end of several months of this regime, he is finally integrated into the center's team.

Once the minimum of theoretical training has been achieved, the candidate may want to go further in undertaking or repeating university studies. He is free to do so, at his own expense. We help by making it easy for him to schedule his work around his classes. It seems we always have seven or eight students at the Center who are pursuing their own studies, most often in education, psychology, and linguistics. We also have had a few medical students, who left us for a time because of the incompatibility between official medicine and our approach. Future specialists in audio-psycho-phonology may very well emerge from their ranks.

Currently, more than 150 authorized centers worldwide accept, or rather demand, our supervision. These centers are devoted to activities which may be classified briefly as follows:

(1) Dyslexia and learning problems among schoolchildren, which comprise half the cases.

(2) Stuttering and other speech and language problems, which comprise 20% of the cases.

(3) Profound personality disturbances such as schizophrenia and autism.

(4) Behavior problems.

(5) Learning modern languages.

(6) Singing.

A little before 1960, speculators hoping to get rich quick set up dubious schemes bearing my name. Most of them failed, but one nearly succeeded. An ex-singer, whose position as General de Gaulle's secretary had given her considerable political influence, was setting up a school of drama in Montreal, Canada and also a college for the correction of voice problems. She expressed eagerness to make my work known in Canada, and I was tempted to make her my official representative in North America. She had already met with a favorable response from the Jesuits and was planning to set up a fine research laboratory. Unknown to me, however, she had also set up a society bearing my name, which had made copies of my machines and which were producing poor results. One discovery led to another until I finally realized there was no basis for collaboration between us. I remained on good terms, however, with the Jesuits and with the University of Ottawa, which also was involved in the project.

In fact, in the mid-1970s, a Child Study Centre was developed under the direction of a psychologist, Agatha Sidlauskas, a professor at the university. This Centre offered treatment and education programs, including our technique, to dyslexic as well as autistic and schizophrenic children. I visited the Centre regularly and was asked to be a consultant on a number of research studies undertaken by doctoral students. Three years later Dr. Sidlauskas retired, and we parted company.

If it is true that "imitation is the sincerest form of flattery," I have been one of the most sincerely flattered men in our profession. I, however, doubt the truth of those words! Systematically, those who plagiarized my work with the greatest impudence were also those who spread the most slanderous lies about me. Of course, they claim to have acted "sincerely" (that is to say, with a perfectly sincere concern to serve their own interests) but that does not provide any great consolation for *me*.

I use the word consolation because some of these intellectual pilferings greatly affected me — not so much because of the badness of the behavior, but because they sprang from people whom I had trusted completely. One of those was a student whom I launched on his career.

One day I received a visit from this student, who was in his fourth year of medical studies. He had come to consult me because he stuttered. As I talked with him, I learned that he had recently discontinued his studies and was thinking of going on the stage like his brothers. All my life I have mixed with theater people, and, although I have nothing against a profession in which my own father achieved renown for more than 40 years, I considered my client's sudden change of purpose to be somewhat flighty and, in fact, to show signs of being a deplorable caprice. When one has chosen to help other people and, in fact, has nearly reached the point where this help can begin, one does not back out on a mere impulse and for the love of applause.

I decided then to take this young man in hand, in a twofold way. On the one hand, I attacked his stuttering problem and rapidly succeeded in relieving him of it. On the other hand, I did everything I could to put him back on the rails of his first vocation. There too I was successful. He finished his studies, specializing in psychiatry, and began to practice as a psychiatrist.

As he progressed, he expressed a more and more eager desire to be initiated into our methods. There was no reason to refuse him. My staff and I, therefore, began to train him in this field.

I should add, for these details are important, that I supervised his thesis very closely (to the point where I was virtually the author of it), and also set him up in practice not far from our center on the Boulevard Haussmann. I provided him with all the clients he needed in order to start his practice. I even organized a reception to enable him to make all the necessary contacts.

I never considered this man to be an "adopted" son; the expression is much too strong. The misfortune was that he really did consider me as a "father," and, in the Freudian fashion, he had nothing more important to do than "kill" his father.

Armed with all that he had learned from us, he began to make his way into the world of audio-phonology and psycho-linguistics. Boldly asserting that he did not know me, even that he had never met me, he deliberately copied one of my machines, one which was no longer protected by a patent and was therefore in the public domain. To better affirm his own authorship of it in the world's eyes, he gave the machine a name, and proclaimed that he was the founder of a new science, one whose direction, he insisted, was the very opposite of my own.

It was this last point in particular that he advertised, knowing full well that it would not be desirable to overemphasize the differences in the apparatus. My ex-protégé gave me the reputation of an investigator from a bygone age, lost in the mists of an outdated science that had been completely outstripped by modern discoveries. He denounced the "absurdities" of my system; at least they appeared as absurdities to him because he had understood nothing of the physiology of the human ear. Finally — and this is no mean paradox on an analyst's part — he described all my ideas about the acoustic relationship between the mother and the fetus as figments of my imagination.

Even after I parted from this jolly fellow, he tried once more to make money out of some illegitimate projection of my discoveries. He went so far as to get in touch with my own patenting agents, who told me all about it. That is the way it goes in this world: everything comes to light in the end.

I had many other imitators, one of whom I treated for a listening problem and then trained in ENT and our Method. He caused a great stir at Annecy. After his start under our auspices, he quickly forgot his learnings about the relationship of the ear, voice, and psychology. We were asked to treat a number of people whose programs he had begun and who were left more distressed than before consulting with him. His ignorance of certain elementary laws of psychology and also his impudent way of starting therapeutic processes had limited if any positive effect in most cases.

I could continue this list for a long time. Not all those who find inspiration in my theories and my techniques are without talent. For instance, there is a Yugoslav linguist, who is sometimes put forward as my chief rival. Initially we were hardly in competition since we were working in entirely different fields. However, after several meetings with me he decided to extrapolate the results obtained with his essentially phonetic machines and extend them into the field of linguistics. His failure to appreciate certain neuro-physiological processes remained a weak point from which to advance, and, in addition, the material which his group used appeared to me in certain ways quite inadequate. For instance, the absence of general prototypical multi-channel gating mechanisms served to render the results obtained incomplete, if not of dubious validity. By contrast, the organization for the dissemination of his work seemed to me a remarkably good one, substantially supported by one of the most powerful ideological frameworks.

My work has been much plagiarized, much plundered, but I harbor no bitterness as a result. I will even go so far as to say that if the counterfeits of the machines I perfected were able to help more clients, I should be the first to commend them. What troubles and grieves me is that the majority of forgers are not content with exploiting someone else's ideas. They want the world to bear witness to their own genius — like a painter who wants to copy the Mona Lisa, then adds a large hat and a parasol because in his opinion "that was a good idea." As a general rule these highwaymen have labored in vain; besides achieving very little therapeutic success, they have not made their fortune as they had hoped. This manifestation of a sort of inherent justice is explained once more by the plagiarists' lack of modesty; they did not have the sense to limit themselves to simply reproducing the model. On every occasion it is this preoccupation with "improvement," founded on a failure to appreciate psycho-physiological realities that has caused their downfall.

However, let me assure the reader that I am not complacent. I am more convinced than anyone that my techniques can be improved. It is our comprehensive foundation, acknowledgement of APP principles, and continued research and engineering refinement that keeps our techniques on the cutting edge. I could not ask for anything better than their further development. But, first, the conditions under which development is possible must be established with great accuracy. To merely slap an alleged "innovation" label onto a machine already a quarter of a century old sets up a "tinkering" process that has no future.

Finally, there is no need to rob me of something I give freely to anyone who asks. Not a day passes by without any number of new ideas crossing my mind. For lack of time I cannot pursue them all. What a comfort, what good fortune it would be for me if young researchers really wanted to take these ideas and bring them to fruition. I would be so pleased if it got to the point where new methods, founded on solid therapeutic and educational principles, could be employed to bring stability and a happy life to people all over the world!

Centers built on our model are operating throughout Europe, Canada, the U.S.A., Mexico, and South Africa. The greatest problem is to train specialist staff. The Paris Centre clearly cannot manage to teach the whole world's supply of students of audio-psycho-phonology! The answer is to develop information/training units for future teachers in parallel with organizations designed to receive clients. Clearly it would be ideal for some of these organizations to be an integral part of the university framework, since this would guarantee strict control.

The relationship between the existing centers and our own activities, whether clinical or investigatory, is not always identical. In some cases, there is constant interaction with them. Others show evidence of greater independence, sometimes to the point of disregarding the guidelines I have laid down. The one point they all have in common is that they have recourse to the Electronic Ear.

The Electronic Ear is manufactured in France and one or two other parts of the world. I personally supervise and control the quality of each and every machine bearing the name "Tomatis" explicitly as authority. That is the least I can do. This represents an extra workload, but I prefer to put up with the burden of providing this warranty, not so much to protect the apparatus, but to assure myself that human ears are not assailed and damaged in my name. In addition, this procedure makes it difficult for greedy businessmen to get near the machines. I have the power to decide whether the apparatus may or may not be put in the hands of someone who requests it. Since I adopted this procedure, the bountiful promoters of "new ideas" have at last left me in peace.

I now have help approving each apparatus put into circulation. A committee, consisting of young qualified personnel, assists me and continues when I am not there.

I am learning to delegate my powers, to use a fashionable expression. My travels all over the world mean that I am away from Paris about four months each year. The day will surely come when I will only be able to give consultations from a distance. I will be engaged in dialogue with men, women, and children who are in difficulty, but I will no longer be able to follow them through to the moment, so satisfying to everyone, when their program is completed.

However, I cannot shirk my obligations as catalyst. In proportion to the faith I have in the methods I uphold and their effectiveness I have to go on being a travelling consultant to spread the word.

To tell the truth, I do not dislike being this kind of *mouthpiece*. I am sometimes led to believe that my principal vocation lies in such activity. The successes obtained from the application of my theories have entrusted me with the mission to spread and share them. I submit all the more willingly to this task, since very positive results are being achieved just as much when I am not there as when I am.

Let me use this opportunity to refute an objection often put to me. "You always take refuge behind your technique and the effects of your machine," people say. "But in fact your whole therapy is based on the personal relationships you maintain with your clientele, on transference phenomena, and on your personal image." I do not know whether or not I ought to be proud that a certain charisma is attributed to me in this way. I am sure, however, that this line of argument is not a valid one. When certain psychoanalysts explain away the success of my "treatments" in this way, I get the impression they would like me to distribute copies of my photograph to my clients so their treatment might be more successful. Well, it is not quite so! And the proof is, all joking apart, that a statistically comparable success rate has been recorded in centers where, after I had given the initial impetus, I never returned, satisfying myself with following cases from a distance or by means of local staff. Many troubled people came to these centers and went away again successfully treated —— without ever having seen me, even in a photograph!

It is true that I move more quickly than some of my pupils, but I do not find any merit in this. It is simply because I myself perfected the techniques and the apparatus (with all the groping in the dark that entailed) so I have a much wider range of experience than they.

However that may be, I have become the pilgrim of audio-psycho-phonology and although this involves a whirlwind existence and 20 hours of work each day (no free Sundays or holidays), I do not complain. I am used to it. This is merely the rhythm of my life, carried on from the early days at Neuilly. It is my good fortune to be healthy enough to bear the burden.

My travels taught me a thousand things. As the saying goes, travels "shaped my youth" when, as a child, I followed my father from town to town during school holidays. Travels also played a great part in enriching my outlook. By meeting cultures different from my own, I came to understand to what extent humanity is manifold and diverse, and how different human groups are in all sorts of ways, ethnic and cultural, grafted on a genetic capital already personalized. All these discoveries fascinated me, transformed my outlook on the world and on mankind. They influenced my theories and therapeutic methods, since I realized that these cannot be the same in every corner of the world.

We established in particular that, according to the cultural background, the average time devoted to each stage of the program (in relation to its total length and to its other stages) varies appreciably. This means that a person's fulfillment, or the "humanization" process, does not take place according to the same rhythms and schemata in every human society. The stages of development do not tally between cultures, nor do the points of delay or fixation. Perhaps someday I will have an authoritative basis for establishing a sort of *Geography of Language Acquisition*, a geography I already anticipate will be notably different. I think there will be great interest in tackling this multiplicity of mental outlooks from the psycho-linguistic angle. The majority of specialists are aware of the problem, but in this very precise field their ideas remain vague, and they must be provided with much more solid scientific support.

I traveled through different regions, societies, and cultures, through the most varied social classes and conditions. In my globe-trotting, I visited every sort of environment. I treated patients who worked in the Air Force arsenals in a veritable inferno of noise, and those who worked at the bottom of mine shafts. My profession also brought me in contact with kings, princes, artists, stage and film stars adored by the public, government ministers, politicians of all parties and holding every variation of moral principles. I met aristocrats and proletarians, productive people and idlers, noble characters and vile ones. I talked with them all. Through them I have learned many lessons. I know now that people of sincere and genuine character are found on every rung of the human ladder. I know, too, that one finds people of very fine quality among those who are hardly educated or not educated at all, just as much as among those who boast the most exalted diplomas. I know, too, that dishonest people exist in every country and race, at all levels of education, culture and talent, and social know-how and success. I often learned this lesson at great cost to myself.

My wife, my closest collaborator, continually shares the time devoted to my work and my travels. It would be very painful for me to be deprived of her presence. Besides, at both the emotional and professional levels, we form a tandem, which only works really well when it is welded together. I believe that by its depth and steadfastness, our understanding is a rare phenomenon among couples, even united ones. The reader should not be amazed to learn that my wife accompanies me on nearly every one of the audio-psycho-phonological "crusades" that I conduct all over the world.

As the years pass, the facts of life and those of my investigations intermingle. Everything that relates to my married life is strengthened and brightened by our exceptional mutual understanding. Each of us expresses what the other is thinking and together we lighten and embellish the hours which slip away day after day.

All the same, this life of travel compelled me to sacrifice something close to my heart: my family life, particularly as regards our daughter, Emmanuelle. The demands of my research and the duties of being a full-time father have been difficult to juggle from the beginning. I was compelled "to choose" with the four children of my first marriage, and, as we all know, to make a choice for one thing is to renounce something else. In reality, I believe *research chooses the person* more than the person chooses research. As for the decision to neglect family duties, one never makes such decisions deliberately, unless one is a monster. It would be fairer to say that one lets oneself be led by events or, more precisely, that one "obeys" (in the true sense of the word) the command "Go towards the voice that is calling you!" The course my wife and I are undertaking with respect to our clients and co-workers, in a way, also demands this. What is to be done when confronted by such a dilemma?

When she was a little girl, as I have said, Emmanuelle was partly brought up by my parents-in-law, in a way that remained exemplary. The quality of her upbringing gave Léna and me some consolation for the impossibility of our providing it ourselves. Later she joined us on our travels and, for several years, pursued her studies by correspondence. This certainly proved an exceptional opportunity for a young girl to open her eyes to the world — up till the day when, having reached the final class, she decided to leave home and fend for herself. She was going to be eighteen years old; she was going to be a grown-up!

Some of my worries are now merely the salt, even the sauce, to my existence. They grow big enough to make me believe I have the devil at my heels. But that is life, I tell myself; it has to be like that. Are we not here, the gospel proclaims, in the house of the prince of this world? The main thing is not to become too enmeshed in worldly concerns. I learned how to take in stride the sarcasm of my critics, and to even be grateful for the stimulus provided by the sound of their voices.

The College of the Order of Physicians summoned me regularly to demand explanations of professional misdemeanors and failures of duty which I was supposed to have committed. How could so many brains be mobilized to legislate so poorly? I tried to defend myself through the medium of eminent men and renowned office-holders, but all to no avail. Those who defended me were confronted by a narrow-minded hostility full of bitterness and venom that never ceased to surprise me.

What should I do? Fight on! Yes, of course, and as often as necessary, but with an honest opponent and for a good cause. That was not the case for me. At each meeting to which I was summoned by my peers, I found myself receiving unbelievable sentences for practicing medicine in such a way as to damage and dishonor it. I remained bewildered in front of these emergency tribunals. They took great pleasure in dealing hard and unjust blows, which might permanently affect a doctor whose only care was to relieve his next patient.

These calls to appear increased from year to year, and only left me short periods of respite between journeys abroad. Clothed in their magistrates' robes, my accusers continued to treat me as a malefactor and to do so with such regularity that even the most steadfast and obliging of my colleagues were exasperated. Finally, in March 1976, I grew weary and decided, in my soul and conscience, to hand in my resignation from the Order of Physicians, an order to which I no longer belonged except from force of habit, since for a long time I had chosen to follow a different path from that taken by the majority of my colleagues. Though I separated from the order of physicians, I stay a physician in my heart and soul and essentially become a researcher who applies what I learn in order to benefit others.

By separating, I acknowledged the predominance of educational activities over medical ones and my desire to teach others about our work when they sought us out. The increase in the number of users is a tribute to the success of the Method. Case studies from every center document the many variables affected in clients and explain why the Method's benefits and observed changes differ from person to person and are difficult to document in quantitative statistical studies. Many physicians now refer clients to our center and some have even become users of the Method themselves.

A page was turned, a sorrowful but necessary one, which enabled me to draw up a balance sheet. As the months passed, I took stock of my situation and set off again towards other horizons, enriched by an exceptional human experience. Especially in regard to my research activities, the balance sheet was positive enough to stimulate me to pursue my goal in the same direction. From the family point of view, harmony reigned supreme. My wife continued to support and sustain me in all our daily undertakings. My children found their niches in life and settled down. Psychology, medicine, and audio-psycho-phonology became the driving forces in their lives.

The uproar caused by my peers during those memorable disciplinary sessions called by the Committee of the Order of Physicians had the opposite effect of overthrowing me; instead, it recharged my batteries. "Recharge" is a word which has come to play an integral part in my recent work. It is a word that develops and explains all the remarkable changes we see every day in the course of program sessions. This is because the first function of the ear is to ensure that the cortex receives sufficient neural energy through the "charging" effect of the ear. If a doctor overlooks this, it is because he is misguided by the generally accepted idea attributing an essentially auditory function to the ear. Indeed, this latter function is very much a secondary one. It is a well-known fact in zoology that the auditory apparatus acts as a charging or energizing dynamo. It furnishes current to feed the brain.

The brain possesses, in addition to an electrical potential, two kinds of sustenance. One of these is ensured by its metabolism: in other words, purely and simply by ingesting food. In addition, it requires oxygen. But a brain may be perfectly well nourished and marvelously healthy and still not be able to think. To remain healthy it must receive sensory stimulation. This is usually in the neighborhood of 3 billion stimuli per second, for at least four and a half hours per day.

For its part, the ear ensures, by means of the vestibule alone, 60% of this electrical charge, by organizing and controlling equilibrium, verticality —— indeed, one's entire anti-gravitational harmony. The cochlea adds 30% to this charge, to the degree it is able to carry out its role as sound detector. Thus one may understand the important part which the cochleo-vestibular apparatus plays in providing electrical potential or energy to the cortex. Delineating the role the human ear plays as a transmitter of energy has been an important object in our investigations; this necessarily leads us to a better understanding of the results currently being obtained in related areas of study on the suppression of noises or the frequency modification of sonic stimulation. Considerable injury is caused today either by the barrage of noise, which assails us in such an exaggerated way, or by certain sound frequency ranges. Sounds have totally different effects depending on the different zones of the ear being touched or stimulated. Either they move over the body without providing it with any dynamic charge (these are the low sounds) or they activate the cortex and thus enable it to think (these are the high sounds).

In this sense, a brain very rich in "neuronic potential" is more likely to use its cognitive functions. Its creativity is enhanced while its essential activity, induced by the dynamics of thought, is aroused. By setting in motion these energizing phenomena, an individual can take command of himself. Moved by will-power, which underlies one's sense of autonomy, he is in position to settle his inner problems. Any success achieved by our methods of training has no other origin. In the behavioral sphere, this harmonizing of the distribution of cortical energy also explains the remarkable results we obtain with clients diagnosed as "depressed." We know how many people are labeled as such, as if the whirlwind in which each of us feels himself carried along condemns some of our fellows to be carried off by the waves without ever regaining the bank. It is also well known that the classic means of treating depression is itself problematical. At the present time, every therapist and every psychiatrist is fully aware of this. That is why research aimed at a revitalization of the whole self by means of the cochleo-vestibular apparatus must be unremittingly pursued.

At present, we rely most on the results of recent years while activating the therapeutic potential of audio-psycho-phonology in the treatment of Ménière's vertigo. The origin of this problem, initially linked to a hemorrhage in the labyrinth of the ear, has been modified in keeping with numerous different ideas. Nowadays, its etiology is connected with hypertension in the endolymphatic liquid. That possibility seems to validate the truth of some measures that have been carried out. But, in my opinion, this is not the cause of vertigo, but its consequence. Still, in my view, it is a matter of an irritative reactionary hypertension. But to what then is Ménière's vertigo due? I believe I have the authority to declare, as a result of the frequent recoveries we have achieved, that we are dealing with an anomaly in the tension of the stirrup muscle. This muscle, which regulates the pressures of the fluid in the labyrinth, can, like every other muscle and especially the facial muscles, be suddenly moved by independent, involuntary movements called "twitches." Each of us has seen or felt one of his own muscles suddenly begin to dance about without his having made any voluntary movement to cause this. Such a twitch often happens on the face, and when one questions those suffering from Ménière's vertigo, one often discovers its co-existence with a facial twitch. In fact, the distribution of the nerves in the facial muscles is similar to that which governs the stirrup muscle. Consequently, under the impetus of the stirrup-plate, which drives itself into the labyrinth like a piston, the endolymphatic liquid is going to be stirred up into a storm, so bringing in its wake a cataclysmic depression. In order to stop such a tempest, everything is put in play to relax this muscle, which is altogether too active. Hence vertigo arises, under the agitated movement of endolymphatic liquids, and so do buzzings (perceived as bodily noises, following the non-regulation of inhibitory phenomena) and hearing loss, as a result of the reduced tonus of the stirrup muscle.

Once vertigo sets in, the musculature no longer is able to easily ensure its normal functioning, and internal irritation triggers off a discharge which in turn brings about hypertension. Through use of the Electronic Ear and its electronic gating mechanisms, the hypertension of the stirrup muscle may be reduced, thereby allowing it to resume its proper balancing role. This is followed by diminution of the buzzing noises in the majority of cases, and finally the restoration of hearing to some degree.

These recuperative phenomena, associated with many others which lie outside the scope of this report, compelled me to revise my ideas on the subject of auditory physiology. Actually, I am not the only one to find myself in the blind alley where every investigator ends up, searching for a more adequate explanation of auditory mechanisms. If it is true that at present many elements may be easily pinned down, it is equally true that many important factors remain unknown. These constitute the stumbling block in the way of generally accepted theories. I revised and rethought my ideas, which are in opposition to the traditional view of how a human ear works, and integrated my discoveries in a more coherent system to offer a way out of the blind alley. A new theory arose from this, one which is still strongly opposed by certain people but which so far no one has been able to confute. Every theory has its limitations. This matters little; the essential thing is that a theory should cause our investigation to progress a notch and thereby push back the barriers of our ignorance.

How then does the ear work? Is my answer best presented here? The explanation is highly theoretical and may seem tedious. Let the reader who really wants to have more precise details immerse himself in a more serious book, *Vers L'Ecoute Humaine*, 1974, Volume 2. But for someone satisfied with images, which I relish myself, let him understand that the ear functions in exactly the opposite way from what is generally believed. In fact, the chain of small bones (hammer, anvil and stirrup) does not carry the sound, as is supposed, like a bridge of bone thrown across two banks, the outer and inner ear. This sequence of bones, due to their position and the play of leverage which they exercise beneath the tension of the hammer and stirrup muscles, has the function of putting the entire cranium into resonance. Sound, picked up by the eardrum, circulates then by means of this osseous route throughout the cranial box which, as a result of its being made to vibrate, implicates the labyrinthine vesicle through its contours. From this point, a balanced interplay of sound distribution and regulation is ensured, because a constant pressure is maintained in the vesicle, which the stirrup muscle is able to guarantee by its movement over its little bone of the same name.

This turns upside down the theories that have been firmly established for more than a century. However, this new approach, which (with the help of widely supported results) brings a complementary dimension to auditory physiology, must not be abandoned. Of course, I shall have to fight rigorously for this theory, which is at least original if not revolutionary, for although some people accept it, others fiercely reject it. Sadly, the majority of detractors deny it in unison without even having full knowledge of it.

One other branch of study is of particular interest to me, that of modifying behavior problems by using certain sounds. As far as minor difficulties are concerned, a normalization of the listening function should bring with it, by restoring the desire to communicate with the environment, a more harmonious relationship with one's family and social milieu. Beyond minor difficulties, there is a particularly alarming syndrome of epilepsy. Yet it, too, seems to have a good chance of being modified by our audio-psycho-phonological approach. A superabundance of medical literature exists in this field, and the sheer weight of documentation makes its study a very complex one. Certainly, the available evidence should not be overlooked. However, certain young clients showing symptoms of epilepsy have been found to improve considerably in the sphere of behavior and socialization after being educated under the Electronic Ear. This has made me wonder whether, perhaps more than has been previously considered, epilepsy in certain cases may be the result of psychological factors.

Of course, there exists traumatic epilepsy from birth, epilepsy resulting from an accident, such as a bar falling on one's head, and indeed, epilepsy related to ailments of early childhood. But there are also all the other kinds that have no explanation, those which have caused so much ink to flow, those which, to give them a name, are adorned with the description "essential." The more I move ahead, the more I believe that in the course of certain improvements and, let us dare to use the word "cures," that the course of the epileptic syndrome always evolves in the same way. From the "Grand-Mal" (or classic "extreme seizure") one moves to short blank spells, then from blanking out to the final resolution, as the doses of medicine are appreciably reduced. I have come to wonder, however, whether the triggering of a Grand-Mal seizure might involve the opposite process. It is as if a particularly sad and painful phenomenon might be cleared up by this blanking out of which certain children are masters. This fabulous mechanism for entering into a state of oblivion enables them to get rid of the emotional turmoil, which makes them suffer. The thunderstorms of the affective brain may in this way, by means of little fits, be eliminated or diminished. But the whole brain becomes engulfed in the flames of the crisis. Self-induced absentmindedness may spread to the cortical level and develop into a "large-scale" seizure. But oblivion is much better achieved when this sensation is repeated and awareness of what one needs to forget is blotted out. In short, it is like a man who drinks in order to forget and then goes on drinking although he no longer knows why.

An epileptic knows in some way how to give himself a kind of electric shock. This medical technique has been properly perfected in order to bring about forgetfulness of obsessional phenomena. Such a theory certainly deserves closer examination, and this is what I am engaged in more and more.

I am also exploring "somatization mechanisms," which are fixations upon one organ or another which become the object of the ailment. In fact, by administering "The Listening Test" one may not only gain insight into the way in which a being relates with the environment, but also discover somatizations in certain parts of the body. Such an assertion deserves some explanation. Let us simply say that the dialogue between the organs and the body as a whole does not always take place in a harmonious fashion. Anxiety, which is itself a form of non-dialogue or non-listening, attaches itself to certain organs, and triggers such ailments as otitis, angina, asthma, thrombosis, and ulcers. More deeply situated at the level of the cell itself — we find cancer which, it seems to me, is also a manifestation of disharmony, of non-dialogue, of non-listening.

It is in these areas, by perfecting tools specially designed to re-establish dialogue between one organ and other and between an organ and one's whole being, that our future work lies. Everything consists of dialogue, of language, and therefore of listening. It is no exaggeration to state that every disharmony in listening brings with it a disharmony in a human being's total integration, whether this manifests itself against some other person or against one's own self.

I spend the best part of my time on audio-psycho-phonology itself, perfecting and embellishing my reflections. I am carried along in its linguistic dimension, whether related to the origin of language, to the meaning of words, or to the aftereffects of sound repercussions themselves as they resonate on the body. We need investigations to determine, on a neuro-physiological basis, the essential structures from which are traced those of language itself. It appears obvious that man's linguistic mechanisms, which formalize thinking in identical ways in the verbal flow of diverse languages, only attain this uniformity of response by reason of an identical neuronic substratum. It is on such a path, leading towards truly applied linguistics, that audio-psycho-phonology appears to me to offer a particularly favorable opening.

12

Death Does Not Exist

In 1976 the first edition of the autobiography was finished and I was the first to be surprised. At the beginning, I must confess, I hardly thought a volume of this size could be created from the principal episodes of my life. At the start, I was pessimistic, and thought that the material collected from my memories would be hopelessly inadequate. After it was completed, I wondered if I had suppressed too much.

In any case, I hope I remained modest, whatever anyone else may have done to provoke revelations of my private life. I do not consider myself a public figure and think that my private life, to which I have referred very sparingly, is of no concern to other people. That is why I often recoiled from this project of writing my autobiography. I originally felt that the only justification for such a recital of the facts was their presentation as the author's "final book." In 1976, at the age of 56, I did not feel ready to draw up a final balance sheet, much less make my last will and testament.

In my work, I felt I was still a long way from achieving the goals that I had set for myself in the beginning. A colossal task remained. When I checked my bearings, I got the strongest impression of being at the start of something, not at the end of it. After so many years, everything remained to be done. After so many pages, everything remained to be said. Can it be that these pages had to be written merely "to clear the ground"?

A long time ago I decided that authorship was an absolute necessity in order to ensure the broad public dissemination of my ideas. If I did not do it myself, who would do it in my place? I had to communicate my experience in my many roles: as neurophysiologist, as otologist particularly experienced in juggling with auditory mechanisms, as specialist with firsthand knowledge of speaking and singing voices, and as linguist capable of throwing some light on the neurological and psycho-organic underpinnings of linguistic structure. My work schedule always included the preparation of books and articles devoted to one or another particular sector of my investigations, so this book was not my first. I wrote several others and published them in different places. My drawers are full of whole chapters of work that I started writing five or six years ago. I need to work on several manuscripts at the same time; it is as if I were building, in parallel shipyards, vessels capable of carrying afar my ideas on laterality, music therapy, singing, applied linguistics, the complex relationships between language and the brain, and other areas.

I also think about articles and in depth studies on Mozart, Beethoven, music in general, music of different kinds, distinctive features of music, and the neuropsychological effects of music. So why abandon these or put off their completion indefinitely? Was I wrong to sacrifice such works, which were considered so vital, just to write about myself when I felt, as I did, that my career was far from over?

In short, I developed a real resistance to this book, which increased the closer I progressed toward completion. I got to the point where I needed twice the time to talk to my editor about the last 50 pages than I had for setting up all the rest! A thousand questions crowded in on me —— questions that placed the project in doubt again and again. By what right does one speak of oneself in this way? In the final reckoning was not the whole project a most presumptuous enterprise?

At other moments, it was the futility of the exercise that plagued me. With pen poised, I challenged myself, "Haven't you done enough? Haven't you spent enough time burning the midnight oil, scribbling away or deciphering what others have scribbled? You enjoy struggling against difficulties; that is a fact. You believe that the obstacles you meet afford the best chance of testing the resilience of this form and matter called a human being. You think these struggles alone enable you to fulfill yourself, or indeed surpass yourself. But have you not struggled enough? Why do you need to involve yourself in this new fight?"

I took myself to task like this, and yet —— I continued. But as I went on, I pressed more and more firmly on the brake.

If I did not stop, no doubt it was because I always held the deep conviction that it is not up to me to decide what tests or trials I should or should not withdraw from. I am not a fatalist, in that I do not attribute anything to the whims of blind fate, but I am one of those who think that one should accept everything which happens to him, simply keeping alert so as to understand all these events properly. Everything that happens has a meaning. In the same way as everything has significance for the person who wants to listen well, everything has meaning for the person who wants to understand well.

The true meaning of this book I discovered accidentally, and as a result of a rather "hard knock." It was well after I had begun to write.

To persist in writing my autobiography, despite all my doubts, I clung to the idea that whereas all my other books were destined for specialist readers —— scientists, doctors, teachers, psychologists and musicians —— this one was for anyone who wanted to read it and peruse it at leisure. (I took care that the technical parts were as easy to understand as possible, provided that oversimplification did not alter their meaning.) I deliberately eliminated everything outside the sequence of events that made me the investigator and educator that I am. All other character traits were ruthlessly censored; otherwise, I am sure I would never have published this book.

But let us return to my initial resistance and the way in which I finally overcame it.

I know today that a premonition guided me. "I feel a repugnance towards writing this final testament," I said to myself, "because there is still work to be done, and my career is not yet finished." Here the beginning gets caught up in the end, and the end is locked up in the beginning. While I was destined to live such an intense life, although at my birth everyone was left to believe that I was dead, so likewise I was to experience the strange adventure of pursuing this book about my life while I was dying.

Perhaps the reader remembers how, while flying in a Boeing over the eastern coast of Labrador in the blaze of a triumphant dawn, I relived the conditions of my existence in my mother's womb and so understood my need for compression, a need which immediately disappeared forever. It so happens that I was also in an airplane when an accident occurred which was to simultaneously put an end to a whole cycle of my life and afford me another conclusion to this work. *I lived through my death*. I crossed the borderline of death and came back again. This is what happened to me in that plane. I belong to the privileged few who have been able to achieve the famous *descent into hell*, so often evoked in ancient classical literature, before receiving at the hands of Dante the inspired treatment that everyone knows.

As usual my program was overloaded, or what I call "well filled." It was September, 1976. In addition to my activities as psychologist at the Centre on Boulevard de Courcelles in Paris and at another Centre in southern Spain, I was assisting the centres at Madrid and Geneva, responding to demands from those in Canada, fulfilling my obligations as a researcher in South Africa, disseminating my conclusions everywhere, and working on various new writings. Besides I had to struggle with the claims of the Internal Revenue, whose complex mesh threatened to swallow me up and pulverize me, and the continued attacks of the Medical Council. The result of this remarkable combat could hardly be doubted. I struggled as much as I could, as if I were upholding someone else's interests, and was defeated all the same.

In short, I was worn out. The only thing that kept me going was my uncommon physical resistance which had never failed me up to this moment. Moreover, it sustained me so well that neither my staff nor I were aware of my true state of fatigue. I was exhausted without knowing it, and it was not obvious, except for an extreme pallor which some of my co-workers observed over the past several months. I was going to have the fantastic experience of dying of exhaustion.

When I returned from Spain, where under the guise of "summer holidays" I presided over a seminar on psycho-linguistics, I set off again immediately to visit different centers. I stayed one or two days at each, giving advice and answering questions from the directors. Then I was expected in Paris, where I had so much to do that during three whole days I scarcely had a wink of sleep. After this brief but severe overload, I left for Switzerland on board a small public service vehicle. I wanted to undertake certain laboratory tests on a group of machines whose manufacture had been put on hold.

I arrived at Fribourg early in the morning and started off again almost at once in order to escort to Geneva a lady co-worker who had to get to Paris. Then I returned to Fribourg where I worked until four in the afternoon. My task finished, I started off again on the road to Geneva with my wife and one of our friends. We were to take a plane to visit The Language Centre in Madrid where forty-eight hours of almost uninterrupted work awaited me.

We were seated in the tourist class section, my wife on my right, our friend on my left, when there was a loudspeaker announcement that Spanish airports were on strike and that landing might not be possible under the circumstances.. I was immersed in thought about the journeys I should have to take after I met my obligations in Madrid. My program had been carefully planned. I knew that people were counting on me during the following days in Geneva, Paris, Metz, Belgium, and then three weeks later in South Africa.

It was about seven o'clock in the evening as we approached the Spanish capital. My neighbor was reading a newspaper which bore the day's date: 17th September 1976. My eye was caught by a front-page article about South Africa, and in particular about various problems arising in the mines. It so happened that I had a good knowledge of this subject as I had often thought about it from various angles, particularly from the linguistic point of view. Furthermore, I was reflecting on my work in that country — at the University of Potchefstroom and the hospital at Witrand — at the moment when the article caught my eye. Better still, the point which was holding my attention was precisely the one I was investigating, about the social adaptation problems encountered by the miners as a result of their different ethnic backgrounds.

What happened? I do not know how to describe it exactly. It was as if this coincidence had triggered off a process of exceptional richness and intensity. At this moment I was nearly asleep. Afterwards they told me that I had abruptly ceased to be present except for my body which had become completely immobile. During this time I had the impression of plunging deep down a mine shaft, strapped in the compulsory protective clothing of such a situation.

I moved with dizzying speed toward the center of the earth. A thousand meters! Two thousand meters! Before my open but fixed and lack-lustre eyes the tangle of geological strata formed crazy images where I soon recognized scenes of hallucinations, replays as it were of all the challenges which had been put before me in the course of my life, no doubt to gauge the resistance of the material.

On the surface of this vast composite image floated, first of all, a representation of the problem which had just arisen unexpectedly at the heart of our home-life. Our daughter, Emmanuelle, following the example of many of the day's young people, had decided on the eve of her eighteenth birthday to break all ties with her family. Next, other difficulties appeared with the Internal Revenue and the Medical Council. The time had come to take stock; I was also able to consider my own attitudes, my behavior, and certain events in which I had become involved. All this was given me in one and the same vision where the different elements, in a most paradoxical way, mingled and yet remained distinct. My whole life was set before me in this kaleidoscopic way, with no detail left out of the picture. I was able to take in with one single glance the film of my past, from the present day to my earliest infancy. My life was then before me, as if engraved on a fresco transforming itself before my eyes. The time lived through in my awareness was beyond ordinary norms, appearing to me then as being both long and short; in the same way the whole experience seemed to unfold in a quick and agitated fashion as well as in a slow and sticky one.

Certain sad or painful facts, which had not altogether disappeared from my mind rose up again with unexpected intensity; I followed the simultaneous unfolding and reanimation of all the memoranda accumulated in forty years of relentless work, studious reading, and multiple investigations. My experience as a human being unrolled before me in a dizzying telescopic panorama of clearly defined but frighteningly mobile segments.

As I continued to plunge deeper into this mine-shaft the scenes of this fantastic visionary theater became more opaque. I entered a more and more viscous, shadowy universe as my fall increased in speed, or rather as *some part of me* continued this underground journey. My body remained on the surface although I was in no way cut off from that fleshy envelope in which I had lived for so many years. The shadows around me became denser and denser. I engaged in hand-to-hand combat with this darkness and oppressive airless atmosphere.

Now I crossed layers of mud. My eyes could no longer see through them at all, and I experienced a certain sense of vertigo. All this was not at all pleasant, and yet I proceeded without distress, as if I were sure of my way, comfortably and firmly clinging onto some lifeline. I got further and further from my body all the time, unaware of any regret since I remained in permanent touch with it. My speed continued to increase until it seemed to me that the final threshold must soon come, beyond which, after time had been abolished, space itself would sink exhausted.

Suddenly in the obscurity, which swaddled me in a layer of blackness thick enough to fill me with mortal agony, I saw a sparkling light towards which I was caught up and sucked in a more and more rapid flight. Happy memories crowded in to the edge of my consciousness. An exultant joy took hold of me.

A blazing light was the only thing I could see. This time I was caught in an upward movement, one that lasted an eternity, and yet moved with the speed of light. I was somewhere else, face to face with light of an indescribable glory and intensity. Nothing could equal the sweetness of such a fire; nothing could equal its radiance. Enveloped in this miraculous aura, I contemplated the image which had just appeared to me, that image which Fra Angelico, too, certainly saw, since he has given such a faithful reproduction of it. I understood at a single stroke that it was this light which had seized me. I understood that life, this life that I had seen pass before me during my fall, was nothing else but the path that led to this light.

Nevertheless, the loss of this purely transitory and precarious state of human existence was not granted to me. I suppose that if I have been given the privilege to cast a glance beyond the death of the flesh, it is to enable me to bear witness to what I saw in the course of my journey. I recall that as I returned to this world I caught myself repeating a phrase that I customarily use with people whom I am preparing to face death: "If you wake up tomorrow morning, it is because your mission is not finished." A voice said to me while I was being reunited with my body, "Your mission is not finished, old friend. You must go on." I recognized my own voice and then opened my eyes. An oxygen mask was on my face, put there by a South American doctor who was a fellow passenger and who worked busily at my side. There was a real clearing the decks for action on the plane. A forced landing followed, and then an ambulance ride.

However, I was perfectly serene after having accomplished this long and complicated journey. The only thing that troubled me was the terrible fright I had caused my wife. She had believed me dead — and, in fact, she was not mistaken. For a certain length of time, all my vital functions had ceased.

Somehow or other I fulfilled my task at the Madrid Centre, after which I went to Fribourg to recuperate, some friends having offered to put me up in a peaceful spot in the Gruyére region. At last I was able to obtain rest and sleep, with the additional benefit of being surrounded by a warm and generous human atmosphere. Everything about this stay was pleasant. There nature has a captivating beauty which renews itself all the time, and the people are polite, obliging, and full of kindness.

The medical diagnosis attached to this incident read "Neuro-vegetative-collapse." Exhaustion was certainly the cause, but for me, there was much more to it and, above all, something much better to be said about it.

This collapse came in the nick of time to help conclude the first French edition of the book and make a coherent whole of it. My autobiography tallied well with an *end*, the end of a cycle, and it is of this cycle that it gives an account. Now it is a question of my catching a glimpse of a new departure or beginning.

In other respects, I have a deep seated conviction that I was granted the grace to encounter the pangs of death so that I could have the experience while still alive of that descent into the abyss which has been so often described. Beyond that, it gave me tangible confirmation of what has always been my deep faith, to know that we never die. Death does not exist. More accurately, that which we call by this name is only the last flight that lifts us up into the plenitude of our being.

The result is that the complex journey of life appears like the series of acts which most people traverse without understanding, insofar as they remain bound by the stratified layers of their education, whether these are familial, social, or cultural. Only a few succeed in making the different stages of life's dynamic process objective enough to decipher them, in going beyond existence to discover the source of Being.

It is by the body and in the body that Being manifests itself. It is by language that it signifies its presence. But it is by means of language, too, that man risks losing himself, if he gets bogged down in the mysteries of a tongue that imposes its structure on him, confusing him in its sayings and suffocating him with its syntax. Hemmed in thus in the web of a cocoon, as thick and dense as a shell, the chrysalis of his creativity wilts, grows thin, wears away, and perishes. Henceforth, man is nothing more than a robot uttering all day long the platitudes that hold him enthralled. Fixed in an unspeakable presumptuousness that he is the master of his own destiny, he acts in blind obedience to the pressure of forces from which all humanity is excluded.

Towards what horizons did this new path lead me? What stages would I next go through? Ready to meet the toughest obstacles, trusting in the image of Life, bathed in its reality, steeped in its revelation, I started off again with enthusiasm towards Him who Exists. Helping some, relieving others, spreading my joy in living, breathing freely, opening my heart to all, responding to every entreaty, understanding more deeply the meaning of this motivation for life and the necessity of making it burn brighter in each person, I left this book to prepare for the next one.

Already I had come a long way. On the road of life I am forever moving ahead of myself and forever running after myself. A light illuminates this space. I am a seeker till I die, and, already, beyond death I feel that I shall not be lost.

13

A New Step

When one's direction in life seems set, it is easy to simply let oneself be carried along. But at each moment we must constantly take into account the reefs thrown in our path, just as the trade winds constantly stirred by the breath of life must do. A firm hand at the helm is required to navigate toward that one goal which alone gives meaning to one's mission. Léna and I continue our long journey with a richness and intensity hitherto unequalled.

The occurrence in 1976 was no mere casual incident and was strongly impregnated with the indescribable emotion I experienced in my trip beyond death. It acted as a renewal, a rebirth, and it seemed to offer no return. But return I did. I was another man, but a man all the same, whose vocation was to continue the journey among my fellow human beings and to tackle new obstacles.

My convalescence was a long one. With my devoted wife and faithful friends beside me, I was able to regain my vital forces and to reanimate the Paris Centre, which had suffered some damage to its internal operation during my absence.

Professionally, I maintained numerous international contacts. Both European and American researchers were becoming more and more interested in the universe of sounds and in the physical and psychological effects music could have on human beings. Studies concerning the action of music in this respect were proceeding at a good pace. I followed all these investigations with caution, knowing the weakness of the theoretical frameworks set up to evaluate them. Few references were made to the apparatus destined to receive this world of sound, the ear. The neuro-physiological basis of the vestibulo-cochlear complex was the subject of works that seemed to me to be on the wrong track. I remained in the music therapy movement and continued to center my investigations on the specific results obtained by means of the Electronic Ear.

My preoccupation with certain aspects of listening and communication problems also continued. Autism, in particular, never ceased to haunt me during my nights of reflection. Also, deep pathological cases grew more numerous among my Parisian clients, and I actually began to plunge into the world of madness — a strange world which reflects above all, in my view, a state of non-listening. The problem was how to get these mad people out of their self-contained world, how to help them to regain a sense of relationship with others. Once more I found myself confronting the source of this essential communication —— prenatal life. Pursuing my research on listening within the womb, I devised new hypotheses. I perfected a prototype of the Electronic Ear capable of reanimating even more strongly the acoustic experiences of the fetus. The technique was improved to better enable these crippled creatures to escape the grip of an abnormal world and to enter a social universe ready to welcome them.

For this purpose I had to work with mother, father, family, therapists, and educators. Nothing was simple. I encountered solid barriers that people had no intention of crossing. No one budged; no one seemed responsible for or appeared concerned with the problems of the child or adult.

In my view, the mother's participation is an indispensable condition for success. More than ever in the Paris Centre as well as the other centers of our network, the mother's help is actively sought. When she submits, the mother herself benefits from a number of sessions of auditory stimulation under the Electronic Ear. It enables her to become aware of the vital role she must play in her child's treatment. Endowed with greater energy and relieved of a part of her anguish, she then can face the distressing problem confronting her.

The father also has a part to play in this common enterprise to help the child. From the first interview and initial history-taking, he is invited to talk with us about the role he feels himself called upon to play in this four-handed *card game* taking place between the child, parents, and therapist. Without detracting from the others, it is the child who must win. The adult participants know that they must give up their prerogatives, priorities, and egotistic tendencies in order to allow the child to take his place in the family constellation and in the social universe.

This is not an easy task for the father. But during the last ten years, a noticeable change has taken place with regard to the father's participation in the problems of daily family life, particularly those which concern the children. In certain ways this has gone too far, making the father into a foster-mother and so causing too radical a change of status within the family. But the dynamics of parenthood have taken a remarkable step forward such that the child benefits from feeling better understood and integrated in his little world.

It is becoming less and less common to see a mother alone bringing her child for consultation. From the first appointment the father is asked to accompany his wife (even when they are separated); nearly always he agrees and is ready to change his engagements in order to fulfill his family responsibilities. This *togetherness* is, for us, fundamental. When both parents feel concerned about their child's problem, we know that we have a good chance of solving it. On the other hand, when the father is opposed to the treatment process, we do not accept the child's case. We know in advance we are likely to meet failure. When the father is merely absent (as with a widow or divorced or single parent), the problem is different and we treat it differently.

In my work outside this deep communication difficulty called autism (of which more will be said later), I found myself facing certain phenomena which particularly concern the child in his school career, but which also concern, to a greater and greater degree, the adult who is engaged in the processes of vocational training and memorization. This is a subject I ought to know well since I first approached it more than 30 years ago. Later I returned to study it in greater depth on the occasion of a Congress on "Learning Disabilities" held in Toronto in 1978. This international conference was the starting point for an adventure in Canada which for several years was to utterly change Léna's and my way of life and, above all, our way of thinking.

Canadian Epic

For a European to tackle the North American continent is not an easy task. To analyze the difference between a citizen of the United States and an Ontarian who seems to speak the same language is not simple. But to work out the essential variations that exist between a French-speaking and an English-speaking Canadian is a fundamental process that must be undertaken if one wishes to understand Canada as a whole.

Léna and I were not prepared for this. For several years we had moved around in the Canadian university milieu of Quebec and Ottawa, so we thought it would be easy for us to transpose to Toronto what we had been undertaking in Montreal. We soon realized that we were in another world.

Since there was growing interest in our special technique in North America, and particularly in Canada, it seemed to us an opportune moment to hold the 5th International Congress of Audio-Psycho-Phonology at Toronto in 1978. The principal emphasis was on learning disabilities and the close relationship between listening and learning processes. "Learning Through Listening" was the theme more than 600 people assembled to discuss.

It was a great debut. Various studies were presented on the potential effect of our techniques on school learning. Some recently completed studies for doctorates in psychology were presented by several University of Ottawa students. An interesting approach involving speech therapy and our Method was presented by a specialist from France. My contribution was to expound on *cerebral integrators*, the vestibular and cochlear ones in particular, which in my view constituted an important advance in the domain of neurology.

The contents of this Congress and the interest it aroused were so substantial that we were approached by a Canadian organization, MDS Health Group Ltd., which had been established in Toronto for some ten years. MDS is a health care company whose main business is medical testing and laboratory analysis. They have a major laboratory facility in Toronto with many branches in the province of Ontario and in several states in the U.S. It was suggested to us that we should focus our attention on the subject of learning disabilities. MDS was not interested in other applications of the Method.

This unexpected and substantial offer lifted our current work into a new dimension, from a small scale craft operation, so to speak, to an almost industrial level. The leap was an important one. Aware of the difficulties awaiting us, my wife and I were full of hope for the future. For once, substantial aid was being offered to us by a high level company. We could not let such an opportunity slip by.

In fact, this was a great chance for us to meet people with broad interests and unequalled human resources, not only for technical improvements but also for research. Unfortunately, some opposition to this alliance existed within MDS. We learned later that certain members were against the offer since they did not see the possible connections between medical diagnostic services and learning disabilities. They could not imagine the relationship that might exist between the ear and learning problems at school, still less those between the auditory apparatus and the nervous system.

Incapable of evaluating the scientific contribution that such a project might bring about, they were unaware of the new prospects that would be created for the benefit of children.

Everything new brings with it this sort of reaction. It could hardly be otherwise. History teaches us that an innovator always disturbs deep-rooted structures, vested interests, and those firmly established in the status quo. An innovator is above all looked upon as a trouble-maker, making people approach problems from a different angle and sometimes forcing them to make a totally new beginning. So it has occurred in every age and every place.

Unaware of the opposition both within MDS and outside it, we flung ourselves with our usual naivety into the marvelous adventure offered to us. The result was a happy one. We experienced moments of exaltation for several years in the environment of an outstanding company, one of deep humanity.

As we divided our activities between Toronto and Paris and kept an eye on the European network, we were literally taken in, looked after, supported, protected, mothered, and sponsored by some members of the MDS Board of Directors. Everything a researcher dreams of was put at my disposal: laboratories, technicians, large-scale experiments, statistics, and research apparatus.

It was beyond my highest hopes. Only one shadow darkened the idyllic picture: the limits set on the field to be investigated. I was used to dealing with several problems all at the same time, all connected with difficulties in listening. Narrowing the application of the Method to one field alone, that concerning "learning disabilities," really pained me.

For the moment I had to turn my back on autism, schizophrenia, epilepsy, depression, Ménière's vertigo, character disorders, psychomotor problems, in short, a whole collection of disabilities that perhaps at first appeared to have nothing in common, but which on more careful analysis proved to be a coherent group. For my Canadian partners it was unthinkable to throw these disorders all into the same bag. It was equally impossible to convince them that the whole group involved a simple but multiform reaction to a unique problem —— the loss or the non-activation of the desire to listen.

Because of the steady determination of my Toronto sponsors I devoted myself for several years to a study of the effects of auditory stimulation on learning difficulties. I soon realized that such a study, even though it involved sacrificing a much wider field, was well worth the involvement. A great deal needed to be learned about the obstacles a child meets at school in the areas of reading, writing, spelling, composition, creative writing, memorization, and learning in general.

The clinical and therapeutic results obtained in Europe over many years satisfied me and allowed me to plunge into new studies. I forgot that I had no statistics —— an unpardonable omission. MDS was aware of this lack and arranged a specific program to remedy it.

It was not a simple matter, I suspect. A genuinely correct procedure had to be established that was capable of adapting transatlantic criteria to European concepts. We trained the North American personnel in the way in which we perceived the problem, while we submitted ourselves to a specialized training course in order to assimilate the American approach. The approaches were radically different.

It was a rich period, but a difficult one. It was rich because it gave us the chance to work with an active and sympathetic group that was particularly dynamic and efficient. It was difficult because the confrontation between two ways of thinking, the American and the European, posed problems with methodology. The restricted framework, more and more limited, eventually totally dried up the very substance of the research. Findings that emerged from the statistics were a long way from representing what we considered to be the real value.

The first steps consisted in building up an internal procedure from the clinical data obtained from the results of our treatment of children with learning difficulties. It was necessary to start tracking down North American criteria capable of being adapted to our Greco-Latin mentality —— not an easy task. However, after 18 long months, we were able to draw up a report on the tests carried out before and after treatment by our Method.

This report was positive, and largely exceeded the scores expected at the beginning, but it did not fulfill the exacting requirements of North American research. Further proofs were necessary, more objective and more accurate ones, involving hundreds of parameters that had to be passed through a computer and interpreted by sophisticated data processors. We had entered the fabulous world of statistics. It is a world one must get to know so that at the desired time one may distance oneself from it and resume an attitude of objectivity of quite a different kind.

We then embarked on a second stage, which led to the official validation of the effects of our Method on children's learning processes. For a start, research protocols were developed and studies undertaken by researchers in three large North American universities, those of Windsor and O.I.S.E. in Ontario and of North Shore University Hospital, a teaching facility of Cornell University in the state of New York. Only Windsor and North Shore brought the work to a successful conclusion.

Each researcher set to work following North American methods and procedures with the aim of comparing our results with those of established remedial programs in Canada and the United States. It was a comparative study — putting our Method in competition with what had previously worked best in North America in the domain of learning disabilities.

Need one emphasize that vast amounts of time were spent preparing and carrying out research studies? A phenomenal sum of money was invested, a sum only America has the power to spend on research of this kind. However, everything was completed in the desired time. At the beginning many different measures of the children's behavior were used by the North Shore psychologists and statisticians. In this way they could assure themselves that all the possible effects of our Method were evaluated, even if this entailed making a selection later on to reduce the volume of results and to tease out the most outstanding.

For the two research projects, which involved children of different ages, the results complemented those already revealed by our previous experiments, with results more or less significant from one measure to another. The more complex the analysis, the less evident the important points became.

Could we have expected a more satisfactory outcome? Certainly not. However, there was a great outcry almost immediately. Based on hearsay and quotations taken out of context, unfounded criticism was carefully directed at our work all the way up to government levels. Groups of speech therapists, who were afraid in the beginning that we were not speaking the same language, put forth the same quarrels we had experienced in France. Although they lacked any proof to the contrary, these detractors were simply terrified by an approach they were unused to, although it was very close to their own work. Panic-stricken at being forced to rethink their own procedures, they gathered up pieces of ill-natured gossip, carefully elaborated them, and passed them on to anyone who might be concerned. Henceforth our experiments — such convincing ones — were opposed by a report, well drawn up from a professional point of view, whose purpose was to warn both the general public and professional colleagues against the program we were initiating.

The conclusion to be drawn from this North American experience is that all the investigations into our techniques were immediately vitiated by mistakes. In fact, it did not occur to anyone in these research teams to see what result would emerge by working in parallel with paired groups of children, one following a normal school program, the other using our Method. On the contrary, the actual comparison was between our techniques and "the best there was in the educational field on the North American continent."

The Electronic Ear itself was ignored, even though it was capable of providing results more than competitive with the weighty apparatus then set up in highly specialized institutions. The existing techniques had some effectiveness, but at what cost! Taking into consideration the professional staff involved over a period of years, the enormous resources deployed, and the investment in premises, their results were very inconsistent. Properly used and with no other help, an Electronic Ear could obtain in six months what entire psycho-educational teams might acquire over several years. The time factor was never considered in these comparative studies any more than the importance of the resources employed, with all their financial implications.

If our Method were adapted to treat educational learning difficulties, thousands of children could be freed from their learning problems in just a few months. A few hundred pupils, on the other hand, cannot obtain the same results in several years by bringing to bear those current methods employing entire arsenals of extremely expensive educational resources. This argument cannot be neglected by responsible people in the educational field.

This being said, I met the same resistance on the North American continent as I had faced several years earlier in Europe. There is no easy passage for the breakthrough of an innovation. It has to make its own way, and the cost is always the same — time. So with this particularly promising venture we were compelled to restrict operations to a minimum for awhile, although a few projects took root. While the statistical analyses were taking place, several Canadian Boards of Education[18] expressed their desire to try our Method. Arrangements were made by MDS for equipment to be set up in several Canadian provinces. Today some of these school programs can look back on a long and rich experience, such as the Sudbury Separate School Board in northern Ontario, which has a home-base center at Sudbury itself and a mobile program offering its services to several schools in the same school division.

In other provinces, too, specialized private schools were equipped with Electronic Ears and benefitted from the same program with very satisfactory results.

In parallel to these educational initiatives, private centers were set up in Toronto, Regina, and Winnipeg. In fact, new projects, with a broader field of action, were under consideration both in Canada and the United States. For some

---

[18] Also known as school divisions, school districts, or education authorities. They administer the publicly-funded schools in a specific region.

it included profound communication disorders, such as autism, and for others, the learning of foreign languages.

Then and now, in North America as in Europe, very thorough training is given to the professional staff who will apply the Method. This training takes place under my supervision, but teaching cadres are organized so the training may take place on the spot in some countries.

While these research projects and various facilities were being set up across Canada, I worked with an engineer on several prototypes of the Electronic Ear and an apparatus for the evaluation of listening, called the Tomatis Listening Test System (T.L.T.S.). I was fortunate to have at my disposal this specialist who was capable of understanding my theories on auditory physiology and of creating out of them a more advanced Electronic Ear and test analysis technology. The test system continues to be refined and developed using different components but always maintaining its original purpose and spirit.

MDS enabled us to make considerable progress and take the important step forward of controlling the most complex electronics through the use of a computer. This approach was not an entirely new one for me since I had previously been called upon to play with computers at the University of Potchefstroom in South Africa. But what I achieved in Canada, both in the design of new Electronic Ears and in the perfection of a number of pieces of laboratory apparatus (filters, densifiers, automatic level-control regulators), was for me a most fascinating adventure. I experienced unforgettable moments with this engineer beside me, asking questions of computers, selecting compatible models, and reassembling the previously used body of electronic data. We combined and shook up the whole, and the machine was created as if by magic. Of course it was not as simple as that, but I must confess that I found this type of work most stimulating.

Successive improvements gave me a taste for going further still on a path leading to more and more sophisticated electronic devices. Tomorrow's machines will enable professionals working with the Method to free themselves entirely to be at their clients' disposal. Already the current machines enable them to cut the length of training by half and sometimes by two-thirds, depending on the person. In 1982, we introduced a new parameter of *precession* in these machines.

Precession and Body Image

Introducing this new dimension of neuro-physiological data was a significant turning point for the Method. New investigations concerning listening mechanisms and the neuronic systems intimately bound up with them are at the bottom of this important improvement.

The listening function, defined in relation to the passive phenomenon of hearing, is an act in which the will plays a part. To listen is to want to hear and then to apply oneself to do so. It is to place the auditory apparatus, adapted to its maximum capacity, to catch what one wishes to receive. It is to pass from mere sensation to perception.

It is, in the strict figurative sense of the term, to prick up one's ear. For this purpose it is necessary to prepare the whole body by means of that sensitive sensory organ, the vestibulo-cochlear apparatus, and in particular to train the musculature of the middle ear and that of the outer ear. Furthermore, the organization of a whole neuronic structure, which depends on this dynamic function, must be set in motion.

This implies that the labyrinth (vestibule and cochlea) is prepared by an act of will. The preliminary *action* that constitutes the desire to listen precedes (hence the term *precession*) a whole collection of neuro-physiological adjustments that bring into play the muscles of the middle ear. The tension of the hammer muscle now has to adapt itself to the tension of the stirrup muscle, the latter taking charge of the functioning of the labyrinth. Then there is also *precession* of the stirrup muscle — and this is important — to the elements that control the mechanisms of the middle ear (such as the hammer muscle, the muscles of the Eustachian tube, and the play of internal air pressures).

The listening function does not affect only the ear. It mobilizes the entire nervous system by means of the vestibular apparatus. By its particular neuronic action, this regulates muscle tensions of the body (both static and dynamic) and relative position of the limbs. In fact, the vestibular apparatus controls everything to do with posture and gesture. This explains how the whole body is called upon when a question of listening arises.

In this way the nervous system organizes cybernetically the ear's response so that it adapts and prepares to listen and catch sound. It is then in a state of vestibulo-cochlear precession. Now the function of the vestibule is set off by means of bone conduction which, in this context, precedes air conduction. This is where the concept of precession of bone conduction over air conduction comes from.

This new approach considerably enhanced the action of the Electronic Ear on speech, voice, and body. Progressively in the studies I subsequently carried out at the Paris Centre, the refinement of precession has become more and more precise in terms of duration. I was led to construct instrumentation for both short precession (from one to ten) and long precession (from ten to one hundred). The latter is particularly useful in cases of autism, stuttering, speech delay (in Mongoloids and certain mentally retarded individuals), and more generally in cases where the body image is poorly integrated.

This idea of precession is a fundamental one in the realm of listening and one that opens up a wide path to new investigations of the ear and the nervous system.

The members of our network and I shared a great adventure on the technical level. It was difficult to learn to handle this precession, to adapt it to the most widely different cases, and to evaluate the results obtained on the body in order that, quite literally, speech, voice, and the elements (which together are called the corporeal schema) may be embodied.

The work is far from finished. We move forward step by step in an area that is thrilling, but difficult to control. The actual turning point does not matter, and precession takes its place among other great moments in the story of the Method: introduction of the electronic gate, bone conduction in parallel with air conduction, and tomorrow, I hope, other discoveries that will enable us to provide swifter and more effective programs for still more of those with listening and communication problems.

This Canadian period was for Léna and me an exceptionally privileged one both in research and in making new friends. Deep bonds were forged between ourselves and some of the people at MDS who were deeply interested in our work and extremely cordial to us. These firm friendships made it possible for us to get to know Canada better —— its culture, arts, customs, and aspirations. We visited its provinces and admired its marvelous scenery, the Rocky Mountains, and the sunsets in the vast plains of Saskatchewan. Experts in Eskimo art introduced us to their subject. The Canadian school of painting, with the Group of Seven at its center, gave us a deep spiritual feeling for this country we were beginning to discover and love deeply.

But everything comes to an end, and since 1983 we once more have been caught up in European operations. We left the Canadian team the task of carrying on what had been undertaken, particularly on the level of school learning. Sad at heart, but also full of hope, Léna and I left our dear friends in Canada to become involved once again with the Paris Centre and all the members of the European network.

The Return to the Fold

The Canadian adventure was truly a departure from the ordinary for us. My inability to contemplate any research except on the subject of learning difficulties was a real *sterilization*. I was so accustomed to letting my mind linger on anything that interested it that it went on working despite my intentions and only detached itself from a problem when it had exhausted or at least thoroughly explored its possibilities.

I had already considered learning difficulties and drawn my conclusions on the topic long ago; sets of statistics could in no way change my perspective. The universe of figures, which is so indispensable for this research methodology (particularly in North America), can only confirm what exists and only if one knows how to discover parameters capable of being translated into numerical form. A great number of subtleties exist that escape this type of investigation. However, for the person who refuses to consider the problem in itself in its deepest dynamics, for fear of being carried away by some theoretical or utopian vision, it may be conceded that statistical criteria lend credibility to a piece of research, no matter what it may be.

Back in Europe I was free once more to explore outside the one small area that had drawn me to Canada. I was quickly reattracted to the European approach, stimulated by its more clinical aspects and by the different questions that bid for my attention. My thoughts were constantly changing direction over a wide range of hypotheses. I was attracted to a deeper study of life in the womb and the behavior of the embryo-fetus. I also found myself increasingly challenged by the problems posed by autism. I pursued a new tact on Ménière's vertigo. I had a thousand occasions to concern myself with unknown aspects of epilepsy. Finally, I joyfully plunged back into investigations of the subject of singing and communication in general.

This whole collection of subjects served merely to consolidate my previous investigations of the ear and its physiology, neuronal networks, links with the brain, and impact on the human psyche. Continuing my many investigations of the last 30 years, I plunged once more into the fabulous universe of life before birth. This study enabled me to publish a work called *La Nuit Uterine* (The Night of the Womb) in 1981.

A Child's Listening before Birth

I was all the more drawn toward a deeper study of life within the womb because of the steadily increasing interest from within scientific circles. In several countries, particularly in Europe, people were busy, each in their own way, rediscovering from the evidence I had set out in 1953-1955 the knowledge that the fetus could hear.

Everyone knows now that I have no doubt that a fetus listens. My insistence in crediting the fetus with this faculty corresponds to my deep conviction that, from the beginning, the power to listen guides man and draws him on both in his biological development and in the course of his human life. In fact, listening is a high level ability that opens directly onto consciousness. Consciousness in turn knows how to use the power of listening to invade the being that abandons itself to it. At this crossroad a dialectic is set up between consciousness and listening, by means of which the one is all the more active as the other grows. The whole framework of human dynamics depends on their interaction.

I now avow with even more insistence and authority that the fetus knows how to listen, and that it does so only to high-pitched sounds. This is where the shoe pinches. If it is true that many investigators now admit the existence of fetal listening, it is no less true that much controversy exists about *what* the fetus is able to perceive. In fact, the majority of those involved in this problem conceive that the fetus hears mainly *low*-pitched sounds.

If such were the case, the infant's life would be a hellish one in the *paradise* of the womb. It would perceive the noisy clamor of the mother's intestine, which surmounts and surrounds the womb; it would be stunned by the ebb and flow of the mother's breathing; it would hear the ceaseless hammering and pounding of the mother's heartbeats; and it would be overwhelmed by the noises its own activity triggers in the amniotic liquid. Its life would be insupportable unless its ear had some sort of protection. By the grace of God, the ear operates and functions like a filter. It is able to sift out all troublesome noises, and it succeeds in this way in suppressing low-pitched sounds. The ear of the fetus acts like a high-pass filter. In fact, it is only towards 2,000 Hertz that fetal hearing begins to take place. This is true for the human ear as well as for animals such as opossums and rats. The elaborate human organism could not allow such an anomaly to be introduced; it would make life impossible for its own fruit before it even ripened in the mother's womb.

It is easy to verify anatomically that the ear of the fetus is not operational in the range of low-pitched sounds. Such a study has in fact been carried out on animals and at different levels. In addition, those professionally concerned with the reactivation of hearing know the beneficial effect high-pitched sounds (filtered mother's voice or filtered Mozart's music) have on reawakening a person. Low-pitched sounds, on the other hand, introduce somnolent or even hypnotic effects. Finally, an observation of a neuro-physiological kind leads us to the same conclusions when we study the child's voice. His voice begins to break in adolescence, a sign of the hearing faculty becoming involved in the area of low-pitched sounds brought about by the already well-known audio-vocal cybernetic loop. At the time the hormonal discharge at puberty causes the voice to break, the auditory spectrum and, as a result, the vocal spectrum take over the area of low-pitched sounds. This extension translates into one octave in boys' voices and a tierce in adolescent girls.

Our investigations showed not only that the fetus hears, but also that it knows how to listen because it is capable of integrating sounds. We also established that the embryo, from the second month of life in the womb, is able to sort out the data that reach it at the level of the vestibulo-cochlear nuclei. At this point the birth of primitive memory takes place, which later will be diffused throughout the nervous system as it pursues its own much slower development than that of the auditory organism. So the *embryo-fetus*, an actual entity as far as listening is concerned, is born, giving a glimpse of structures being prepared that lead to the human being, by implication already alive and vibrant since the moment of conception.

A Plea for Pro-Life

I am well aware that this approach goes against the current opinion that defines the fetus as a *non-being*, and so allows some specialists to cut up fetuses into little pieces to extract the active ingredients capable of treating *real children*. This increasingly widespread movement led me to take part in a 1984 conference held at Strasbourg under the aegis of "The Association Against the Exploitation of Human Fetuses." Doctors and legal figures were to meet to discuss the possibilities of making a stand against this trade in unborn babies. I was the only physician to attend, the others having disappeared in route for reasons I did not spend time in discovering as I had other things to do. The distinguished personage who was to preside over this conference also was absent. Only the lawyers and theologians faithfully attended. Full of courage and daring, they expounded competently and sincerely upon the statutes and decrees that conferred genuine rights upon the child from the moment of conception. They did not hesitate to bring into the full light of day the international traffic of this *product*, which had occurred for several years under the indifferent gaze of public authorities and medical circles. Thus whole wagon loads of human embryos and fetuses arrived at certain hospital laboratories and cosmetic companies.

Where did they come from? Doctors and experimenters did not know. They received *the goods*, but chose to be ignorant of their origin. Besides, that was not their business. The important thing for them was to be able to extract *live* organs, glands, and active ingredients from these parcels of human flesh delivered to them —— at a price, of course.

The mothers who had been carrying these exploitable children before their birth were knowingly prepared by professional abortionists who carried out caesarean operations. The pregnancies were ended at a definite date, a date which was postponed further and further —— up to six months and more in order that the fetus could be really *alive* before being dissected.

The courageous movement against these barbarous practices continues in spite of the conspiracy of silence of which we are well aware. Articles, radio interviews, and public appearances by lawyers are regularly canceled, curtailed, or hidden from view. As far as we are concerned, a human being is *listening in* from the moment of that first spark of life marking its conception; during its period in the womb it has experiences of the highest importance for its future as a human being.

At a time when the contraceptive pill has thrown birth statistics into confusion, when efforts are being made to manufacture test-tube babies, and when decadent morals are destroying the whole family constellation, it seems important to us to re-establish certain essential ideas about life itself and the potentialities it contains.

Should not society make and enforce laws which protect and respect the rights and responsibilities of women as child bearers? Does not society let us down, by not valuing the mother or child, and instead making of each a dehumanized object?

Yet, should we not make every effort to help the child prepare for his birth and to allow him to live comfortably and above all humanely after his entrance into the world? Should we not do everything possible to lighten the burden of the baby-at-the-breast in its suffering and distress (particularly that experienced by the premature infant), deprived of the nirvana of the womb, sometimes as early as the sixth month of normal development?

The Premature Infant Hears Its Mother's Voice

Plunged abnormally early into a universe for which it is not prepared, suddenly deprived of its intrauterine communication, the premature baby is and remains one who lacks everything. The very specific stimuli only the voice of the mother can bring him are totally absent, all the more so as he is surrounded by the inadequate atmosphere of the incubator. This milieu is full of low-pitched sounds, which plunge the baby into a state of total debility. To counteract these unsuitable low-pitched sounds it occurred to me to modify the sounds surrounding an infant placed in a incubator, particularly by introducing filtered sounds, especially those taken from his own mother's voice.

I conducted such an experiment with the help of Professor Klaus Riegel of the Sick Children's Hospital affiliated with the University of Munich. In his clinic we gained fundamental information concerning the essential relationship of mother and child. Because women using birth control pills give birth to numerous twins and triplets every year in a continually increasing proportion, studies can be made of those children who have shared a womb for a shorter than nine-month period as is the case with premature babies.

In this study, triplets weighing about one and a half pounds and in a situation of serious distress were selected to meet certain experimental criteria. The first was placed in his incubator in normal conditions, while the second benefitted from some music by Mozart, broadcast in the register of filtered sounds. Finally, the third was plunged into the sound of his mother's voice, also filtered to enable him to re-experience fetal perception. The reactions of each triplet were observed, with an additional control of a respiratory and cardiac monitor.

The first infant, totally deprived of stimulation, remained motionless in his incubator, making painful efforts to survive. The one exposed to Mozart showed clear signs of activity, with fuller and quicker breathing and a pulse rhythm varying between 140 and 160. Finally, the third, the happy one who was drinking in the filtered sound of his mother's voice, showed his pleasure in living and tried to move himself with some force. More than that, he smiled. His deep regular breathing was accompanied by a regular and lasting pulse rhythm of 160. It should be noted that without the filtering and gating effects provided by the Electronic Ear, Mozart's music and the mother's voice had no effect whatsoever.

All this certainly confirmed what we had been asserting for more than 30 years: the mother's voice has a vital impact when it is perceived in the way the fetus perceives it. Such facts, now established, should challenge all those in pediatrics and gynecology who are responsible for seeing that premature babies survive. Surely a situation can be envisaged in which these children are literally bathed in such a sonic ambiance.

Is there not, in fact, an imperious need for this *affective feeding* just as much as there is for urgent medical aid? Every clinic for premature babies ought to be equipped in this way so that this type of stimulation, on which the fundamental organization of the nervous system depends, can enable the principal areas of the brain to be put in working order.

This finding needs to be acknowledged. The infant whose life before birth is dramatically cut short by several weeks from his nirvana-in-the-womb needs intensive treatment, some of which must address his emotional life and especially his vital relationship with his mother.

The Embryo-Fetus, A Whole Human Being

Our investigations of fetal hearing enabled us to reinforce the theories that claim for the fetus a very intense psychic and sensory life. In fact, it is during the nine months of fetal life that the infant stores up the greater part of its human experiences, those which will weave the web of its post-natal existence.

Such an idea seemed absurd only a few years ago, but not today. Specialists in many different disciplines have obtained proof to support the theory we have put forth since 1954 — that the fetus takes an active part during the mother's pregnancy in setting up a dynamic relationship with her.

It is now commonplace to state that the fetus feels, perceives, memorizes, and integrates. It is also admitted that the fetus hears from four and a half months of prenatal life. Our research indicates that it perceives well before this moment and that it gathers numerous memories and establishes an outline of psychic life from its sensory experiences of communication within the womb. A whole universe of relationship is established *in utero*, which opens up an unsuspected field of investigation to all those who wish to plunge into the mysteries of the beginnings of life.

Our investigations over 30 years reveal a convergence of clinical data that makes the existence of a prenatal psychology an undeniable fact. Moreover, anatomical, embryological, and physiological evidence show that the origin and development of the psyche in the embryo-fetus is also a well-founded fact.

My analyses in these different areas enabled me to paint a picture of the manifold sensations the infant is called upon to try out within the womb's cave. Among these, listening to the mother's voice remains the most fundamental perception. It constitutes the very basis of the desire to communicate.

Numerous investigations carried out before or parallel to mine in the areas of phylogeny and ontogeny proved the priority of the human ear in relation to the rest of the body. They made it clear that the inner ear is the organ that undergoes the most rapid and amazing changes in the life of the embryo. They emphasized the part played by early development of the vestibular system and the resulting effect on corporal dynamics and on the shaping of one's body image. They proved that the maturation of the nervous system, joined to the vestibulo-cochlear apparatus, is fully developed at birth, whereas the entirety of neuronic connections is only fully functional at the age of 42. There is precocity for you!

The human ear in its quest for listening prepares its kingdom from the very first days of conception. It is the first in every respect to show life in its dynamic of communication and communion. It prepares its whole neuronic network in order to record and memorize to maximum effect the fetal experiences that will be the very basis of the human pathway upon which the child will tread after its birth.

On this anatomical and physiological foundation, essentially a living and active one, a psycho-genetic framework is established from which subsequent psychic activity will build its own basis. It is on this level that developmental psychology puts down its roots. There is nothing unusual about that. As far as the embryo-fetus is concerned, it is normal to think that an intense psychological dynamism, both emotional and relational, is very quickly organized.

Moreover, if one searches carefully for the source of habitual human behavior, one is quite surprised to discover how the most archaic structures known to be rooted in our innermost being are related to experiences acquired in the womb. From this primordial dwelling, this envelope that has enclosed every human being, many archetypal memories find their ultimate origin.

Already an important relational dimension develops between the external world, the womb, and everything for which it stands from the aspects of nutrition, communication (both sound and touch), and the organization of spatial exploration. Henceforth, every further fetal development will be a repetition of these fundamental frameworks. One witnesses a real *detelescoping* of various stages that seem to overlap, and so they are in their programming: the embryo emerges from the egg, the fetus is born from the embryo, and the fetus produces the new-born infant. It is the same process for the primitive cell right up to man in the last stage of his life. Every early integration forms the pattern on which every subsequent psychological activity rests, reproduces itself, and becomes more and more complex.

We can observe this projective symbolism and rediscover traces of this primitive experience by using certain psychological tests, for example, the house-tree-person drawings technique. These tease out of integrated drawings underlying archaic themes related to a person's earliest prenatal recordings.

In addition, sounds of the mother's body (her heartbeats and respiratory rhythms) and those of the fetus itself are so many sound-sensations gathered in, filtered, and perceived solely on the level of rhythm. The repercussions of this sonic experience may have very important consequences in the course of post-natal life — on the psychological and even on the psychiatric level. Though external noises and sounds on the abdominal wall also have their effect, absorption of the mother's voice is the major factor that influences all subsequent affective and emotional structure. The filtered sound of the mother's voice makes a considerable impact in the development of the desire to communicate.

Clearly this relational dynamic must be properly established and supported by the relationship with the mother. This deep, affective, primordial communication, which puts the mother and unborn child in harmonious touch with one another, is emphatically important. No intimate relationship can be so intense as the one established during these nine months when mother and embryo-fetus experience a genuine symbiosis that enables them to fulfill their potential of becoming mother and child. By its presence from the very first moments of its insertion in the womb, the embryo-fetus changes the woman who bears it. She is another person, and her spirit vibrates with a specific love duet, which is quite different from all the usual emotional outpourings. Henceforth, she vibrates on the same frequency as the life she transmits. To be with child awakens in a woman her dimension of potential procreator. Nothing can replace this experience.

Man in his spirit of destruction knows how to cut off, damage, demolish, annihilate this essential intimacy that allows him to encounter life in the first place. He is enclosed in an existential logic that makes him lose his way in the winding paths of an evolution settled by his predecessors. Therein, he is sometimes forgetful of his own essential being, that essence from which emerges the true dialogue and the exceptional relationship between two beings who merge in perfect trust. Only pregnancy can set up this mutual amorous intimacy, in the noblest sense of the term, which is a dependence freely consented to and presided over by an attentive mutual listening.

The psyche does not develop without the mother's total involvement. In spite of man's destructive frenzy and even in spite of the most hostile and rejecting attitude of a woman towards her pregnancy, a maternal vibration exists in her innermost being. But while a woman with this hostile attitude is giving life, she is also introjecting death, and this involves her own psychic self-destruction. Thus one can foresee the whole subsequent psychological structure and its deviations that will form the child's psychic universe and on which will be grafted the universe of the adult.

Listening leads the fetus toward assuming its task of becoming a human being. Listening calls not only on the ear, but also on the whole cutaneous sensitivity, even deep visceral sensitivity. It means stretching out one's whole body to the other in order to listen, but it is also to confront one's own existence by means of this same relationship. It is impossible to listen without involving oneself, and listening begins with one's own self-listening in organizing the relationship with the other person.

Life's journey begins with this primordial relationship with the mother. It proves all the more genuine and authentic if it is stripped of all emotional and affective distortion. Then it will more clearly represent the development of being. We know that what happens is not like this, but I remain convinced that an in-depth study of the dynamic relationship established during life in the womb would be a rich source of information to help us understand and direct all human behavior. Moreover, education could derive some fundamental principles from this source. In this way the embryo-fetus is our teacher.

The universe of the womb, so fascinating and vast to explore, so valuable for research on the reconstruction of being, and so rich in providing therapeutic answers of all kinds will doubtless hold our attention for many years to come, for our generation and the next. But to plunge into such a universe can only lead us to study one of life's saddest problems, the problem of total isolation of the being from its environment and chiefly from the mother who has given it life —— autism.

The Autistic Child —— Storming the Fortress

Autism is a generic term with many facets. Certainly a common core exists, but a thousand and one details produce as many different clinical pictures as there are autistic children and show evidence of as many disorders in relationships as there are families involved.

The pathology of autism is obscure. It provides great dialectical material for specialists' dissertations, too often to the detriment of both the child who is actually at grips with the situation and the sorely-tried family. In fact, the whole family structure is confused, distorted, and dramatically disturbed in such a context.

The Autistic Child Does Not Listen

We find ourselves confronted by a clinical situation where an important signal may be discerned as a major element — the autistic child does not listen. It is not always possible to determine the precise causes of this. What we are sure of is that the autistic child *hears* — at least he seems to show us this is so — but he deliberately refuses to *listen*.

Consequences follow swiftly. To refuse to listen is to refuse to integrate language, so the child will live in a sonic universe where the word is excluded. This is a particularly painful situation, equally as trying for the child as for the family, which is totally without recourse when confronted by this refusal of all communication.

The autistic child lives, intensely and paradoxically, in a world of sound and hearing where all meaning is eliminated. Although he can hear an insect flying around, he is not able to recognize his own name even when it is called out right beside him. Everything happens as if a cleavage has taken place between sensing and perceiving. The passive attitude leaves him immersed in sounds, sometimes even in an exaggerated way. The step forward towards alertness, from which consciousness emerges, does not take place.

A mechanism is absent. Whether it has been lost, has never matured, or is nonexistent, the fact remains — it is not there.

In consequence, autistic children are assailed by all sorts of stimulation, but without any framework that may be categorized. They hear, but do not listen. They have eyes, but do not look. They have a mouth, but do not speak.

Under this definition, autism is much more widespread than was believed. The cases we refer to here are extreme cases.

The universe surrounding autistic children is a paradoxical one, without connections and without any synthesis as far as the sequence between one event and another. They get over their misgivings in their own way by certain stereotyped actions or rituals that fixate them on themselves and at the same time give their behavior an appearance of reality.

The world appears to them to have no unity, no development. Their vision is composed of a succession of widely separated stereotypes. Sounds strike them like repetitive sequences, without any one of them having any reference to spoken words. In fact, if the meaning of a single word were actually understood and its effect felt, the syndrome would disappear forthwith.

Faced with such a problem, what can we do? Unfortunately, it is not merely a question of *training* a child to pronounce words, as one sees done so often. All educational attempts based on this type of system are doomed to failure. The only eventual result lies in the utterance of dozens of words, and this after months or even years of efforts.

We suggest, above all else, a *listening program*. After working with a large number of autistic children, we have come to believe that the desire to communicate, especially with the mother, was not born in these children.

It seems relevant to recall that the ear is an organ that matures early and on which is grafted the most ontological desire — to communicate. A human being is an eminently social creature, and his sense of communion with the group is only conceivable if the listening faculty is quickly used.

Listening shows itself in a precocious way because the human ear is fully developed as an anatomical organ from the first months of life in the womb. *The embryo-fetus is already a listening entity.* The whole neuronic apparatus attached to the vestibulo-cochlear ensemble is operational from the fifth month of fetal life. Moreover, the auditory-temporal lobe of the brain is fully developed at birth.

This remarkable precedence of the ear in relation to every other formation explains why the desire to listen is a human's most ontological desire. This desire to listen calls the unborn child to be a human being. Since his communication is here and now established, listening reveals to him his membership in the surrounding world of sound. The ear of the fetus perceives the mother's voice in a remarkable way. There exists an inter-communication, a real communion, between the mother and her child. Mothers know this very well. They speak and sing to the child they are carrying.

In this intimate, daily, permanent relationship where low-pitched visceral noises are happily eliminated by the working of the cochlear filtering, the fetus is already living a wonderful experience, aroused by the gentle rustling of its mother's voice.

With the mother's voice and nowhere else begins the desire to listen.

If for some unsuspected reason the desire to listen is not sparked or it dies in the ovum, deep communication troubles will appear, the consequences of which are known. They are serious consequences for the child, who shuts himself in his ivory tower, which is nothing but a prison. Is he not, in fact, enclosed in a space where there are no reactions, in a time without any continuance? He seems not to obey the psychic laws of gravity. Nothing attracts him; all relationship is absent or of very poor quality. Alone in an enclosure with no way out, he turns round and round within the boundaries he never wishes to cross. Does he feel desire of any kind? For us, autism is a field in which the psyche plays a leading part. The results we obtain only derive their effectiveness from the fact that organicity is put out of play.

We attempt to awaken an autistic child's desire to listen by means of the mother's voice, heard as the fetus hears it, that is, by means of filtered sounds. It is astonishing to see the ease with which autistic children, so strongly disinclined to accept the universe of language, are immediately caught up by the desire to understand this new message. The filtered sounds risk either reminding them of a time *already lived* or provoking in them the desire to listen.

This could appear obvious to those who accept the importance of awakening the listening faculty, which is surely the most astonishing acquisition of all dynamic human structures. But the program we are undertaking on the child can only be contemplated if we simultaneously invite the mother, and if possible the whole family, to follow the same program.

In fact, when an autistic syndrome lies at the heart of a family structure, the entire dynamic of relationships is profoundly disturbed since no normal means of communication exist. Any attempt to begin changing this situation is immediately obstructed and rejected, sometimes with notable violence.

So we ask the family, and specifically the mother, who has agreed to give us her voice for the child's benefit, to undergo a listening training program. Clearly, if the opportunity exists to use the grandmother's voice, results are achieved more rapidly because the autistic child's mother herself benefits from sessions of listening to the filtered sound of her own mother's voice.

Certain reactions on the child's part show us that we have set in motion certain structures that had been previously inert. At first, they are situated at the neuro-vegetative level (sleep, appetite for food), then at the behavioral level. At this moment, the mother must be helped to accept these changes. She has been used to non-typical and unusual reactions from her child. In fact, by his disconcerting attitude, the autistic child becomes the object of his mother, she herself having become the child's object. The web of tension set up between them may hinder the process of reintroducing the child into normal life.

The father, as we already said, is not excluded from this program. We explain to him the part he must play in the heart of the family. In fact, he must reassess his attitude towards this child who has never been his, one might say, since he has never benefitted from any meaningful language; indeed, it is language that makes a child into his father's son. We are talking of quite specific language, that where information is exchanged and rules are established. The father's role is not one of scolding but of explaining and guiding, of expounding the rules until they are actually accepted. It is up to him to ensure that they are applied. If the father himself is able to undergo a listening training program, results will follow more rapidly still.

It is certainly difficult to achieve complete articulateness within the different family relationships. The first step is to lead the child to a genuine meeting with his mother. He will have to *grow-up* to discover her; he will have to become an adult to love her.

This is not to say that the mother's heart will be ready to respond to such a leap of love since she has remained for so long the prisoner of the fetus she has been carrying, inside her and outside her at the same time.

If one wants the child to transform himself, to grow up, the father and mother must each play their part. The stake, of course, is the child. The mother offers him her heart, and the father offers him language. The mother alone has the right to the child's love as he makes his way to a more and more adult state, while the father sees how his attitude affects the child's growing process.

In this atmosphere of relaxation, the child will begin to want to communicate, to express himself. We often have the opportunity to be present at the birth of speech, which builds up through a babble. It may shock the family unless they have been prepared for it.

At this point more than at any other time, the mother and father must be helped to curb their desire to move ahead too quickly. The desire to listen is a fragile one, slow to become strongly established. The desire to communicate needs to be firmly fixed. It must not be jostled, and it is fatal to wish to accelerate the process. If the parents are over-urgent, if they push the child to repeat words, they risk compromising everything that has been gained.

It is noteworthy that in the presence of a normal infant who wants to bury himself in babble, then in speech, everyone respects his capacity, even admires it. On the other hand, faced with an autistic child, or one embarked on a course of refusal and backwardness, people often tease him unceasingly and keep asking him to repeat things. They harass him in order to see him react like a performing animal in a circus. But a circus animal is better off. If the child is suspicious of all this distorted activity, he refuses to take part in it. He will control the entire family by releasing only the words that he wants to when he wants to, or by refraining from speaking and refusing to do what is demanded of him.

The child wins at this game — true enough — but his desire to communicate dies all over again. When an autistic child begins to speak, one should accept what he says quietly and lovingly, make a note of his progress, and draw up a list of what he has gained.

The initial stages are the most difficult. Afterwards, things move more quickly. As speech grows, eye contact increases. The child's look becomes expressive. Words beget more words, and later whole phrases occur.

In this way the child enters the world of communication step by step. His speech becomes more normal, and his socialization both in the family and at school is built up and becomes more successful and harmonious.

Results we classify as positive are obtained in 60% of the cases we treat. The remaining failures continue to challenge us and to show us that the task is by no means finished.

In fact, there is much yet to be done in the realm of autism. Investigators all over the world must multiply their efforts in order to release these children from their hell. Is this fortress in which they are imprisoned an empty one? I do not think so. It is filled with a being whose only wish is to express itself, to participate in the life surrounding it. But the fortress remains and a breach must be made in its walls.

The distressed infant who is knocking on the door must be taken in hand.

We must acknowledge that he exists and that he is a person. We must make him aware that he belongs to the human race.

The Year of Music

Apart from the problem of autism, many other subjects held our attention during these ten years of research. Music and singing were, of course, favorite subjects, particularly during 1985, which was designated "The Year of Music."

Owing to many events in various countries, music regained a select place in the field of human activities. It seemed only just to dedicate a year to music, 1985, and to organize cultural and scientific events in its honor.

Top level performances occurred everywhere in the form of concerts with soloists or choirs. Some brought together hundreds of singers or sometimes thousands of children belonging to many ethnic groups. Conferences were held like the one that took place in Paris on Gregorian Chant. I place great value on this form of musical expression and reserve an important place for it at the heart of our Method. There were also other educational and cultural activities, particularly in the realm of creativity. They marked this auspicious period with an indelible stamp.

I was not able to respond to all the speaking requests from France, Canada, Norway, and elsewhere, but I did address several conferences, and once more drew attention to the power of sounds and the neuro-psychological effects of music. I emphasized once again the postural reactions to acoustic phenomena, the correlation between the architecture of sound and the structure of the human body, the benefits of song, and the educational power of vocal practice. I stressed what I had affirmed nearly 40 years before concerning the effects of music and song from an educational and therapeutic point of view.

The important place singing once held in the field of education has been forgotten for several decades. Today, initiatives on the part of both musicians and teachers are aiming to reestablish the proper value of singing, which is such an essential element in humanization. Teachers in both nursery and primary schools should become aware of this necessity; they should rededicate themselves to learning to sing, read music, and play an instrument.

The school timetable does not have enough periods devoted to the teaching of music. Talk abounds of developing body image, bettering psychomotor skills, and improving posture, but people forget that the vital factor that can mobilize the body in a correct and effective way is sound, and in particular, song. Not any kind of song or any old music, of course. One has to bear in mind the potentialities of the nervous system of the child being educated, and also of the finality of the exercise he is required to perform. His body must be prepared to be an instrument for learning, memorizing, expressing, and communicating.

Teachers today do not always know how to sing properly. In some cases their speaking voice is poor, low-toned, and harsh. It fatigues those who listen to it. Instead of stimulating their pupils, they send them to sleep, demotivate them, and lessen their powers of attention and concentration. They speak as poorly as they sing.

Modern means exist today, based on the latest scientific discoveries and techniques, which are capable of training adults in a very short time to listen and sing properly by permitting the audio vocal circuits to operate correctly. Today it is easy to train a voice, to open up its potentialities by means of a cortical charge, and to improve its tone, quality, and melodic power.

Educational decision makers must be convinced that nursery and primary school teachers should be given thorough musical training. I am not talking about preparing them to become virtuosos, accomplished instrumentalists, or choirmasters. It is merely a question of making genuine teachers of them, capable of guiding the children towards well-constructed speech by means of counting songs and other children's songs. To make children sing a language is to go to the very source on which it is built neuro-anatomically. This prepares the listening faculty necessary to learn the mother tongue.

The necessity of getting little children to sing can never be overemphasized. Besides, everyone knows how happy children are to express themselves in this way. Zoltan Kodaly introduced this vital idea and set up an outstanding musical education program. His approach is now well-known all over the world. Other musicians, too, have developed effective methods that take into account learning processes involving the operation of neuronic circuits, triggered by means of visual and acoustic corporal integrators. (These are discussed elsewhere.) The work of Willems should be acknowledged in this field. It enables children and adults to fully enter the fascinating world of music. During the Year of Music, I had the privilege of meeting the teachers and some of the instrumentalists who had assembled at Lyon under the aegis of the Willems Association directed by Jacques Chapuis and his wife, Beatrice.

So music is gradually gaining ground once more among educational activities both at school and in the daily life of one and all. Bearer of harmony and energy, alertness and creativity, music begins at the very source of mystery; we learn by intuition that the world of sound is called upon to interpret by its living response the vibrating melodies of the underlying silence. A particular kind of music, in fact, is capable of putting humankind in sympathetic vibration with the universe. By its modulations, music fashions human beings in their physical, mental, and spiritual components. By its tones, it can free from bondage the man who is caught in the nets that life has weaved around him. It is the very basis of the song which chants liberation for the being who is a prey to the agony of life. It is a free gift, a strange and marvelous offering, which enables man to raise himself to his true human condition.

I cannot conclude this short passage about music without warning parents and educators alike against certain deviant compositions that are real sonic drugs deliberately intended to enslave generations of young people. Blasted out at top volume, modern pop and rock music is very damaging to the ear. Some injuries can be irreversible. It can sometimes totally destroy a nervous system.

Little portable tape recorders, increasingly popular, produce a sort of collective autism by isolating human beings from their environment and shattering any desire to communicate. The frequency content of their sonic messages is relayed through earphones and favors low-pitched sounds, that is to say fatiguing sounds, which bring the listener towards a state of inertia that often precedes a depressive syndrome. To all this is added the very important factor of the volume of sound, which destroys the ear and all its faculties — listening, concentration, energy, and creativity.

Some people wanted to use one of these portable tape recorders with filtered music in place of the Electronic Ear. While some users describe benefits of this focusing of their ears to specific frequencies that may or may not be missing from their individual listening experience, it is not the same as using the Tomatis Method. The inference that the two experiences are the same ignores what we know about the neuro-physiology of the ear and gives a false hope for extensive gains. Also, a good assessment of someone's listening is necessary to create a proper program. It is also necessary to monitor the changes that occur during the program to effect the maximum gain to accomplish a particular goal. An Appendix in this book includes a description of the *authentic* Tomatis Method so that all the components included in our comprehensive approach may be known.

Another method received considerable attention using loud filtered sounds of any kind *but* Mozart. Changes have been reported with autistic children using such a method and one has brought attention to the frequent finding of hypersensitive hearing with many, indicating they lack defense against sounds and an ability to adapt their listening. Though the method uses filtered sound to focus the ear it may require the child to listen to painful, loud sounds and not address the changes required in the communication environment. The goal is to improve hearing and no emphasis is on speaking. We, however, continue to insist that communication is two-way, self and the other are involved. To work with the ear and not the voice leaves half the work undone. Likewise, to go to the voice before the ear is ready will cause a problem.

Deviations always exist in this world. They pass and die out while the truth remains unchangeable and eternal. Music, with a capital M, distances itself from these deviations to preserve its universal character and lead humanity to the lofty spheres of creative harmony.

While making this foray into the field of music and song, I also made a thorough study of certain themes: stuttering, body-image, symbolism of drawings, and family dynamics considered from the point of view of mutual listening. What a godsend to have a specialty that touches on so many things! In the face of the vast panoply of subjects our Method incorporates, many people are frightened, others are amazed and dumbfounded, and some intensify their skepticism. It is a great pity from their standpoint. Fixed in a kind of mental straightjacket that prevents them from imagining a synthesis of many problems collected together, they remain resolutely in their own positions. If one follows their way of thinking, two different phenomena could not be attributed to the same cause. How can one claim that the principle of gravity that governs an apple falling to the ground is the same principle influencing a satellite such as the moon to revolve in orbit? How can one connect the attraction of the ear to material bodies with the attraction by which all material bodies are drawn to one another? The same kind of breakthrough thinking is required when considering the ear's role and its control over various mechanisms that are indicative of the many facets of its activity.

Autism is subject to the ear, as are all communication problems. These problems are various manifestations of the inability of the organ of hearing, usually for psychological reasons, to function in the ideal manner for which it was conceived. Other cases of faulty functioning affect the ear itself in its activity, like Ménière's vertigo. We discussed this earlier in the book and commented on the psychological origin of such a syndrome. The medical theories presented today do not adequately explain these phenomena or respond at all to what we have regularly been able to establish by means of auditory training using the Electronic Ear. The usual anatomical/pathological diagnosis of such a syndrome is in need of total revision. It is now well-known that the problem is not one of a hemorrhage of the inner ear. In our judgement, the hypertension established is only the result of a secondary irritation, which is set up by a faulty action of the middle ear, and in particular of the stirrup muscle.

In view of the consistently positive results obtained over several years, the publication of a book on the treatment of Ménière's vertigo (*Vertiges*) provides answers to the problems of this widespread and particularly handicapping disease. We now collaborate with specialists who apply the same principles as we do for tackling the treatment of problems in the vestibule of the inner ear.

One Is as Old as One's Power to Listen

These ten years also led me to reflect on the process of aging. As people become more and more preoccupied with life's third and fourth ages (the post-retirement years and those beyond 80), they paradoxically seem to ignore the problem of how to enter these stages of life with joy and enthusiasm.

More than at any other stage of the human adventure, the brain needs stimulation during these years. The ear plays a fundamental part in providing such cortical recharging so the dynamism of both body and spirit is ensured.

But, in real terms, what do we offer these men and women who have grown old in order to prepare them for their final meeting with Creation, just at the time when they usually are disengaged from life's little problems? Nothing, except a retirement that is often premature, badly organized, poorly understood, and unattractive, supported by some sort of pension scheme. Instead, what *should* be done is to nourish and stimulate his or her cortex, filled as it is with knowledge and enriched by a lifetime of experience.

Energy through sound is an inexhaustible source of power and joy in life. It confers on those who receive it a renewal of activity, a potential for one's whole personality to be taken over in an often remarkable way. From the moment the ear resumes or first begins its role of dynamization, in fact, from the moment that it recovers its desire to listen by means of the techniques described in this book, it becomes easy to ensure that these processes continue. It is enough for the person who is *reanimated* to listen to classical music, in particular to Mozart's violin concertos or Gregorian chant. He could equally well consolidate this renewal of energy by reading aloud for 30 minutes a day, taken in one or several sessions.

If experts in gerontology were willing to take into consideration the potentialities of the human ear and orient themselves towards this process of dynamization by sounds, they would surely involve themselves in our technique. Besides cortical stimulation, endocrine processes, which are themselves often in a state of malfunction, are certainly affected. Such a dynamization is capable of diminishing and even eliminating signs of aging that often strike people in the third and fourth age (or even in the seventh age referred to by Shakespeare). I am thinking particularly of how loss of memory, from which most old people suffer, could be powerfully diminished by means of new techniques. In the same way, the faculties of attention and concentration, which usually grow weaker as the faculty of listening does, could also be revived with the help of program sessions using the Electronic Ear.

The International Network

After setting up and then dismantling the network woven for more than 25 years by the users of our Method, I regrouped a certain number of specialists who were capable of correctly applying the techniques we had perfected and of seriously pursuing the development of the investigations undertaken by the Paris Centre team. This effort depended as much on the quality of the personnel as on the reliability and improvement of the machines. To obtain results of any value, our standards had to be strictly adhered to. It was because of deviations from these exacting demands that we have had problems with the trademark of our Method. *Forgers* still exist who copy certain machines that have fallen into public use and then circulate them after a half day of training. Perhaps they have more talent than we do since we spend many months training experienced specialists and even then demand that all certified users attend refresher courses on a permanent basis. Additionally an entire group of people describe their method as that of Audio-Psycho-Phonologie, when in fact they have limited their use to our early technique and philosophy and not kept current.

For this reason, we issue a current *Certificate of Agreement* to all members of our international network. This declares they are fit to apply the Tomatis Method according to standards taught them during their training period and the updating seminars. If the name "Tomatis" is not present, they are not part of our network. If they are linked to the Paris Centre by agreement, it entitles them to receive information useful to them in the course of their practice.

We have established a high-quality network, composed solely of professionals who are psychologists, speech therapists, audiologists, teachers, kinesiologists, physicians, professors of music and singing, and linguists. Annual conferences and seminars bring them together to study their results and propose new working hypotheses.

As for the forgers, it is certainly easier to construct machines than to train competent personnel. But a piano is not much use if one does not know how to play it. (And it must be said that an Electronic Ear does not have the same aesthetic charm as a piano!)

Saint-Yves

All our achievements in technique, methodology, neuro-physiology, and electronic machines have not been, for me, the essential point of the ten years ending in 1986. The reader may already suspect this. The journey I undertake with my wife at my side is of quite another kind; this journey does not nullify what came before, but rather gives it another dimension.

During this decade, moments of both shadow and light occurred. Among others, there was a dark period in a literal sense when I became practically blind with a rapidly developing bilateral cataract. A whole year without being able to read is a long time for a bookworm. Léna became my official reader and my private chauffeur. I was spoiled.

This passage through darkness was a turning point for me. I continued to practice without being able to observe the faces of the children and adult patients who entered my consulting room. My assistants read me their case histories, and in the shadows, after listening to everything, I delivered my diagnosis. This was an interesting experience. It enabled me to comprehend the nature of the listening world as well as that of the visual world — two quite different universes, but how they complement one another! One discloses a thousand and one details by posture and gesture. Normally one can observe how a person moves his body in order to express himself. But during this period I could no longer observe anything. Only listening was available, a very special kind of listening that enabled me to reconstruct what sight once brought me.

I became a much more sensitive listener than before. I learned that to perfect listening, it is almost essential that one not be able to see. I plunged deeply into this profound listening with a morale always equal to the situation.

"For you, the darkness is not dark,
And the night is light like the day."

As I plunged into this universe, I experienced once more the reality of the refrain in Psalm 139:

"Thou didst knit me together in my mother's womb."

After a very painful operation on my face and jaw that put me in a state of enforced rest for several months, my left eye was finally operated on at the Evreux hospital. I acquired 9/10 vision, something I had never had. In fact, I had suffered from severe farsightedness since childhood, which caused a doctor at Marseilles to predict that I would be blind by the age of 12.

My return to the world of light was a marvelous occasion. What thrilled me most was rediscovering my books, those travelling companions that so faithfully marked out my career as a researcher. I could read again, even without eyeglasses. But what surprised me most of all was the rediscovery of whiteness of which I no longer had any idea. Gradually and before total darkness overcame me, everything had become grey, dull, without any vibration. Imagine my joy to see light again, along with colors and shapes — and Léna's beautiful eyes, which for a long time had sparkled only in my memory. I realized, too, that these months of trial had whitened her hair and engraved some wrinkles on her always smiling face. She had lost some of her joy of living and her smiles had become less frequent.

We sought a way to rebuild the glowing palace of our life together, which had been temporarily overshadowed by this long journey through the tunnel. The best way was by resuming our activities at the Paris Centre and elsewhere, while keeping time for ourselves at our house in Bec Hellouin where I had spent my convalescence.

This house is situated in the middle of a village in Normandy, and was christened Saint-Yves by Mother Elizabeth, founder of the monastery of Saint Françoise Romaine that adjoins the Abbey du Bec. Father Yves Cossart, a missionary in Japan, was sponsored by this monastery, and it is in his memory that the house was named. Accidentally drowned at the age of 40, Father Yves left deep impressions of his ministry in Japan. The nuns of Bec remain faithfully attached to him and have just celebrated the fortieth anniversary of his death with a great service of meditation.

Our house at Bec, admirably restored by Bernard Cossart, Father Yves' brother, has undeniable charm and enables us both to relax when our professional work becomes a little too much for us. Still vibrating with the prayers of monks and nuns and impregnated with an exceptional silence that is stirred regularly by the sound of the Abbey bells, this little house has profound repercussions on both of us.

We have known the monks of the Abbey for many years, especially the Abbot, Dom Grammont. From 1976 we stayed often at Bec because one of our former collaborators (whom we consider our adopted daughter after her dying mother entrusted her to us) took her vows as a nun in the Monastery of Saint Françoise. Sister Emmanuel Marie became a powerful link between the Abbey and the Monastery.

Providence offered us Saint-Yves at the desired moment, and so we live there between our trips abroad and our stays in Paris. While Léna provided a harmonious atmosphere, filling the house with flowers and music, I set up my laboratory and library. In the calm of this dwelling, I devote myself to one of my passions, writing, acknowledging that the time has come to transmit to my successors the fabulous riches I have been given. The list of works taking shape grows longer every day.

We spend our time at Saint-Yves with a very particular approach to life: existence only has real meaning for us if it opens onto God Himself. It is very difficult to imagine a world without His presence, and it is all the more astonishing that so many people are content to live without believing in Him. How can they fail to do so when confronted by a universe that reveals more of its depth and amplitude every day, when they see a flower opening, or a child being born? How can they remain unaware of the life that is given us and that animates everything that exists?

Really enormous efforts must be made in order *not* to believe, to think of oneself only with despair, and to satisfy oneself with the vanity of being what one is. Nevertheless, one can be great when one is nothing, although always on condition that one is a *listening* nothing, one of those nothings who can detect the universe and feel oneself being crossed with the thoughts offered to it. Positive actions are possible when one is a nothing who abandons oneself, whereas the opposite is true when one attributes actions to oneself alone.

Heaven also guided us to Mesnil Saint Loup, desert cradle of the monks of Bec. In the midst of dry Champagne, where silence reigns, burns a hearthside fire lit more than a hundred years ago by Father Emmanuel, founder of the

Monastery of Saint-Esperance. Following some of the monks of Bec who had returned to their original monastery, we were drawn to this brotherly community. There, religious men clothed with a deep faith chant praises to God in a place where the Holy Spirit breathes with a special intensity.

In this friendly atmosphere, I began to offer again those courses I used to give at the outset of my career as a specialist in voice disorders. They consist of a theoretical and practical exposition of the basic principles of the audio-vocal act. My students now are often monks; in the old days they were usually lyric artists. Sacred chant is gradually returning to holy places, and Gregorian chant is regaining its role in the church, which it never should have lost. In certain cases, various attempts to introduce French chant have made people forget the fundamental laws of religious chant or simply of chant itself. Gregorian chant, elaborated over centuries and put back in its correct form by Dom Gajard at the Abbey de Solesme, has carefully preserved these laws. That is why after having been temporarily abandoned, it is once more becoming the preeminent sacred chant in countries ready to make it part of their liturgy once again.

The Opportunity to Grow Old

Years have slipped by and time has made its mark on the faces of those around us and on ours, too. Some friends have left us. George Massié has departed to rejoin the Father's house. Others are living a life of retirement, deprived of all struggle and all effort, with more or less success. Most of them are childhood friends or working colleagues who have recently relinquished activities that gave their life meaning. At age 45 I declared that one should never retire; people find such a proclamation strange. Yet the problem is an acute one in many cases. Society today is challenged not only by the economic consequences of retirement, but also by the very idea of this stoppage of activity, which crushes energetic men and women when they are at the very height of their powers.

It is God's will that man should work, or as is more precisely written in the Hebrew Text, "Man should cultivate," with its underlying implication, "cultivate himself." That is why I continue to undertake, with great pleasure, all the responsibilities inherent in my different activities around the world. That may be why I preserve within myself an impression of eternal youth. And perhaps the best way of remaining young is never to be afraid of growing old.

It is essential for someone ending his earthly journey to pass through the different doors that lead to the ramparts within (those very doors which, paradoxically enough, seem to be more open to the infinite the more deeply they are hidden within one's innermost being). There time crystallizes into eternity, and space into infinity. There is no longer anything but life and light. Death vanishes and darkness is dissipated.

In this boundless temple our oneness with creation becomes obvious. We are invited to sing the glory of God whose presence makes itself ever richer in meaning and enfolds us more and more. Growing old is merely a conscious acceptance of Him, which enables us to step quickly forward into the hidden places of the infinite universe. Whatever the anxieties that may arise from the first attempts at this incursion and however numerous the obstacles may seem, one must never step back. True, it is easy for someone who has seen the sparkle of this interior light, even if only once and only for an instant, to let himself be absorbed by it, even when an eclipse happens to take place.

Who has not seen this metaphysical flame shining within himself? Who has not been invaded at least once in the course of his life's journey by this state of being filled with a sudden and sovereign clarity?

As age advances, the adventures that mark the course of human life take on a quite different color. They become saturated with a quality of tone that reflects a mission to be accomplished. Each of us can then grasp the reason for his life's journey and, more than that, foresee the end. Everything is centered on what is essential, this essential source of life, an incessant flow of energy, which modulates our thought, fashions our spirit, and causes our soul to vibrate. When the years have passed, our soul catches once more its first rhythm, wiping away the constraints that darkened it or at least surrounded it with mist and greyness. Henceforth the soul becomes the expression of life. Life sings permanently just as the soul does; it is in resonance with it. It begins to pray without ceasing.

Finally, everyone knows that the soul sings and that, in this world, everything is done to prevent it. As age advances, the soul sings naturally. It is made for this purpose, and the only cause of all its suffering is the suppression of this deep respiration of praise for the universe, for the great omnipresence to which it belongs.

To grow old, then, is to pass beyond what shackles this vibration of the soul. It is to reach the level of wisdom where everything falls into proper proportion in relation to human activities and the reckoning of their vanity. It is to reach the level where the futility is revealed of things that once seemed so indispensable. It is to see the disappearance of everything that is hiding the presence of God.

It is true that I myself was particularly favored after my adventure of passing the boundaries of everyday life. My experience in Spain represented a genuine foretaste.

In another respect, my adventure allowed me to meet men who have discovered dwelling places of dazzling light where God is present in His splendor, men whom we call accomplished and who by means of a humble and solitary life have discovered the grandeur of God. I am thinking particularly of the Most Reverend Father Abbot Dom Grammont of Bec Hellouin. He is and remains for those who know him the model of shining vigor, a man with an unfailing sweetness and an infinite understanding. To have drawn near him is to understand what prayer means; to come close to him is to understand what is the abiding presence of the Word made flesh.

I am also thinking of Father Dudeban. He enabled me to cross the threshold towards which my faith led me, but which many scruples forbade me to approach.

As I recall the vital stages of my life, I acknowledge an equal debt to Father Michel, Prior of the monastery of Mesnil Saint Loup. By his genial brotherly love, he welcomed Léna and me to a world where God alone reigns in glory. Thus, places such as Le Bec and Le Mesnil are for both of us wellsprings that guide us toward a transformation more and more affirmed by our way of life, already carefully structured, and which enable us to understand our daily activities from quite a different angle.

Within the very framework of my activities I feel most deeply the repercussions of this conversion. It has become clear that, while it is easy to treat those who have difficulties of communication, what really matters is to save them. That is essential. There is no point in existing without joy in life. But it is true that one cannot reach this primordial state without having discovered life itself, without knowing the path that leads to it.

This chapter provides a conclusion and the beginning of a new stage. Every quest, every search, and every piece of research (however scientific it may appear to be) only has value in so far as it leads to the divine. Every discovery has a purpose only within a context that draws together into a greater understanding the relationship that should exist between the human condition and the infinite grandeur of the Creator. At this level, man is not shut up in his human body; he is part of an infinity which encompasses him and carries him in his sidereal course, to sing in unison to the glory of the Absolute. What matters in human life is the opportunity to discover God Himself.

14

Conclusion Without End...

Léna and I are fortunate in living so many good and successful years; we continue to enjoy life. In the context of the first English language edition, we once again prepare a last chapter, a conclusion without end, this time incorporating a metaphysical dimension while bringing the reader current with what has happened since Robert Laffont published the last French edition of this book in 1986. Since life continues to take us along on its endless path, it must mean that our mission is not yet over. We enjoy and appreciate the opportunity to continue our work. We do so with as much enthusiasm and fervor as ever, pleased with how well it is turning out. Moreover, we freely surrender ourselves to what feels like the ardor of an indefatigable youth, literally caught up in the perspective of this new stage.

The past four years have yielded progress in research and teaching as well as travel. Our activities have included numerous trips to attend the openings of centers around the world. At present a new center opens every eight to ten days. This accelerated rate is quite the opposite of the fate of slowing down which confronts us as we age. Fortified with a good dose of vigilance and a realistic outlook acquired over the years, we prepare to greet the challenge of expansion. We have paid our dues along the way and, fortunately, have managed not to fall into a tyrannical obsession, created by doubt and suspicion.

We have reached the age where it is customary to be invited to inaugurations. At least that is what we like to say since it is a good, though unnecessary, excuse for our travels. Rather than tiring us, the trips energize and revitalize us, often to the amazement of many of our contemporaries. Some of them do their utmost to convince us that we must be exhausted, which we are not in the slightest. At times, their insincere compassion reveals their secret desire to also be so busy. These people tell us it is utterly absurd to be monopolized by a job, one they see as burdensome, and that we would be so much wiser to wholeheartedly enjoy a well-deserved partial or complete retirement.

How can we convince them that it is not really work to us? In fact, we do not even like the word *travail*, or *work*, because of its etymological association with the word *torture*. Their unsubstantiated arguments are impossibly lost in illusions and a state of mythical nirvana where nothing of any consequence happens, especially coming to grips with the meaning of one's life and facing the existential assessment, the final reckoning. Such illusions prevent these people from advancing past boundaries beyond which lies the challenge of reevaluating their lives.

Also from this perspective, they do not want or are not able to admit that an essential part of our work is to respond to the solicitations that initiate our diverse activities. On the bright side, many eagerly want to be informed about the Tomatis Method and to follow us in our work. Still others who are already settled into their own work just need a little encouragement. These collaborators come from many professional areas and orientations. Some are in the field of health service while others are in colleges of medicine and psychology and such paramedical fields as speech, physical, and somatic therapies. Those in the medical field are interested in all of the energetic dynamics, which are easily discovered when one remembers the dynamizing effect the inner ear has on the vestibular-cochlear system. Some others are in related fields throughout the social and human sciences. At universities, the colleges of arts and human sciences are the most interested, especially those departments involved with general linguistics and research in modern languages.

Whether we are called upon to help found a new center or to provide information to either the general public or the professional world, we respond with equal delight, moved by a never-ending desire to serve. It would have been a real pity to so passionately have done this work if we had lacked passion for it or not used it for the benefit of others. The clear development of our expertise, consolidated through more than 45 years of constant practice, allows us to believe that we were meant to spread our ideas and their implications to all areas of the world where conscious ears are listening. We are dedicated to this work both to be true to ourselves and to assure that the work will continue in the future.

This continuation of the Method is one of Léna's and my most basic concerns. It has preoccupied us continuously for many years, often against great odds. In this difficult and on-going battle we daily discover and know the other in a marvelous way. It gives us singular joy to know that we are united in the same spirit, working towards the same objective, and engaged in the same research without ever feeling the slightest tension. This is a true blessing, one that should be savored with each passing day and throughout the years. I like to tell people that, as a united couple, we have the strength of a regiment. But one must always be on guard to protect this state of grace. We consider as indispensable the daily renewal formulated from the vows that started our marriage.

The force of our combined strength makes it easier to navigate through the storms encountered in our lives. This strength also allows us to install a network of solid collaborators along the way and to provide top notch professionals in whom we have the utmost confidence as to their dedication concerning the authentic implementation of the Method. The Method survives well, although some unsound and false reports have hurt certain people in the network. Some have increasingly been left behind, finally overwhelmed by their own inadequacies. Their inability to hold on to the everyday theoretical, clinical, and technical information as well as the constantly changing innovations have left them stranded on the side of the road. But this situation is not surprising and, in fact, characterizes all noteworthy research.

Regardless of how quickly changes occur, a consistent effort to keep pace is required by members of the international network and those who aspire to take part in this work. Fortunately, many members have become outstanding performers even as they have built their skills in related areas. Some have turned out to be true leaders.

The actual creation of such a dynamic organization proves to be a real challenge. It took us over ten years of persistence and obstinacy to reach our current status. We endured many tiresome, useless, and costly meetings with experts of many kinds in that time. I could draw up a list of the most impressive of them, but what good would it do? Though each was well paid and feigned an unconditional affection for us and interest in our work, they offered only incompetence.

Everything happens in its own time. Every event, no matter what it is, cannot take place until the conditions permit a crystallization. Previously, it was too soon. Afterward, it will certainly be too late. One should not infer from this that we are zealous fatalists, for we are not. Nevertheless, we are convinced of the need for a sudden convergence of what was once a thousand and one elements into something comparable to a perfect coalescence, congealing *en masse*.

To succeed in these well-defined conditions, everything must be analyzed, especially the moment in which the event unfolds, and more precisely, the instant of the inception of the event and its difference from the moment that preceded it. Whether one looks at modern physics or social events, the responses are identical. In our case, we may have had some inkling of what was to come from the appearance of some of these super experts, but their impact was only discovered later through hindsight. Our sole regret is having paid copious amounts too early instead of awaiting the most opportune moment.

One day we noticed around us a new group of collaborators, real fighters who came to us to reinforce those who came before. Since then we have been surrounded by a hard-working group of loyal, professional, and respectful collaborators. One of them, Dominique Cavé, is a very highly qualified consultant. She has been with us for more than 18 years and has learned more from our clinical teaching than any other. And who does not remember Dominique Huneau, who has been with us for 25 years? You could not forget her way of working with severely handicapped children. Possessing such a warm attitude and lifestyle, she never shows impatience with the children; she always creates joy and comfort around her. We also could talk about the more than 30 other collaborators and assistants of the Paris staff. They have a range of diverse qualifications. Among them are psychologists, educators, aides, and the technicians who run the Electronic Ears, which provide the foundation of the work at the center. We also have a necessarily large administrative office staff.

The Paris Centre is responsible for training people who are interested in opening new centers and applying our techniques. One department takes care of all the training and theoretical instruction. One management team, assisted by several colleagues, organizes each comprehensive training program. Several training stages are organized so people can first understand and then directly apply theoretical knowledge with clients. A practicum, internship, and probation period provide important firsthand experience for people before they open a center. It also gives us time to get to know them and discover their strengths and abilities.

Each member of the network devotes him- or herself to spreading and strictly adhering to our techniques according to his or her aptitudes and personal knowledge. Each is taught to use the Method in a particular professional setting.

Though we cannot mention the names of all our colleagues, they all know that they are in our hearts and we are sure that none of them doubt that we have anything but the warmest regard and appreciation for them. For many years, the thousands of clients who have been served in the Paris Centre have told us about their rewarding experiences with the staff.

We have benefitted from watching how the new organizations around us have expanded and molded with what was already in place. We also have seen an integration into the heart of various activities we had kept at arm's length for decades. In particular, having a consolidated management team has liberated Léna more and more from the administrative worries she previously handled. The unified management team fell in place right on time, and with the impetus of the Board of Directors, we established a workable structure that allowed us to multiply the scope of our activities. Several independent departments were established and competent managers were hired to enable the proper development of the entire system. Each unit is responsible for its own financial and organizational aspects.

We eagerly introduced our plan for Tomatis International with the objective of creating a unified and truly operational global structure. It took many months to put the internal structure in place. None of us, neither Léna nor I nor even any of those who worked with us, could have imagined how long it would take to reach our goal.

The highly-regarded board chosen to design and build this administrative center was also surprised that it would take so long. Its analysis addressed two of our long-held personal concerns: first, the perpetuation of our work and, second, the selection of board members to take charge of all aspects of business, which was not our area of expertise.

A total reorganization established an overall pattern for future organization and expansion. The results were so positive that the board members were fascinated by the universe opening up in front of them. Without a doubt, the social implications of our research interested them the most. They also were very impressed with the immense possibilities of our research in education, psychology, neurophysiology, audiology, linguistics, speech, and, in short, any humanistic concern. Certainly, the importance of their feedback to our daily work laid a solid foundation for our future plan. Their dedication and their complete immersion in the battle that we had carried on for so long meant a great deal to us.

So, without hesitation, they began to manage the practical and beneficial application of our work. Léna and I devote our energy to teaching, research, writing, conferences, and visiting new centers.

The impending breakup of the old organization caused visible changes at the heart of the new structure. It was a matter of redefining the direction of the team. It was not easy and, in fact, it took a lot of tact to achieve the anticipated outcome. The goal was partially reached by simply distributing responsibilities differently.

The board members, whose mission it was to install a well-defined structure, acknowledged their utter astonishment at the enormity of what Léna and I had been doing. They realized how so much was accomplished only when they recognized us for what we were: two fanatics who went in many directions, without respite, continually working on a thousand different projects at once. For three or four decades we had surmounted our worst difficulties because of our irresistible love of life and our desire to be of service to others. We remained strangers to despair by being endowed with the greatest hope.

So these last few years were quite constructive: the organization improved, new centers opened, and our scope became more creative and much more effective.

New structures are being established in the international network, also. In Spain, for example, under the guidance of pediatric physician Dr. Cori Lopez-Xammar and her husband Joan Viñas, another network has been founded with its epicenter where they work in Barcelona. Armed with all possible qualifications to integrate our techniques at a high level, Cori is at one and the same time well-grounded in neurology and psychology. Embodied in this one woman are all the qualities needed to assure a definite propagation of our ideas. She has been able to assimilate all these ideas in order to apply the Method as a whole. By her side is her husband, who is an active member of the administration of Tomatis International and the promoter of the Tomatis Method in Spain. He has been completely responsible for the Hispanic delegation. Under Joan's leadership, expansion has continued and the structure has become solid. It is working so well in Spain that it is used as a model for new ones in Switzerland, Italy,

Greece, and Germany.

While Europe moved ahead, the world across the Atlantic experienced a slower, almost lethargic period. Numerous causes affected the opening of centers, especially in Canada. As I have already mentioned, it was difficult to proceed amidst the opposition and resistance we encountered. Nonetheless, in hindsight we drew several conclusions from our experience with MDS. First, the orientation of this powerful organization was based on a dynamic medical model and, as such, could not lead to a humanistic structure. This was very clear and quite understandable. Also, the *social-missionary* crusade, which I have lived for such a long time as a researcher and which keeps me going even today, was not in harmony with such a well-oiled system. Finally, the impact of being centered solely on academic problems produced a reduction in the holistic power of our work.

However, the venture taught us a lot and produced some mild successes. Also, without a doubt, the MDS organization opened the door for us to an extraordinary exploration of an almost unknown universe. Léna and I continue to be very much committed, filled with the mutual admiration and profound respect that, for us, remains the epitome of precious human collaboration.

The seed has been planted in North America, and, even though it had a rough start, it has taken hold and is blossoming in the desert of Arizona. A center that opened only a few years ago is now firmly in place and spreading our ideas further. Under the professional directorship of Dr. Billie Thompson, soundly supported by her husband, Dr. Kirk Thompson, the Tomatis Center of Phoenix is well on its way. Billie brings her competence in the field of education to our work, while Kirk offers support with his expertise in electrical engineering as well as in the fields of computers and management.

Billie, who holds a Ph.D. in Education, is well-versed in all fields related to education. Many organizations have already profited from association with her. The center, which is already quite active, has begun to answer the demand for information and education in Phoenix and across the United States. It seems that the time has come to approach the New World once again. We are hopeful and confident that we will meet more teams who share and uphold our ethics. If it is true that hope does not betray us, we can affirm with some degree of certainty that its roots remain in us at the greatest depth of our sanctuary where God resides. This solidly anchored conviction provides the strength and courage to start again after 30 years with as much hope as we had before. Even if we are thought of as quixotic by those who live only to maintain their social status, we take our swords of knowledge in hand to joust with the New World.

In spite of all the extra work required to restructure the organization, our research in various fields was not slowed down. Advances in electronics, in particular, enabled us to create new prototypes to further improve the performance already achieved and to keep up with recent technical advances. Research on the neurophysiology of the human ear also took a great deal of our time. One knows that the ear plays a large part in our activities, and we are convinced that it cannot be separated from the integral psychological dimension. It is no secret to anyone that the psychological dimension is determined by the audiological apparatus through the process of listening.

Quite suddenly, and thanks to the structure we had put in place, an exceptional opportunity arose: a laboratory was put at my disposal. This was a dream of mine, one that had lain dormant for many years, in fact, ever since that unscrupulous charlatan shamelessly took for himself the monies that should have been devoted to research. No matter how long the wait, however, it is always with delight that I receive what comes, thankful for the patience and willingness to continue in the face of great adversity. In the past, such an attitude probably would have been judged as the consequence of being oblivious to everything. Maybe now this attitude can be viewed as a form of wisdom.

Some people have said that Léna and I have been lucky because everything has just fallen into our laps. But rather than dumb luck causing things to go our way, our good fortune is the result of paying constant attention to quality, to doing the job well. Our continual activity, which appears to be a state of constant agitation to some people, is based on my firm conviction that we are being carried along. By this I mean that I feel *led*, as if supported and protected by an interior dynamic from which I derive inner strength and energy. These are new discoveries, although I think they have always been present in my deepest convictions.

The activity in the lab is a two-fold occupation, which makes things doubly exciting. I am doing the fundamental research and also manufacturing the equipment used in the Method. I no longer have to rely on subcontractors, which in the past has made us completely and intolerably dependent on others.

The new structure also permitted greater dissemination of my writings. *L'Oreille et La Vie* was published by Éditions Robert Laffont in a revised edition with a chapter to bring it current to 1986. *La Nuit Uterine* (The Uterine Night), published by Stock Editions, experienced huge success in Germany after the remarkable translation done by Rowohlt Editions from Hamburg (*Der Klang, Des Lebens*). The success of this work resulted in many German editions, including a soon-to-be-published paperback edition. This testifies to the growing interest of German speakers in issues related to life before birth.

The Greek translation of *L'Oreille et La Vie* was presented to us at the opening of the Tomatis Center in Athens. Although the center has been open only since 1988, we are not surprised by its rapid growth due to the extraordinary and lively team involved there. Tony Evangelopoulou is the driving force, assisted by her husband, Likas, who also is dedicated to the administrative activity of the center, which fortunately harmonized well with his own professional occupation. Tony is able to use all her skills, especially those in the field of educational psychology. Because of the rapid growth of the center and the organizational efficiency shown by them, we accepted their invitation to organize and host an International Congress to regroup all of the network members from Europe and North America. This was bound to be successful, but it even exceeded our expectations.

During a marvelous cruise through the Greek Isles, we spent hours sharing and studying even as we observed our own ethnic moments of meeting. Like Ulysses, we peacefully traversed the luminous expanses of the sea; the trip was very conducive to thinking and creating vision. Transported from isle to isle, each more beautiful than the one before, we actually set foot on those sites, filled with the poetic mystery of ancient Greece, that continue to beckon to this day.

During this unforgettable journey in the country of my distant ancestors who left Crete in the 12th and 14th centuries to settle in the Piedmont and Carrare regions of Italy, we became better acquainted with and more appreciative of the young couple, Billie and Kirk Thompson. In this wonderful setting we had the opportunity to have an open and relaxed dialogue and we discovered many shared interests and qualities worth knowing.

Because of this dialogue, I find myself once again extending and updating this autobiography. It seems healthy to look the past directly in the eye and recognize it for what it is. Our purpose is not necessarily to contemplate the ground covered, but more to prepare the reader for what is ahead in the near and distant future. To write just to write and blacken the paper does not interest me. We are convinced that we have valuable information that should be transmitted in as many languages as possible; to do so, we must take note of the most important facts in our progress.

This summation, which certainly is not a conclusion, is being written at the request of our new partners, Billie and Kirk Thompson. It is for the American edition, which they valiantly decided to produce in the spring of 1991. Obviously they realize that the publication of such a work will do much to spread information about the Method. Numerous editions in France have contributed to the diffusion of our ideas. The decision by Billie and Kirk to bring this book to the North American public bodes well with us. It builds a solid base for future collaboration and constitutes a very favorable component for beginning and promoting new centers. This book will be a support for all the people who will benefit from the Method both in the Tomatis Center in Phoenix and in those centers that will be founded across the United States. One must dare to dive into new situations, and Billie and Kirk have not hesitated to engage in the struggle. To do a book for potential clients takes a lot of courage.

The Tomatis Center Phoenix is becoming the core of the structure on which we are laying many hopes. The desert of Arizona will henceforth be like a magnet. We look forward to seeing the gigantic Grand Canyon on one of our upcoming trips. In this region where the sun puts out such an unusual energy are other states that we hope to make aware of the potential of the Method. Pilot studies are being done to determine a strategy of expansion across North America. With the Phoenix Center at the heart of the American network will be a permanent training center, following the guidelines of the Paris training center. All of this work will be done in collaboration with the training department of the Paris Centre, beginning in March 1991.

Undoubtedly, the stepping stone to America, with a strong organization in which we have confidence, is well in place. This seems to predict favorable expansion. Léna and I feel very committed to spreading to a new continent this work that has done so much good in Europe. This work will be much bigger in the U.S. because of the size of the country. A young, competent, bold team is needed, a team ready to fight. And more than a team, we have a couple and the efficacy of such a tandem cannot be beat. All I see are good omens, setting off on this new adventure with the same enthusiasm and dynamism. Dare I say with the same youth? Why not? In our hearts, we are eternally young.

Four other books have come out recently. One was published in 1987 by Éditions Robert Laffont, entitled *L'Oreille et la Voix* (The Ear and the Voice) while the other three appeared almost simultaneously from Ergo Press in 1988 and 1989. The publisher handles such diverse topics as scholastic problems, vertigo, and prenatal life.

There was a real demand for *L'Oreille et la Voix* from the public and from professional singers and actors. It is out now and has been well received. Nothing is more natural than talking and singing, and yet what difficulties we have when trying to express ourselves! This book attempts to clarify audio-vocal technique with the ear as the great verificator of vocal emission and controller of all processes related to phonation. As I have said before, *we sing with our ear*. It is therefore necessary to readjust the entire vestibular-cochlear apparatus to be assured of a good voice. These ideas, patently obvious yet not well known, are beginning to gain acceptance and to spread not only into artistic spheres, but also into educational, political, and socio-cultural circles. The voice is reclaiming its rightful place in the world of communication. In response to the ever increasing demand by those who are conscious of its value, I continue to offer a practical audio-vocal class one week per month in our training department in Paris.

I am concentrating now on research, teaching, writing, and consultations. When I do the latter, they are sometimes in the presence of apprentices-in-training.

In regards to research, we are concentrating now on the training problem in schools. We talked at length about our experience in the Canadian system both here in this book and, in a simple and amusing form, in the book *Les Troubles Scolaires* (Academic Problems). From the beginning, the response from the general public and certain areas of education was very encouraging. The media got involved with a series of articles, followed by numerous radio broadcasts and some interviews on television, all of which served to spread the word. The book was so successful that following several hard-cover printings, it came out in a soft cover. It was promoted to a wide audience and was well-received by teachers. In spite of being terribly busy, teachers are fully conscious of the enormous problems that come with having to educate the children who are entrusted to them. The parents themselves are grappling with the difficulties their children are experiencing. One can see how many young students in school settings are completely discouraged when faced with anything that smells of academia.

We undertook an extensive campaign so that a large number of unfortunate people could benefit from the available technology. Fifteen schools, both public and private, throughout the world are equipped to do the Tomatis School Program. This is only the beginning, but because of the fantastic results, the program merits continuation. We are also introducing, in an educational context, the analysis of part of the listening test to evaluate elementary through university level students' strengths and weaknesses for language acquisition of one's native language or of certain foreign languages. The same test could be given in conservatories of music and singing in order to determine the best instrument or voice range potential of a student.

The recent book *Vertiges* (Vertigo) addresses a topic that was close to my heart for a good many years; it allowed me to proclaim my conception of the vertigo syndrome of Ménière. In the first place, the book provides a new diagnostic definition and dimension. It also offers a real therapeutic solution for resolving equilibrium problems. At the same time, the solution allows the attainment of great improvements with the associated symptoms of buzzing in the ears and of deafness. I am greatly committed to and have also largely developed the psychological dimension concerning the foundation of this ailment, as far as I deem it essential.

Secondly, this book interested me because it provides to a wider audience of readers my ideas about a new concept of hearing. Research requires that the driving force must be stronger than steel, for one needs a good dose of obstinate perseverance with a great deal of courage to confront the unconfrontable force. The proof for these new concepts dates back to 1953, the year when I presented them to the members of the Association of Acousticians of the French Language, headed then by the chief of telecommunications, Mr. Chavasse. He was particularly interested in me as a young researcher and provided enough encouragement that I continued. I initially was too naive and idealistic to believe that more work would be needed in order to prove what I considered to be foremost findings, findings I felt would certainly become well known and stand on their own merit.

Later I stopped deluding myself and realized it would take more time. I put my legendary patience to the test. In fact, as time passed, I found myself increasingly prone to quietly wait for the opportune moment, just as it is normal for one to reap the fruits when perfect maturity is attained. This particular moment of harvest is not comparable, as some commonly presume, to *the idea* which suddenly follows the spark of intuition. The germination and ultimate realization that follow require an incubation period. With hindsight one comprehends the problem as viewed in reverse order. Then the evidence rises as if by magic. Moreover, it takes on the authenticity of truth at the exclusion of all analogic comparisons. From this perspective, the usual manner of approaching the problem is completely stripped of realism, and in one fell swoop it loses all its credit.

What can be said about this reversal of point of view? Where are the mature fruits? And finally, what are they? They are no more and no less those that must *mature* in order to finally accept the proposed change. Growth is indispensable, but it can be long in coming and subject to sudden leaps or even blocked by obstacles. Are not the obstinate at odds with their simple personalities, those in which they have invested so much and have settled within themselves? They think, no matter what happens, that all is well and good in their universe. Nothing is to change or exist beyond it. Their know-how is like a house of cards that would crumble if they accepted a modification to the rules of the game.

Fortunately, people have more or less similar characteristics, which create some uniformity, mentally, and behaviorally. Yet, if it were possible for each of us to perceive ourself through the multiple facets of our personality, it would be bewildering to find oneself, in some ways, still quite distant from the afore-mentioned maturation level.

Another recent book was also well received. Its title evoked, beyond an indisputable curiosity, the quest for a mysterious universe in which an archaic memory survives deeply in every being. Of course this is a memory one would like to rediscover, so much so that *Neuf Mois au Paradis* (Nine Months in Paradise) provided real echoes in the innermost depths of everyone. This book makes available to the general public concepts that I brought forth in the 1950s. Now they are considerably more documented and reinforced by a long personal experience that ten years earlier must have stimulated much research in all corners of the world.

Studies about prenatal life are now abundant, though not all are of equal value. Many are nothing more than compilations of previous discoveries. It is amazing how many pseudo-scientists boast about proving what was demonstrated over 40 years earlier. The fascination with intrauterine life reminds one of veins leading to the gold mine. One often wants to dig up the wealth of fame while ignoring the hard work it takes to be a pioneer. Besides presenting new ideas about embryonic and fetal life, I was simultaneously able, within the scope of this work, to set the record straight. It provided me with an opportunity to give credit to other researchers for their own individual research, which cost them many long and tedious years of research. I was well positioned to be the spokesman.

I began to view these publications in a radically different way. In fact, it became apparent to me that I should have written directly for the audience who would be served rather than trying to convince those who refuse to listen. Just as one cannot force a donkey to drink when he is not thirsty, one cannot persuade someone who does not want to believe something to believe. Medical education is regulated by a remarkably finite set of rules, good and bad, that retard the diffusion of information addressing the basis of this need. By not acknowledging perceptions and experiences that are counter to others they have had, some people continue to block growth and change.

The diffusion of my ideas seems to follow the normal course —— man wants to be completely and expediently educated. There must be ethics, though. While trying to make the Method more generally known, I cannot allow a debasement of the message.

I survived a difficult period, which seemed to me overly long, during which I was barely able to transmit my ideas. They appeared only in scientific reviews, mostly medical, or in books destined for specialists. It seemed impossible to adequately reach specialists via the professional literature, so I jumped ship. I introduced to the general public that which previously was thought to be only in the domain of specialists. One should not assume that only specialists need information!

Just as the pace of expansion of the Method accelerates, so too does interest in reading about it. Numerous publishers urge me to write more, which I do with pleasure. One of them even proposed that I edit a collection. So the tide has changed. It appears that people are now ready to seek out and accept such ideas, to branch out in new directions that will continue and one day surpass us. The world is in constant flux, following its course from stage to stage, from maturation to maturation.

Currently I just finished two books for release this year. The first is titled *Nous Sommes Tous Nés Polyglottes* (*We are All Born Polyglots*). It discusses linguistics, especially the learning of modern languages. The second book fulfills an old dream, while also systematically explaining our auditory training programs in which Mozart's music is used almost exclusively. *Pourquoi Mozart?* (*Why Mozart?*) states the specific and singular characteristics that make this music an exceptional choice.

While I write, Léna prepares my work for publication. I know that it is difficult to follow me, but she does so wholeheartedly and with competence, energy, and constant good humor. We continue to move along with an identical cadence. There is no slowing down.

Besides the pleasant time spent writing and teaching, I continue to create new prototypes of the Electronic Ear and to further improve it. Eventually, they will become fully automatic, which will simplify working with them. This also will change the amount of time the educator will have to work directly with the client. The client's perception will be that he receives more support from a person, rather than first from the machine. Yet he will not fall into the trap of a transference relationship causing dependence upon the therapist. While we acknowledge that this form of therapeutic power exists, it is not at all necessary for our auditory training to occur. What is important is not only knowing how to listen to one's interlocutor, but also permitting oneself to communicate with oneself to finally succeed at listening. The former is not easy, but the latter is even more difficult. So if a transfer does occur, and it could, it should be a transfer of the self in the integrated present to the evolving self.

For those not familiar with our work, this discussion may not make much sense. No doubt it might be considered part of the linguistic panoply of the psychologist who is used to playing with an exclusive nomenclature, perpetuated by the chosen few who believe that they alone understand. There is no need to criticize the use of specialized language, for every field has one. Yet, negative consequences exist because the objectives remain hidden and hardly have a chance to ferment, thus risking being lost in the next generation.

Therefore, listening to others must be developed in tandem with listening to oneself. Though this should be obvious, it is often difficult to accept. Actually, how long can one pay attention to another's discourse? Our thoughts quickly wander. Is one not already preoccupied by what answer will be given, and when we give our answer, are we really saying what we mean? In terms of our delivery, does it transport the subtleties of the word and give it any impact? Is not the paralanguage as important as the language itself?

But what control, for all these linguistic mechanisms are not even necessary! Nothing is so difficult to completely master as the human machine when seen from the perspective of being a wonderful instrument. The dialectics established within the human being between thoughts penetrate and inhabit the self on the one hand and the body taken as a whole on the other. It is not an easy thing to understand let alone to manage. However, for one who would bury himself in his metaphysical dimension the realization that shows the result of the expressed aspiration requires an intimate knowledge of the body and its reactions. At the level of its motivations, needs, potential, and reserves, one's list of assets and liabilities should be sincere and genuine. It pleases everyone to agree on the all-too-often illusive possibilities, while it is with a certain repugnance that we take an honest look at our own limitations.

Finding out what one is truly capable of doing is a very difficult undertaking. In fact, it requires a good deal of *realization* paired with a certain amount of abandon to *Providence*, a word we deliberately write in italics. This Providence is nothing other than a consciousness about one's vocation that is subtly perceived as a distant voice and that shows the way to those willing to accept the message. If one at least lets go of the ego, one would find the means to catch a glimpse of the horizon as defined by one's own limits and from then on they would be clear. This stage that is so evident is nevertheless very rarely attained, so great are the barriers set up at each level. They arise in the family, complemented by those set in place at school, and are further complicated by the societal structure itself. We could easily come up with a whole list of reasons for imposing restraints upon ourselves, which then hinder the true liberation that is only gained by loosening the hold. One freely longs for a state of grace whereby things would work out how they normally would anyway. Normalcy is so rare that it paradoxically is considered to be an anomaly or an exceptional occurrence.

And all the while life goes on, carrying us along on an existential path that does not characterize reality except when we follow the path we have chosen. It is nothing but a contrived reality, realized and supported by the mask we have chosen to adopt and have believed in for some period of time. This scenario is quite fragile and can be overwhelming when we find ourselves confronted with the truth. Truth causes the veil that hides our true being to fall away. Being is not seeming or appearing to be. Confronted with the truth, we uncover the real difference between the person and the personage. In the former, you know you are nothing; in the latter, you appear to be someone. *To be someone*, in the strongest sense, means being able to let the intimate perception that one is nothing show through. But the presumption about a personage, one who appears to be someone, is that he undertakes life's path with a propensity to measure its degree of difficulty, which is experienced as exasperation with the ego.

Events mark the passage of time and some provide transitions to new stages. As we enter some stages, we take up the challenge full speed ahead, without thinking of obstacles. Some stages renew our energy and provide a boost. Other stages are melancholy and plunge us for a time into distress, back into the sad reality of some gloomy area. Then, in the midst of this black hole, all our strength is mobilized, mustered as if to set us back on track to let us discover our nettle and measure the extent of our faith. We are confronted with a true test of faith, a death followed by rebirth in our lives, which never fails to unsettle us, despite our deep conviction that such stages are necessary as we march toward the heart of the dark night of death.

The loss of a dear friend of ours, Dom Grammont, ushered in a feeling of uncertainty for us, a time in which pain and joy are strangely mixed. To be sure, the pain is the greater emotion at first, hiding the rejoicing that one should feel for the rebirth that was promised, expected, and foretold. It takes time for the heartache provoked by the sudden breaking off of the relationship to lessen. Slowly there is a clearing, and I realize that the true essence of our friend who is gone never really disappeared. From that moment on, his essence expands in space where time itself melds with the eternal continuum, to the place where *never* has no meaning, to the place where *always* is fully realized throughout eternity.

Must we be confronted by death in order to rediscover the meaning of life? Yes, I am sure we must. I am convinced that this death was a necessary part of the metamorphosis, allowing his essence to take flight from the encasing shell of the chrysalis. From that moment on, a peace settles in our hearts. It allows the uneasiness that encompasses us to shrink, establishing and spreading a quietude over us, and thus freeing our affective recollections in the midbrain and making way for memory. The recollections affect us; the memory summons us to answer. Recollections corrupt the clarity of memory. They cause us to lose touch with reality by living so much in the past. Some people create an unattainable, uncertain universe full of anguish that offers only some escape, such as evasion and illusion. How many times do we feel helpless, as if being human means we must be forcefully dragged along in a stream of uncertainty? In the uncertainty, it is hard to dispel our inner essence unless we are in just the right place at just the right time. But whether or not any transformation to a permanent change takes place, due to our strong resistance to change, within freedom lies the ever-present fear of abandonment.

As I have just described, a period of mourning can throw us into a period of reflection. We have been greatly concerned that a whole web of misunderstandings would be woven around this conclusion that would only bring up more questions. In fact, our friend, Dom Grammont, the Holy Father of the Abbey Bec Helloin must have died an agonizing death. Why? Why was he not spared from such a death? Would not his greatness, which in many respects bordered upon saintliness, protect him from the agony of death? A year has passed already, and it seems normal that his grandeur met with so many difficulties, so many obstacles that only he could face, go beyond, or assume. He had to pay the price for involving himself with those whom he deeply loved and for being strangely betrayed by some who went so far as to risk compromising his life's work. He died disincarnate, his arms crossed, full of hope to face his *true love*, his Lord and Master, thanking the Lord for allowing him to participate in the sacrifice of Christ.

A storm allows one to appreciate the calm that follows. Following the three year storm that had been brewing long before it started, the heavens again were peaceful over Bec Helloin. The crisis should have ended when Dom Gramont reached the age of 75 and resigned his duties, as is customary among the Benedictine monks of Mount Olive, the group to which he belonged.

While the whirlwinds of the tempest died down, a calmness settled in this high place and the proper vibration, which only the spirit can inspire, was recovered. As the traces of the commotion unleashed by the upheaval gave way in a show of power, a radiance only God can grant newly enveloped the atmosphere. Liturgy was restored to Bec.

At the beginning of September 1990, Léna and I announced that we were changing our course. It is good that we know how to change direction regularly and do not rest merely on our laurels, becoming creatures of habit. If one gets into doing routine *assembly line work*, instead of quality work, no matter at what level, one risks deviating from the path of destiny. Everything in this universe is in flux, and we should never subject ourselves to that fundamental law that would seemingly inflict its conditions upon us, but instead should adjust ourselves to it.

We have recently established a priority and are dedicating more time to it. In regard to publication, we are providing the much needed writings that will pass on the knowledge we have gleaned over the years. Through training, too, we are responding to the same demands, again supplying what has been requested.

Clearly the most precious gift we have received and the thing we feel is most important to share with others is the infinite love of life that resides within us. This seems to have provided the enduring quest in our existence. More precisely, this will have been the prime motivating factor in our carrying out our research as far as we have unto the end of our existence. All of our medical knowledge would have no meaning except through the discovery of this truth. Emanating from this truth is the need to spread and share it. We know that we are anchored fast to this tenuous but existing cord, extending toward the unknown, coming from the unknown, identified with life itself, in which the ultimate expression is none other than love.

Appendix A

The Authentic Tomatis Method

In the past several years, we have received an increasing number of inquiries about individuals and organizations promoting sound therapy techniques that claim they are the Tomatis Method or a variation thereof. Often the public is led to believe that these sound therapies employ technology or cassette tapes approved by Dr. Tomatis. Considerable confusion has resulted since these techniques are not approved by Dr. Tomatis nor do they approximate the Tomatis Method developed by him.

Claims have been made by the proponents of these techniques which, to the best of our knowledge, have not been substantiated through systematic documentation or research evaluation. Furthermore, it is our opinion that any self-administered sound therapy may present risks when undertaken in the absence of a diagnostic assessment and systematic follow-up to monitor the effects. This is especially the case for those who may have undiagnosed hearing losses or hearing disorders.

The Tomatis Method is practiced in authorized facilities throughout Europe and North America. You can determine whether the service being offered is the authentic Tomatis Method by the following:

(1) The Tomatis Method will be supervised by a professional trained and <u>certified</u> (certification is renewed annually) by Dr. Tomatis.

(2) The Tomatis Method includes a specific battery of diagnostic procedures, ongoing supervision and progress evaluation by certified professionals.

(3) Users of the Tomatis Method employ the most advanced electronic equipment which meets current standards established by Dr. Tomatis. This equipment includes specially modified headsets and play-back machines linked directly with an Electronic Ear™.

(4) The Tomatis Method consists of both active (singing, speaking, sounding) exercises as well as passive ones (listening to tapes). These active exercises, carefully monitored, are essential for long-term improvement.

(5) The Tomatis Method includes both individual and family counselling as an integral part of the intervention.

(6) The application of the Tomatis Method in North America has been geared toward developing and improving listening, language and

communication skills in persons with normal hearing as a primary goal. Beware of any claims which suggest the "curing" of hearing disorders and "restoration of hearing loss."

(7)   The Tomatis Method's efficacy and beneficial effects are supported by a growing body of systematic documentation and scientific research evaluation.

(8)   A group version of the Tomatis Method is used by school boards and private schools in Canada, the United States and Mexico. Through this Tomatis School Program for schools, the authentic Method is made available to hundreds of children each year at no direct cost to their families.

We have found, after nearly 35 years of research and practice, that the Tomatis Method is a powerful and effective program of auditory stimulation and counselling. It requires careful, professional supervision to produce positive and lasting benefits. Users of alternative techniques of sound stimulation should proceed with caution.

Appendix B

Patents Held By
Alfred A. Tomatis

Patent #	Date	Title
3,043,913	7/10/63	Apparatus for the Re-education of the Voice
3,101,081	8/20/63	Apparatus for the Conditioning of the Auditory Lateralization
3,101,391	8/20/63	Apparatus for the Acoustic-Ambience Conditioning of a Medium
4,021,611	5/03/77	Electronic Hearing Apparatus
4,212,119	7/15/80	Audio-Vocal Integrator Apparatus
4,327,252	4/27/82	Apparatus for Conditioning Hearing
4,615,680	10/07/86	Apparatus and Method for Practicing Pronunciation of Words by Comparing the User's Pronunciation with the Stored Pronunciation

Appendix C

Works of Alfred A. Tomatis

Audiologie et phonologie expérimentales et appliquées. Cours à l'Ecole des Psychologues Praticiens, 1959.

Audiométrie objective: Résultats des contre-réactions phonation-audition. *Journal Français d'Oto-Rhino-Laryngologie*. Lyon: Imprimerie M. Gautheir, 1957, 5/6, 379-391.

Conditionnement audio-vocal. *Bulletin de l'Académie Nationale de Médecine*, Tome 144, n° 11/12. Communication présentée par M. Moulonguet, 1960, 3.

Considérations sur le test d'écoute. Publication du Centre Tomatis, Paris, 1974.

Correction de la voix chantée. In *Cours International de Phonologie et de Phoniatrie* (Faculté de Médecine de Paris). Paris: Librairie Maloine, 1953, 335-353.

Education and Dyslexia. Translated from original French by Louise Guiney. Fribourg, Switzerland: A.I.A.P.P., 1978.

Education et Dyslexie. Paris: Editions E.S.F., 1971.

El Fracaso Escolar. Barcelona: Edicions La campana, 1989.

Incidences observées dans les lésions articulaires constatées chez le personnel des bancs d'essai et les professionels de la voix. *Bulletin du Centre d'Etudes et de Recherches Médicales de la S.F.E.C.M. A.S.*, 1952, 9.

Inconscient et conscience. Publication du Centre Tomatis, Paris, 1979.

La dyslexie. Cours à l'Ecole d'Anthropologie. Editions Soditap, 1967.

La Libération d'Oedipe. Paris: Editions E.S.F., 1972.

La Musicothérapie et les dépressions nerveuses. Rapport au IVème Congrès International d'Audio-Psycho-Phonologie, Madrid, 1974.

Là musique et l'enfant. Communication faite au ler Symposium Régional de la Musique, à Pierrelatte, 1972, 5, 11-14.

La musique et ses effets neuro-psycho-physiologiques. Conférence donnée par le Dr. A.A. Tomatis lors du XIII° Congrès de l'I.S.M.E. (International Society for Music Education) à London (Canada), August 1978.

La musique, notion indispensable et pourtant supposée superflué. Extrait de la revue *Diapason*, 1980.

La Nuit Utérine. Paris: Editions Stock, 1981.

La phénoménologie de l'écoute. Publications du Centre Tomatis, Paris, 1984.

La rééducation automatique. Ecole Polytechnique de l'Université de Laus-anne. *Annales du G.A.L.F. (Groupement des Acousticiens de Langue Française)*, 1958, 9.

La rééducation de la voix -- les differentes methodes de traitement. *La Vie Médicale*, 1974, n° 20, 5/4.

La résonance dans les échelles musicales -- le point de vue du physiologiste. *Annales de l'Institut de Musicologie* (sous la direction de M.J. Chailley). Conférence prononcée le 9.5.1960. au cours du Colloque International sur la "Résonance dans les Echelles Musicales" à l'amphithéâtre de l'Institut d'Art et d'Archéologie.

La Sélectivité auditive. *Bulletin du Centre d'Etudes et de Rechercheses Médi Médicales de la* S.F.E.C.M. A.S., 1954, 10.

La surdité. Conférence faite à la demande de la Caisse d'Allocations Familiales de Paris. Editions Soditap, 1965, 11, 17.

La surdité à la D.E.F.A. *Le Médecin d'Usine*, 1955, n° 8/9/10, 401-404.

La surdité professionelle. Rapport au Congrès de la Société Française d'Oto-Rhino-Laryngologie. Paris: MM. Maduro, Lallement et Tomatis. *Librairie Arnette*, 1952.

La surdité professionnelle. Revue "Travail social." *Revue de la Fédération Française des Travailleurs Sociaux*, 1956, n° 2, 39-42.

La surdité professionnelle à la soufflerie de Vernon. Rapport des journées des médecins de la D.E.F.A., *Direction des Etudes et Fabrications d'Armement*, 1955, 5, 16-18.

La vie psychique et sensorielle du foetus. Traduction de *La vita psichica et sensoriale del feto.* paru dans *l'Enciclopedia della Scienzia e della Tecnica*, 7° édition, Milano, 1984.

La voix. *Revue Musicale*, édition spéciale consacrée à "Médecine et Musique," 1962.

La voix chantée. *Bulletin du Centre d'Etudes et de Recherches Médicales de la S.F.E.C.M. A.S.*, 1953, 7.

La voix chantée -- sa physiologie -- sa pathologie -- sa rééducation. Cours à l'Hôpital Bichat, March, 1960. Cours d'Orthophonie et de rééducation de la parole.

L'arbitraire dans le langage. II° Congrès National A.P.P., Pau, 1976.

L'audiométrie d'usine. *Bulletin du Centre d'Etudes et de Recherches Médicales de la S.F.E.C.M. A.S.*, 1953, 10.

L'audiométrie de dépistage en usine. *Bulletin de la Société d'Hygiène et de Médecine du Travail de Normandie.* Le Havre, 1958, 5.

L'audiometrie dynamique. *Bulletin du Centre d'Etudes et de Recherches Médicales de la S.F.E.C.M. A.S.*, 1953, 9.

Le begaiement, essais de recherches sur sa pathogénie. *Bulletin du Centre d'Etudes et de Recherches Médicales de la S.F.E.C.M. A.S.*, 1953, 6.

Le chant et la musique: Leur importance dans le développement de la personne. Rapport au Congrès Kodaly, Aylmer, Canada, octobre, 1982.

Le défi de l'audio-psycho-phonologie. Symposium d'Audio-Psycho-Phonologie, Université de Potchefstroom, avril, 1980.

Le dépistage de l'enfant dyslexique à l'école maternelle. Conférence faite à l'Université de Potchefstroom au cours du Congrès National de la South African Society for Education, 1976, 21-1.

Le langage -- examen clinique -- pathologie -- traitement. Société de Médecine de Paris. *Revue d'Enseignement Post-Universitaire*, 1970.

Le phonème, sa projection psychosensorielle, sa réponse psychomotrice. Proceedings of the Fifth International Congress of Phonetic Sciences, Münster, 1964.

Le rôle de l'oreille dans la musicothérapie. Rapport au Congrès International de Musicothérapie, Paris, 1974.

Les aspects médico-psycho-pédagogiques de l'audio-psycho-phonologie. Conférence d'ouverture au Congrès International d'Audio-Psycho-Phonologie, Montréal, Mai, 1978.

Les bases neuro-physiologiques de la musicothérapie. *Bulletin de l'I.S.M.E. (International Society for Musical Education)*. Exposé fait aux Journées d'Information sur les techniques psycho-musicales. Conservatoire de Grenoble, 1974, 4, 1-3.

Les nuisances du bruit. Revue "Le Médecin d'Usine." *Revue Pratique de Médecine et Hygiène du Travail*, 1957, 11, 605-624.

Les pouvoirs du musicien. *Revue Musicale*: "La face cachée de la Musique Française Contemporaine," 1979, N° 316-317, 3.

Les réactions somatiques et psychiques au bruit industriel. *Archives des Maladies Professionnelles*. Tome 20, n° 5, 611-624. Communication faite au cours du Vème Congrès International de Médecine du Travail. Lyon, 1958, 10.10. Revue de *la Médecine Aéronautique*, 1959, 2ème/ 3ème trimestre, Tome 14, N° 2-3.

Les Troubles Scolaires. Paris: Ergo Press, 1988.

L'électronique au service des langues vivantes. Conférence donée à l'U.N.E.S.C.O., 1960, 3, 11, Parue dans le *Bulletin de l'Union des Associations des Anciens Elèves des Lycées et Collèges Français*, 1960, 3.

L'intégration des langues vivantes. Editions Soditap, 1970.

L'interprétation du test d'écoute. Rapport au III° Congrès International d'Audio-Psycho-Phonologie, Anvers, 1973.

L'O.R.L. devant les problèmes du langage. *L'Hôpital*, 1964, n° 747bis.

L'oreille considérée comme capteur. *Les Cahiers de la Méthode Naturelle en Médecine*, 1974, 9.

L'oreille directrice. *Bulletin du Centre d'Etudes et de Recherches Médicales de la*

S.F.E.C.M. A.S., 1953, 7.

L'oreille directrice. Editions Soditap, 1967.

L'oreille et l'enfant. Conférence donnée par le Dr. A.A. Tomatis à l'Université d'Ottawa dans le cadre du "Festival de l'Enfant," 1979, 3, 16.

L'Oreille et la Vie. Paris: Editions Laffont, 1977, 1986.

L'Oreille et la Voix. Paris: Editions Laffont, 1987.

L'oreille et le chant. Conservatoire de Musique de Berne, Suisse, August, 1980.

L'Oreille et le Langage. Paris: Editions du Seuil, 1963.

L'oreille musicale. *Journal Français O.R.L.* Imprimerie Gauthier, 1953, 2 N° 2, 99-106.

Neuf Mois Au Paradis. Paris: Ergo Press, 1989.

Nous Sommes tous nés polyglottes. Paris: Fixot, 1991.

Nouvelles théories sur la physiologie auditive. Rapport au IIéme Congrès International d'Audio-Psycho-Phonologie, Paris, 1972.

Ontogenesis of the faculty of listening. In T. Verny (Ed.), *Pre- and Peri-Natal Psychology: An Intro-duction.* New York: Human Sciences Press, 1987.

Oreille et difficultés d'apprentissage. Conférence donnée par la Dr. A. A. Tomatis au Congrès de l'A.Q.E.T.A. à Montréal, Mars, 1979.

Porquoi Mozart? Paris: Fixot, 1991.

Pour information sur la surdité professionelle. *Bulletin du Centre d'Etudes et de Recherches Médicales de la S.F.E.C.M. A.S.*, 1954, 10.

Psychophysiologie des troubles du timbre et du rythme dans le langage. Cours professé à la Faculté des Sciences, dans un cycle de conférences sur les "Problèmes de Psychophysiologie Acoustique," sous la direction du Docteur Busnel, à la chaire de Psycho-Physiologie de la Sorbonne, February, 1959.

Recherches sur la pathologie du bégaiement. *Journal Français d'Oto-Rhino-Laryn-*

gologie, 1954, 3 N° 4, 4, 384.

Relations audition-phonation. *Revue Promouvoir*, 1960, 9, n° 1, 7-10.

Relations entre l'audition et la phonation. *Annales des Télécommunications*. Cahiers d'Acoustique, 1956, Tome II n° 7/8.

Rôle directeur de l'oreille dans le déterminisme des qualités de la voix normale (parlée ou chantée) et dans la génèse de ses troubles. *Actualités Oto-Rhino-Laryngologiques*, 1953.

Vers L'écoute Humaine. Tome 1: Qu'est ce que l'Ecoute humaine? Paris: Editions E.S.F., 1974.

Vers L'écoute Humaine. Tome 2: Qu'est-ce que l'oreille humaine? Paris: Les Éditions E.S.F., 1974.

Vertiges. Paris: Ergo Press, 1989.

Voix, audition et personnalité. Revue *S.O.S. Amitié*. France, 1974, N° 48, 9.

Appendix D

Alfred A. Tomatis

Born: Nice, January 1, 1920

Doctor of Medicine, Université de Paris, Otorhinolaryngologist (Ear-Nose-Throat Physician) Specialist in Problems of Hearing and Language

TITLES

- Professor of Audio-Psycho-Phonology, The School of Anthropology, Paris
- Professor for Psycho-Linguistics, School for Practicing Psychologists of the Catholic Institute of Paris
- President of the International Association of Audio-Psycho-Phonology
- Ex-Director of the Laboratory of Acoustic Psycho-Physiology of Le Centre d'Essai des Propulseurs de Saclay
- Honorary Member, Dorstmundt-Institut, Munich
- Member of GALF (French-Speaking Acousticians Association)
- Member of the Board of Directors of La Société des Grandes Conférences Scientifiques
- Honorary Member of the Department of Psychology, University of Potchefstroom, South Africa

DISTINCTIONS

- Chevalier de la Santé Publique (1951)
- Médaille d'Or de la Recherche Scientifique - Bruxelles (1958)
- Grande Médaille de Vermeil de la Ville de Paris (1962)
- Prix Clémence Isaure (1967)
- Médaille d'Or de la Société <Arts, Sciences et Lettres> (1968)
- Commandeur du Mérite Culturel et Artistique (1970)

RESEARCH

- for the French Ministry of Labour: various Commissions on noise, professional deafness and voice; studies on the legislation and the classification of occupational deafness

- for the French Ministry of War and the Air Force: work on the effects of sound trauma; studies of damage resulting from exposure to noise; development of an automatic audio testing device

- work on voice and vocal production emphasizing the feedback mechanisms between ear and voice, later named the Tomatis Effect (introduced at the Académie des Sciences and at the Académie de Medicine by M. Raoul Husson in 1957)

- development of a range of electronic instruments designed to measure and treat:

  - learning disabilities (reading, writing, spelling, calculation)
  - problems with speech and language
  - problems with lateral dominance, handedness
  - problems with the singing voice
  - hearing problems (from hyperacousia to deafness)
  - behavioral problems (attention, concentration, memory, aggressivity, hyperactivity, regressive tendencies)
  - difficulty in learning foreign languages

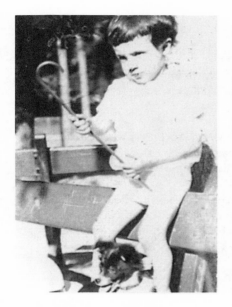

Tomatis at age two, 1922.

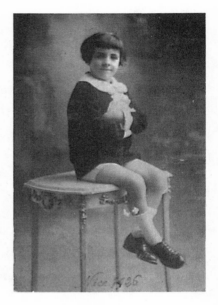

Tomatis at age six, 1926.

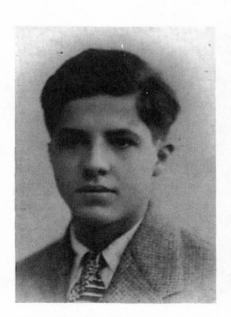

Tomatis at age 14, 1934.

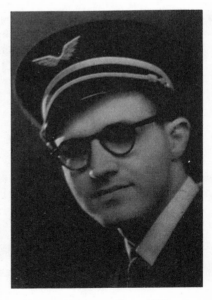

Tomatis in Air Force uniform, 1940.

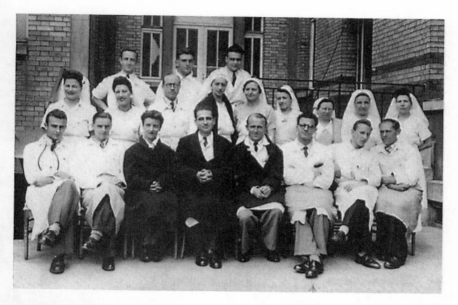

Tomatis and colleagues at the Hospital Bichat, 1944. (Front row, third from right.)

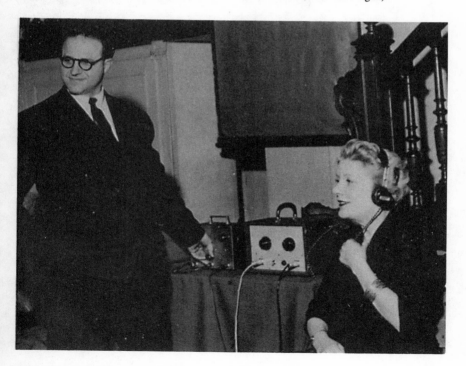

A demonstration with one of the first Electronic Ears, 1950.

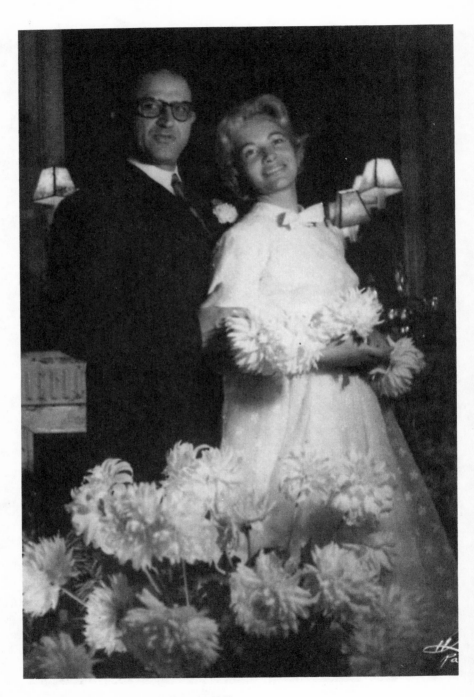

The wedding of Alfred and Léna Tomatis, 1958.

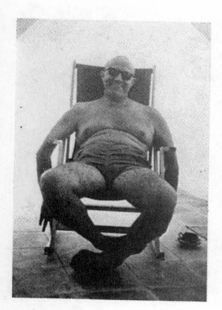

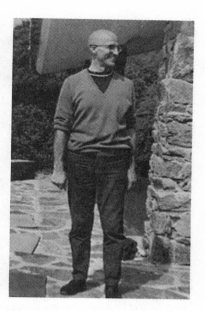

Tomatis before the diet, 1963.

Tomatis after the diet, 1964.

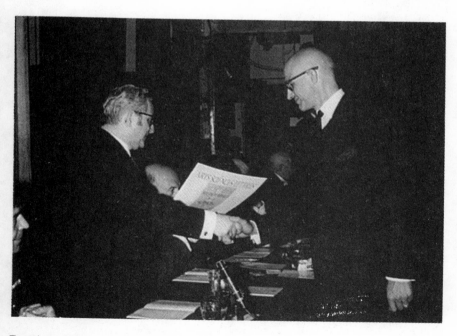

Tomatis receiving the decoration of Arts, Sciences, & Letters, 1968.

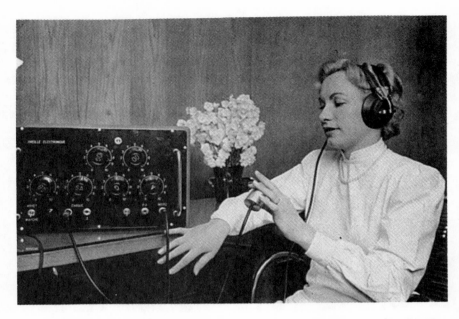

(Above) Léna with one of the first Electronic Ears, 1958.

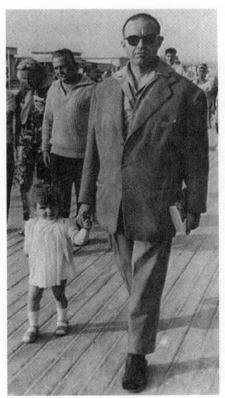

(Left) Tomatis with daughter Emmanuelle on the Boardwalk of Deauville, 1962.

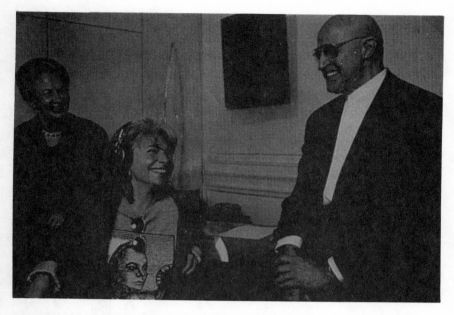

Tomatis with Léna and Catherine Lara, a famous rock singer, 1989.

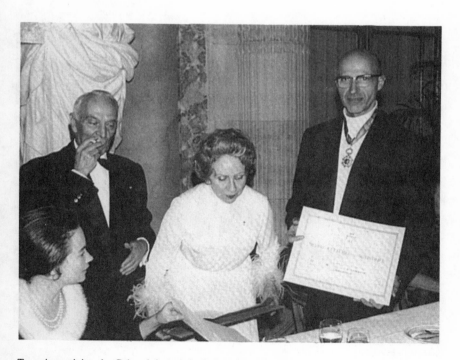

Tomatis receiving the Cultural & Artistic Order of Merit, 1970.

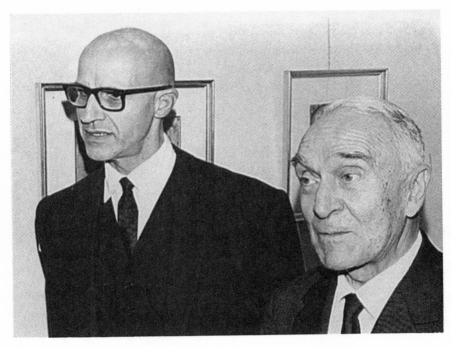

Tomatis with George Massié, Director of the Department of Fine Arts in Paris, 1976.

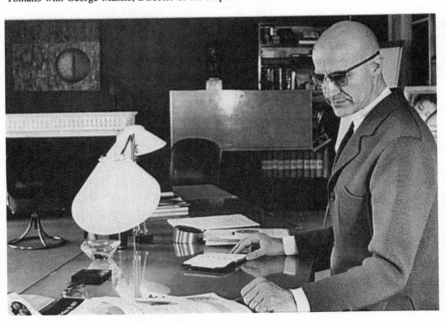

Tomatis in his office on Boulevard de Courcelles, 1972.

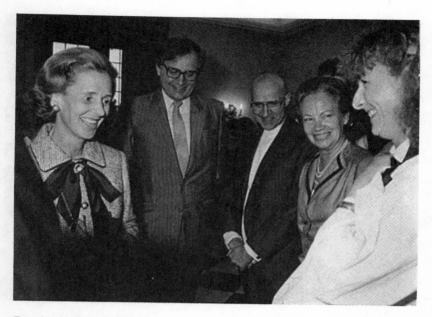

Tomatis with Queen Fabiola of Belgium, during a conference about birth in Brussels, 1985.

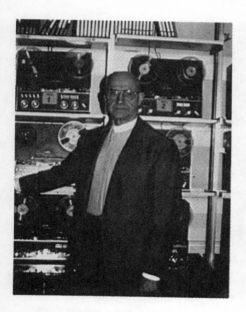

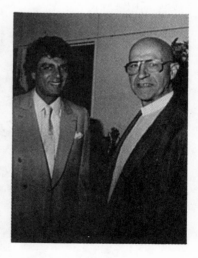

Tomatis with Enrico Macias, a famous variety singer, 1987.

Tomatis in his Paris laboratory, 1988.

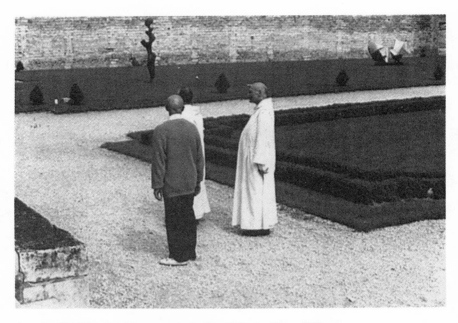

Tomatis with Abbot Dom Grammont at Le Bec Hellouin Abbey, 1987.

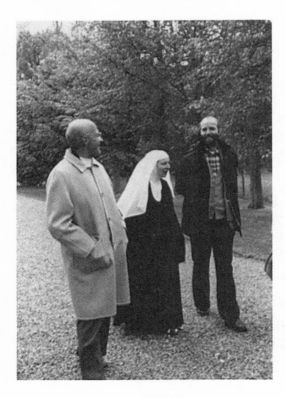

Tomatis with his adopted daughter, Sister Emmanuel Marie, and son, Christian, 1982.

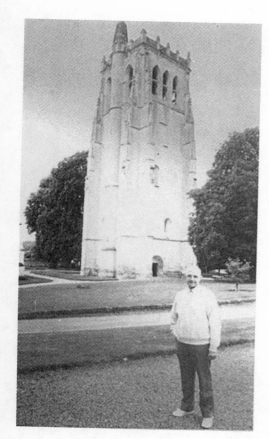

(Left) Tomatis at the
Abbey Notre Dame du Bec, before
the "Tour Saint Nicolas," 1988.

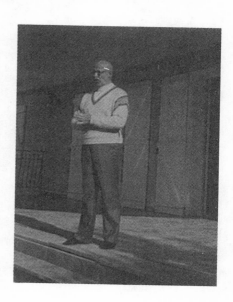

(Right) Tomatis singing in Murcia,
Spain, 1982.

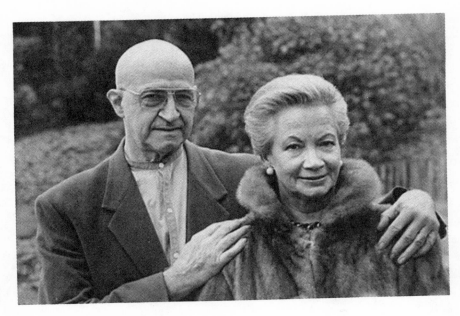

Dr. and Mme. Tomatis, 1990.

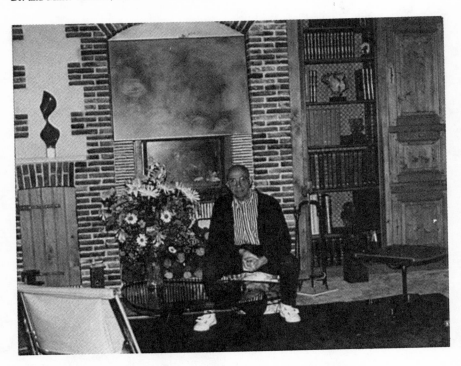

Tomatis in his living room at Saint-Yves Le Bec Hellouin in Normandy, 1988.

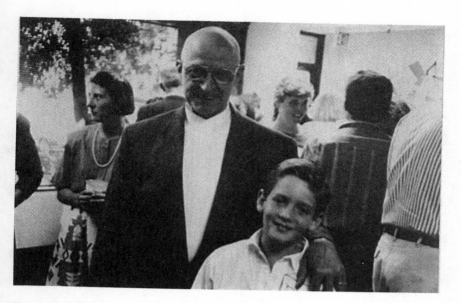

Tomatis at a reception in the Phoenix, Arizona Center, 1990.

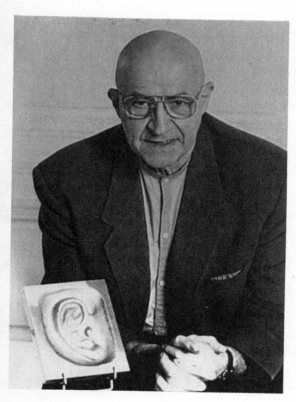

Tomatis, 1990.

About the Tomatis Program

If you would like additional information about the Tomatis Program or training, you may contact the following:

Tomatis Center
2701 E. Camelback Road
Suite 205
Phoenix, AZ 85016
(602) 381-0086

- or -

Tomatis International
2, rue de Phalsbourg
75017 Paris
(1) 43-80-92-22

Acknowledgements

Many people have read, edited, and in numerous ways encouraged the publication of this book in English. Léna has provided her constant support and been an intimate partner in preparing the book and sharing my life. Special thanks go to George Quasha, who took a personal interest in getting the work out to others, and to Billie Thompson for finding the publisher and editing the final copy to be inviting to the reader. Stephen Lushington provided an initial translation, and Tim Gilmor, Rob Roy, and Paul Madaule provided early assistance with editing Lushington's translation and seeking a publisher.

Index

Names and Subjects

Music and Your Mind
Listening with a New Consciousness

DR. HELEN L. BONNY & LOUIS M. SAVARY

The power of music to effect significant changes in consciousness has long been known, but it was Helen L. Bonny's pioneer work in the field of music therapy that first offered a specific method—using guided imagery—for altering our state of awareness. This updated and expanded edition offers step-by-step descriptions of twenty-five listening experiences designed to open new doors to creativity, insight, and self-understanding. With the author's new survey of developments in the field of music therapy, and with an extensive updated discography, this is an essential volume for teachers, therapists, music lovers, and anyone interested in breaking through to new levels of awareness.

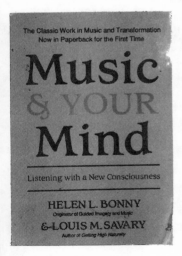

Helen Bonny's book has to be considered the classic in the area of music and healing.
> ROBERT GASS, Ed.D, Harvard; composer, therapist, recording artist

A user-friendly guide to exercises and a discography that is both timely and timeless.
> STEVEN HALPERN
> Recording artist, author of *Sound Health*

HELEN L. BONNY is a professional musician, educator, and founder of The Bonny Foundation: An Institute for Music-Centered Therapies. A Doctoral program on her teachings is offered at NYU.

LOUIS M. SAVARY is the author of *Getting High Naturally*.

$10.95 paper, ISBN 0-88268-094-3; 192 pages, 6 x 9, notes, appendix, tables, updated discography.

Music and Sound in the Healing Arts
An Energy Approach

JOHN BEAULIEU

Music is patterned energy. Here at last is a book that shows us in depth how to make use of this energy as a healing force. The result of such conscious use of sound and music is enhanced life-energy and wellness. Richly illustrated with pictures, stories, and the author's experiences as composer and therapist, this book explores the history and practice of healing sound from ancient philosophies to the practical applications of therapy, religion, and art: mantra, toning, voice evaluation, tuning forks, and music listening. It also contains guidelines and exercises for teaching and an evaluation of music therapy today.

An invaluable resource for teachers, students, and practitioners in all the healing arts.
ELISABETH MACRAE, M.D.

Artfully done and maintained by a well supported and cohesive systems view.
JAMES Z. SAID, D.C., N.D.,
President, American Polarity Therapy Assoc.

JOHN BEAULIEU, active as a composer, pianist, music therapist, and naturopathic doctor, is the founder and director of the Polarity Wellness Center and the Sound School of New York. He has studied acupuncture, polarity, cranial therapy, ayruvedic medicine, nutrition, and psychotherapy.

Special discount, $15.95 cloth, 0-88268-057-9; 160 pages, 6 1/2 x 9 1/4, illustrated, photos, charts, notes, bibliography.

BodyStories
A Guide to Experiential Anatomy

ANDREA OLSEN
with Caryn McHose

Thirty-one days of pleasurable learning activities help readers directly experience their anatomy in an entirely new way. For two decades an international dancer and teacher of anatomy, Olsen now shows how attitudes about the body can affect well-being, and demonstrates methods of bodywork to promote physical efficiency and healing. Her work with other teachers in experiential anatomy and in Authentic Movement also shows how movement patterns and memory are part of our physical and cultural heritage. Amusing personal stories ("bodystories") enliven the discussion. The works of twelve visual artists, childrens' drawings, over 100 photos, medical illustrations, and multicultural images are included to broaden our way of looking at and listening to the stories of the body.

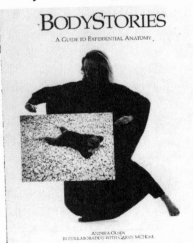

The perfect book for anyone who wishes to understand anatomy in more depth through their own inner journeying. BONNIE BAINBRIDGE COHEN, Co-Director and Founder of The School for Body-Mind Centering

It should be required reading for all dance students. SUSAN WALTNER, Professor of Dance, Smith College; Director of the Five College Dance Department

ANDREA OLSEN is an Associate Professor of Dance at Middlebury College in Vermont and has taught anatomy and kinesiology since 1972 in workshops and colleges.

CARYN MCHOSE practices bodywork in Vermont and Maine.

$19.95 paper, ISBN 0-88268-106-0; 8 ½ x 11, 164 pages, 100 b & w photos, adult and children's drawings, medical drawings, bibliography, index.